Kampala Women
Getting By

Wellbeing
in the time
of AIDS

Eastern African Studies

Revealing Prophets
Prophecy in Eastern African History
EDITED BY DAVID M. ANDERSON
& DOUGLAS H. JOHNSON

Religion & Politics in East Africa
The Period since Independence
EDITED BY HOLGER BERNT HANSEN
& MICHAEL TWADDLE

Swahili Origins
*Swahili Culture
& the Shungwaya Phenomenon*
JAMES DE VERE ALLEN

A History of Modern Ethiopia
1855–1974
BAHRU ZWEDE

Ethnicity & Conflict
in the Horn of Africa
EDITED BY KATSUYOSHI FUKUI
& JOHN MARKAKIS

Siaya
*The Historical Anthropology
of an African Landscape*
DAVID WILLIAM COHEN &
E. S. ATIENO ODHIAMBO

Control & Crisis in Colonial Kenya
The Dialectic of Domination
BRUCE BERMAN

Unhappy Valley
*Book One: State & Class
Book Two: Violence & Ethnicity*
BRUCE BERMAN
& JOHN LONSDALE

Mau Mau from Below*
GREET KERSHAW

The Mau Mau War in Perspective
FRANK FUREDI

Squatters & the Roots
of Mau Mau, 1905–63
TABITHA KANOGO

Economic & Social Origins
of Mau Mau 1945–53
DAVID THROUP

Penetration & Protest in Tanzania
*The Impact of the World Economy
on the Pare 1860–1960*
ISARIA N. KIMAMBO

Custodians of the Land
*Environment & Culture
in the History of Tanzania*
EDITED BY GREGORY MADDOX,
JAMES L. GIBLIN & ISARIA N. KIMAMBO

Jua Kali Kenya
*Change & Development
in an Informal Economy 1970–95*
KENNETH KING

The Second Economy in Tanzania
T.L. MALIYAMKONO
& M.S.D. BAGACHWA

Kampala Women Getting By
*Wellbeing in the
Time of Aids*
SANDRA WALLMAN

Uganda Now
Changing Uganda
Developing Uganda*
From Chaos to Order
EDITED BY HOLGER BERNT HANSEN
& MICHAEL TWADDLE

Decolonization & Independence
in Kenya 1940–88
EDITED BY B. A. OGOT
& WILLIAM OCHIENG'

Slaves, Spices & Ivory
in Zanzibar
*Integration of an East African
Commercial Empire
into the World Economy*
ABDUL SHERIFF

Zanzibar Under Colonial Rule
EDITED BY ABDUL SHERIFF
& ED FERGUSON

The History & Conservation
of Zanzibar Stone Town
EDITED BY ABDUL SHERIFF

Being Maasai
Ethnicity & Identity in East Africa
EDITED BY THOMAS SPEAR
& RICHARD WALLER

Kakungulu & the Creation
of Uganda 1868–1928
MICHAEL TWADDLE

Ecology Control &
Economic Development in
East African History
The Case of Tanganyika 1850–1950
HELGE KJEKSHUS

Education in the Development
of Tanzania 1919–1990
LENE BUCHERT

* *forthcoming*

Kampala Women Getting By

Wellbeing in the Time of Aids

SANDRA WALLMAN
Professor of Social Anthropology
University of Hull

IN ASSOCIATION WITH

GRACE BANTEBYA-KYOMUHENDO
VALDO PONS · JESSICA JITTA · FRANK KAHARUZA
JESSICA OGDEN · SOLVEIG FREUDENTHAL

James Currey
LONDON

Fountain Publishers
KAMPALA

Ohio University Press
ATHENS

James Currey Ltd
54b Thornhill Square
London N1 1BE

Fountain Publishers
PO Box 488
Kampala

Ohio University Press
Scott Quadrangle
Athens, Ohio 45701, USA

First published 1996
1 2 3 4 5 00 99 98 97 96

British Library Cataloguing in Publication Data
Wallman, Sandra
    Kampala women getting by : wellbeing in the time of AIDS
    1. Self-care, health - Africa. 2. Health behaviour - Africa
    3. Women - Health and hygiene - Africa - sociological
    aspects
    I. Title
    362.1'096

ISBN 0-85255-242-4 (James Currey Cloth)
ISBN 0-85255-241-6 (James Currey Paper)

Library of Congress Cataloging-in-Publication Data available

Typeset in 10/11pt Baskerville by
Long House Publishing Services, Cumbria, UK
Printed in Great Britain
by Villiers Publications, London N3

Contents

List of Photographs, Sketches, Maps & Figures   viii
Acknowledgements   ix
Notes on Contributors   x

1 *Introduction*
Preamble   1
The Problem   2
Uganda Setting   4
    Recent history – Repercussions in the health sector – A short note on local government and Kamwokya
Analytical Background   8
The Development of African Cities   9
Health Care in the Household   11
Varieties of the Urban System   13
The Form of the Book   15

2 *Kamwokya*
Preamble   17
The Physical Setting   20
    Time perspective – Land prices, landowners and landlords – Roads, tracks and pathways – Dwellings and other buildings – Water and sanitation – Communal, commercial and service premises
The Urban System   28
    The distribution of difference – The movement of people

3 *People in Place*
VALDO PONS
Preamble   47
Introduction: Kampala and Kamwokya   48
    Population growth and declining sex ratios – Composition by age and sex – Household size – Places of birth and the migrant nature of the population as a whole – Religious and ethnic affiliations – 'Activity status' and occupations – School attendance
Conclusions and Comments   69

4 *Community Life I*
    Observers' views
Preamble   73
The Market and Shopping   75
Activity around a Protected Spring   77
Sunday Morning   79
Football   82
Drinking   83

Contents

An RC Court Case   85
Neighbouring   88

5 *Household Wellbeing*
Ethnographic & Women's Survey Responses
Preamble   90
Income Potential   92
Conditions of Housing, Hygiene and Sanitation   94
Illness and Disease   98
Immunization of Children   104
Fertility and Childbirth   104
Support and Advice During Illness   106
Feeling Good about Kamwokya   108

6 *Treatment Options*
Preamble   111
Theoretical Perspectives   112
    Modernization – Economic approach – Homophily
Treatment Sources Survey, Kamwokya II (1993)   114
    Personal characteristics of the treatment providers – Therapeutic situation –
    Payment – Symptoms treated
Observations of the 'Visible' Health Units   122
    Clinics – Drug shops
Interviews with Ten Traditional Healers   129
    Profiles

7 *Home Treatment*
JESSICA OGDEN & GRACE BANTEBYA-KYOMUHENDO
Preamble   142
The Household as the Locus of Health   142
The Home Treatment Process   144
    Drug shops, clinic dispensaries and pharmacies
Illness as a Moral Category: Invisibility, Stigma and Secrecy   148
Health and Agency: Home Treatment and Autonomy   150
Conclusion: Implications of Home Treatment   151

8 *Children's Illnesses*
Mothers' definition & management of 'serious enough' symptoms
JESSICA JITTA
Preamble   152
Introduction   153
Findings   154
    Common perceptions and beliefs about acute symptoms in young children –
    Home treatment of acute symptoms of children – Factors mothers
    consider in determining severity of symptoms – Treatment options and
    factors influencing choice of treatment – Perception of treatment outcomes –
    Respondents' recommendations for improvements in caring for sick children
Conclusion and Recommendations   165

9 *Private Disease*
Perception & Management of STD
FRANK KAHARUZA & OTHERS

Preamble	166
Links Between HIV and STD	167
The STD Situation in Uganda: Treatment Provision	168

Specific diseases – Clinics – Findings and recommendations

The STD Situation in Kamwokya: Treatment Seeking	175

Summary of treatment seekers' views on STD – Treatment and diagnosis –
Why delay? – Treatment seekers' views: notes from Focus Group discussions –
A few words about 'discipline'

Appendix: Local Glossary and Symptomatology	187

10 *Six Women*
Individual women's accounts of treatment seeking
GRACE BANTEBYA-KYOMUHENDO & JESSICA OGDEN

Preamble	189
Case Study 1: Betty	190
Case Study 2: Rose	193
Case Study 3: May	195
Comparison and Analysis of Cases 1, 2 and 3	196
Case Study 4: Mary	198
Case Study 5: Sally	201
Case Study 6: Ann	202
Comparison and Analysis of Cases 4, 5, and 6	204
Conclusions	205

11 *Community Life II*
Participants' views (The video project)
SOLVEIG FREUDENTHAL

Preamble	206
Introduction	
The Ethnography of the Video Production Process	207

Stage I: Planning – Stage II: Shooting – Stage III: Editing –
Stage IV: Viewing of Kamwokya 1994

The Making of a Commentary	
Concluding Remarks	224
Epilogue	225

12 *Summary & Conclusions*

Preamble	226
Scientific and Technical Objectives	226
Results and Interpretations of Findings	227
Last Words	230

References	236
Index	241

Photographs, Sketches, Maps & Figures

Photographs   *between pp.* 6–7

Sketches by Abraham Kafeero   *between pp.* 37–46

Maps

I	Uganda	16
II	Kampala with zones and parishes	18
III	Kamwokya and surrounding parishes	19
IV	Kamwokya II, 1991: Buildings, roads and footpaths	30
V	Communal, commercial and service premises	31
VI	Kamwokya II: Population densities in each enumeration area	32
VII	Ethnic groups (by region)	33
VIII	Housing tenure	33
IX	Income levels	33
X	Cityscapes	33

Figures

1.1	Recent events in Uganda	5
2.1	Time chart showing highlights in the growth and development of Kamwokya II (1960–94)	20
2.2	Ethnic distribution, Kamwokya, 1993	29
2.3	Place of other origin: 'home area'	29
3.1	Population pyramids for Kamwokya II and Kampala in 1991	51
3.2	Population pyramid for Kamwokya, 1993	54
3.3	Population pyramids for Kamwokya II in 1969 and 1991	54
3.4	Population pyramids for the migrant and market areas of Kamwokya II, 1991	57
3.5	Population pyramids for the migrant and permanent house areas of Kamwokya II, 1991	57
3.6	Population pyramids for residents of the migrant area born in Kampala and elsewhere	61
3.7	Population pyramids for residents of the market area born in Kampala and elsewhere	61
4.1	Court case layout	86
5.1	Reasons for coming to Kamwokya	108
5.2	Other reasons for coming to Kamwokya	109
5.3	Household types: Status of children in relation to parents	110
5.4	'Where the heart is'	110
10.1	Treatment-seeking diagram	190

Acknowledgements

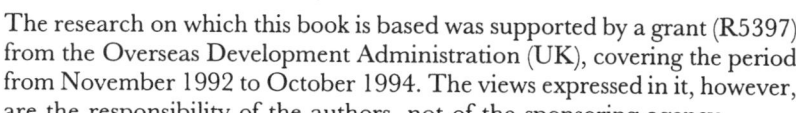

The research on which this book is based was supported by a grant (R5397) from the Overseas Development Administration (UK), covering the period from November 1992 to October 1994. The views expressed in it, however, are the responsibility of the authors, not of the sponsoring agency.

We have been grateful for administrative support from the implementing institutions – in Uganda the Child Health Development Centre (CHDC), Makerere University, Kampala (through the work of Augustine Mtumbwa and his colleagues), and in the UK the Department of Sociology and Anthropology at the University of Hull (particularly, in their respective offices, from Greta Charlesworth and Margaret Pullar).

More specifically, this book has benefitted from the professional expertise of people not listed among its associated authors. Each has been central in a particular sphere: Yvonne Dhooge in the training of local interviewers: Catherine Barasa and Achilles Ssewaya in organizing field operations; Jesse Busuulwa and Elke Konings in quantitative data management; Maia Baker in the analysis of 'informal' resources; and Velories Figures in discussions with the local traditional healers.

A team of Makerere University students assisted most ably in the preparatory mapping and 'Broad Brush Survey' of Kamwokya, and in the de-briefing of residents acting as interviewers for the various surveys. Invidious as it is to name some but not all, the art work of Abrahim Kafeero (whose sketches appear later in the book) and the research assistance of Eva Nantongo deserve special mention.

Last, but not least, we are grateful for the generosity of the RCs and people of Kamwokya II – both as individuals and as a community. Their energy and enthusiasm and critical commentary sustained the project from the beginning, and they are crucially responsible for any of its successes. Its failings, on the other hand, are our own. We apologise for inaccuracies or misrepresentations which may have crept through their friendly filter.

Notes on Contributors

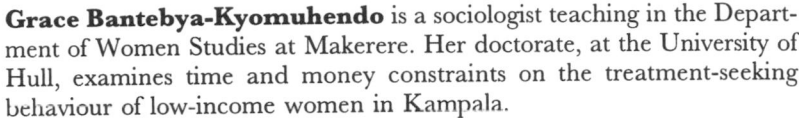

Grace Bantebya-Kyomuhendo is a sociologist teaching in the Department of Women Studies at Makerere. Her doctorate, at the University of Hull, examines time and money constraints on the treatment-seeking behaviour of low-income women in Kampala.

Solveig Freudenthal is a film-maker and social anthropologist, seconded to IHCAR, Karolinska Institutet, Stockholm, from Stockholm University. She has made prize-winning short films and continues to explore 'participatory video' as a development strategy.

Jessica Jitta is a paediatrician and director of the Child Health and Development Centre at Mulago (teaching) Hospital in Makerere University, Kampala. CHDC, under Dr Jitta, was host institution for the project in Uganda.

Frank Kaharuza, also based at CHDC and a medical doctor, is a clinician who has specialized in the diagnosis and treatment of sexually transmitted diseases (STD) in various parts of Uganda.

Jessica Ogden is a social anthropologist who now works in the London School of Hygiene and Tropical Medicine. Her doctorate, completed at the University of Hull under the title *Reproductive Identity and the Proper Woman* (1995), is based on fieldwork done for this project.

Valdo Pons is an urban sociologist, now Professor Emeritus at the University of Hull. He first came to Kampala to teach at Makerere in the 1950s, and is the author of *Stanleyville* (1969), a pioneering work on another African city.

Sandra Wallman is professor of social anthropology at Hull. She works on Europe as well as Africa, and is interested in parallels between them – notably in the effect of options offered by inner city slum areas on the economic and identity resources of their residents. In this respect Kamwokya echoes the findings for Battersea, published as *Living in South London* (1982), and *Eight London Households* (1984).

One

Introduction

This book is set in 1994. It is about 'getting by' in a small and densely populated area on the outskirts of Kampala, the capital of Uganda. In 1969, as old people remember it, Lower Kamwokya (pron. Kam-oh-tcha) was no more than a handful of houses below the Kira Road. It began to burgeon with the disruptions of war, displacement and civil unrest which Uganda suffered over the twenty years leading to 1986, and continues to grow — now popular with people from many backgrounds for the range of options it offers whether for housing, getting by or for the treatment of illnesses.

Because the settlement is largely unplanned and thus without municipal benefits, well-being of every kind depends on the ingenuity of ordinary men and women who live in it. At the same time, the diversity and openness of the Kamwokya urban system ensure both that the informal economy flourishes and that people have relatively more scope for putting a livelihood together in this than in other parts of the city. However meagre their material and social resources, residents on the whole expect to get by here as well as, if not better than, in a home village or other Kampala suburb.

A positive atmosphere does not, of course, deny the fact that this is a community under stress. Given the constraints on resources and the compression of diversities in Kamwokya, getting by depends on existential as well as economic compromise. Each set of beliefs, boundaries and norms will inevitably have been challenged by encounter with many others, and everyone's traditions transformed by more or less painful bricolage.

Because the following chapters report the essentially creolized ways of life that result, some of them bear little resemblance to earlier accounts of culture and livelihood in Uganda. Furthermore, being multi-disciplinary, the book's narrative line is less consistent than that conventionally expected of a single subject monograph — whether ethnographic, economic or medical in intent.

The first objective here has been to freeze-frame a still changing community to see how it deals with epidemic and other crises now, so that well-intentioned intervention may be designed to enhance local capacity rather than ignoring or suppressing it. The second has been to grasp as a single system, in the way real people must, the many dimensions of context which impinge on the general business of getting by in these turbulent times, and on the specifics of women seeking treatment for acute illness in their children and venereal infection (STD) in themselves. These are the practical foci of the book.

Health is an aspect of wellbeing (in Luganda the same word represents both) which tends to be the special concern of women. Women, after all, are everywhere defenders of the household's moral and economic boundaries. And if this is true even when there is a responsible man in charge, it applies all the more where there is none. In Kamwokya more than a quarter of the households surveyed are run by a woman – whether as sole adult, or as head of a household with other adults in residence.

Different proportions of men and women in particular age bands, occupations and neighbourhoods are functions (sometimes as cause, sometimes as effect) of the realities of risk and opportunity in Kamwokya. The disruptions of Uganda's years of turmoil demanded extraordinary resilience of all its citizens. But while HIV and the collapse of the formal economy increased, in their different ways, the hazards and hardships facing everyone, circumstances seem to have evolved to create 'extra' possibilities for women. We cannot judge whether these new opportunities are actually gender biased or are simply made to appear so by women's 'extra' capacity to exploit – as much as they are exploited by – the informal economy. It is only clear that men and women residents differ in their relation to work, to health – and to Kamwokya itself.

The Problem

This book maps and discusses the informal economy of health as it affects treatment-seeking and health-care decisions of women in a densely populated urban setting in Africa.[1] It is based on a two-year multi-disciplinary study of Lower Kamwokya parish in Kampala. The study distinguishes city, neighbourhood, household and individual levels of analysis[2] to assess their separate relevance to two steps in the decision-making process: What combination of cultural, clinical and economic/environmental factors constitute a set of symptoms 'serious enough' to be taken for treatment outside the home? And on what basis is choice among the treatment options available then made?

The primary concerns of the book are the factors affecting the response of 'ordinary' urban women to their own symptoms of sexually transmitted diseases (STD) and to acute symptoms of illness in their children under the age of five. Among the factors documented are the resources and infrastructure of the study area as a whole; the treatment options available within it, and the accessible alternatives outside it; women's assessments of how good/kind/shameful/feasible/private/appropriate those options are;

[1] The project was sponsored under the title *The Informal Economy of Health in African Cities*.
[2] The research strategies and methodological frames used at each level are indicated throughout the volume, but only briefly. They have been documented at length elsewhere and will be replicated in further studies. On this basis Kampala can be systematically compared with other cities, and findings based on this study generalized and applied to disease control in other parts of Africa.

local perceptions of the symptomatology and aetiology of 'serious enough' infection; women's access to the resources necessary for health care (including time, information, confidence, autonomy) and the characteristics making for more or less capability to cope:- i.e. power structures and other-things-happening at household and local level which assist or impede that capability.

Although the aims of the study are quite specific, this framework has made it possible to address four distinct problem areas:

(i) Relative to men, women are often disadvantaged by lack of economic and jural authority at community and household level. Nevertheless, the woman is largely responsible for the management of illness in all members of the household.

(ii) Among them, children under five are particularly at risk in Africa at this time. While their vulnerability is a matter of extreme concern at all levels, it is women in the domestic sphere who must take the first crucial decisions about their care when crisis symptoms occur.

(iii) Where adult health is concerned, endemic STD in Africa has long been the cause of chronic morbidity, reproductive incapacity and social stress. In this era of AIDS its effect is made more dramatic by association with HIV: persons with (other) STDs, particularly those characterized by skin lesions, are hugely more vulnerable to HIV infection (Green, 1992; Lal & Kennedy, 1988; Laga *et al.*, 1991). The proper treatment of curable STD is therefore a significant AIDS prevention measure (Moses *et al.*, 1991; Grosskurth *et al.*, 1995). Further to our focus in this book, it should be noted that women tend to be more susceptible to, and to be blamed as the source or the cause of, both infections (PANOS, 1990).

(iv) The complexity and inaccessibility of social process in dense and highly mobile populations in tropical cities prevent effective targeting of scarce health resources. Much economic and health-relevant activity is therefore in the so-called informal economy – by definition unenumerated and widely assumed to be incapable of enumeration (Gregory and Altman, 1989).

There are implications for intervention to be drawn. They are indicated in different parts of the book, notably in the conclusions (Chapter 12), but it may be helpful to signal them in outline here. Identifying factors which make STD/HIV prevention infeasible, or which impede early and effective treatment of STD, will allow the sharper targeting of prevention and intervention efforts. It also allows the question 'What (most) needs doing?' to be realistically asked – e.g. does it make more sense to give priority to transport, better clinics, more drugs, economic support for women – or to provide more STD information and better health education services? Our view is that even if once-for-all prioritizing is not feasible, a full and 'thick' description of what goes on in the arenas of illness and treatment is itself useful, and that we have certainly provided. In addition, by combining medical and social perspectives on the whole range of 'informal' treatment options and the ways they are merged, by treatment-seekers, with 'formal' biomedicine, the book offers a holistic picture of problems of and opportunities for health care in Kampala and similar settings.

One more justification: effective multi-disciplinary work on STD/HIV is still scarce, and this volume reports a number of new elements which together make a particular contribution to the field. Among them is the fact that it is urban community based; that its focus is on women as ordinary citizens, selected by residence and not by reference to known medical conditions or high risk behaviour; that it specifies the dimensions of context whose effects are analysed and compared; and that its field strategies involving training and employing residents within the research project have had the effect, here as elsewhere, of encouraging local informants to become active participants in the definition of local problems and their solutions (Busuulwa *et al.*, 1994; Wallman *et al.*, 1980).[3]

Uganda Setting

Parallels for much of what is said in this book about social contexts of health and disease in low-income Kampala could be found in another – perhaps in any other – tropical city. But media coverage of AIDS in the last ten years, encouraged by the country's pioneering candour about the extent of HIV infection in the region, led to Uganda being especially closely identified with the epidemic. This prominence built on and revived international memories of the national experience of divisive and brutal regimes. The combined effect has been to associate Uganda, in the general reader's mind, with decline and disaster – negative images overshadowing descriptions of it as 'the pearl of Africa', the very real achievements of the current regime, and the remarkable buoyancy of its people.

In fact Uganda is both like, and unique among, low-income countries in sub-Saharan Africa (LISSA). It ranks as better-off than many on certain authoritative league tables (*The Economist*, 1994), and by some measures the picture is brightening. For example, although for the years between 1975 and 1984 Uganda's economic growth (at 0.2 per cent average annual increase in real GDP) was the seventeenth slowest in the world, for the period 1985–92 it was in the fastest top third, at 4.2 per cent well up with Ghana and Kenya. (Among European countries, only Israel and Luxembourg rank among the top forty by this measure) (*ibid*.: 26–7).

We cannot here go into anything like detailed accounts of Uganda's recent history; the collapse of the formal economy; or the operation of the new local government system, all of which impinge on Kamwokya in significant ways. But the rest of this section offers a brief sketch of the main issues, and provides references where they may be followed up at length.

---

[3] Results were first presented at an open meeting on 7 August 1993 by Achilles Ssewaya.

4

Introduction

Recent history

The introduction to *Uganda Now* acknowledges the uniqueness of Uganda's crises since independence, but argues that in many respects its recent history also mirrors 'a dilemma currently shared by many other black African countries' (Hansen and Twaddle, 1988: 9). Its typicality in tropical Africa remains a matter of some debate (cf. Wrigley, 1988). The sequence of political crises, however, is not in doubt, nor are the parallel changes in the country's economy. Brief paragraphs on the economy and society in the 1960s, 1970s and 1980s flesh out the skeleton history of Uganda since independence. which is shown in Figure 1.1.

(a) Political sequences			(b) Economic overview
1953–5	British Kabaka conflict		Steady state
1962	Independence		Boom
1966	Kabaka/Obote crisis	—> Obote 1	Obote 1 era
			Political but not economic turmoil
1969			until Amin. Turmoil developed quickly in his era. But late 1970s before disaster.
1971	Amin Coup	—> Amin	
1972	Asians expelled		
1978	Invasion by Tanzanian Army		
1979	Collapse of Amin	—> Obote II	
1979–85			'Struggle to live'. Theft, fraud, rip-off, corruption (*magendo/mafuta mingi*) in formal economy plus development of informal/second economy
1985	Collapse of Obote army	—> Museveni	
1986	RC system established. NRA in Kampala		Museveni clamps down on corruption and/but formal economy fades out altogether, only the 'informal' left.

Figure 1.1 *Recent events in Uganda*

Jamal (1991: 79) refers to the relatively good economic situation in the 1960s, the first Obote period. 'Uganda had already passed the phase of import substitution...' etc. Similarly, Edmonds (1988: 96) claims that 'between 1963 and 1971, the economy performed impressively', and Lateef (1991: 21) makes the point that with inflation as low as 5.6 per cent 'Uganda's economic and social performance in ... 1965 73 ... compared very favourably with that of LISSA' etc.

But we know that problems were developing politically, and with unfavourable trade balances. Southall (1988: 5) refers to 'the inexorable deterioriation of the Obote regime'. The economy, however, apparently continued buoyant. There was rising productivity based on labour-intensive technology, and the division of labour remained much as it had been pre-independence, with Asians and Europeans as entrepreneurs and Africans as farmers and wage-earners. Wage-earners including the greater part of the urban labour force were still the 'labour aristocracy' and doing relatively better than African farmers (see Jamal, 1991: 81).

By contrast, the 1970s (roughly the Amin period) were marked by 'economic collapse', although 'the full impact of Amin's mismanagement was masked by the great boom in commodity prices that occurred in 1977...' By the time of Amin's downfall 'the economy was well on its way to ruin' with the main 'free fall' occurring in 1978–80 (*ibid.*: 79). But the 'economic collapse' had many aspects to it. Not merely was there a decline in real wages but the whole structure of the urban economy changed (*ibid.*: 86–7, Table 5.4). Migration into the city slowed down and 'reverse migration' to the countryside became increasingly common (*ibid.*, fn. 13, O'Connor, 1988: 92). The *magendo* economy, which combined black marketeering in foreign exchange, overcharging and more or less petty corruption, began to flourish. Obbo (1991) describes it as a trend towards things increasingly being done 'in the private sphere', despite the continued existence of the public service. She also notes the growth of 'interstitial jobs' (p. 100), an element in the occupational pluralism referred to in Chapter 5.

Most writers on the period discuss the development of *magendo*/parallel/ informal, etc. economies by dwelling on fundamental changes in people's living situations. A point of particular interest is that in the overall process of economic collapse and *magendo*-style living, wage-earners in the formal economy 'lost their viability as a group' (Hansen & Twaddle, 1991: 11).

After Amin the years 1979/80 were unstable and chaotic politically, economically and socially. But the period 1981–5 (Obote II) saw some early indications of success, particularly in dealing with the *magendo* economy (see Belshaw, 1988; Edmonds, 1988, 101ff., 108). GDP rose and inflation fell, but continuing political turmoil and social unrest were followed by what several writers refer to as 'the second economic collapse' in 1985: by July 1985, in terms of inflation and to a lesser extent the balance of payments, the situation was once again similar to that of December 1980 (*ibid.*: 109) and continued this way until the Museveni era (*ibid.*: 109, 112–14).

Repercussions in the health sector [4]

According to Hansen and Twaddle (1991) there was no serious structural adjustment in Uganda until May 1987 when the NRM regime began its current programme of economic recovery (NRM Secretariat, 1986). But although the country has since registered increased industrial investment and improvement in physical infrastructure (especially roads), at the micro level there is a growing realization that these achievements have been at the expense of equity, growth and economic transformation. In particular, severe cuts in government social spending have dealt a crippling blow to

---

[4] This section was prepared by Grace Bantebya-Kyomuhendo.

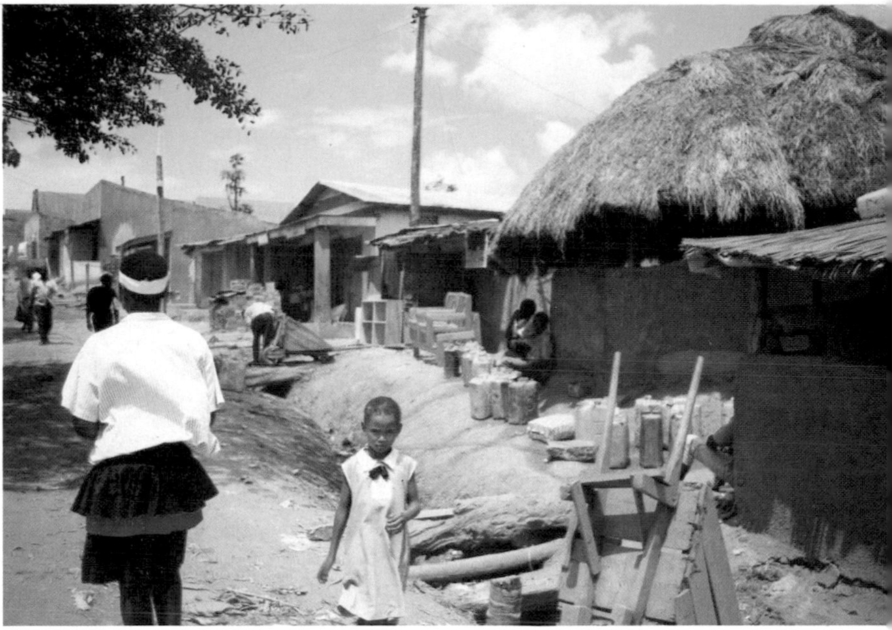

Street scene: water sellers with their jerry cans and wheel barrows, furniture for sale and traditional thatched drinking hut.

Street scene: drying millet for brewing, locally made beds for sale, shops, and dishes put to dry in the sun.

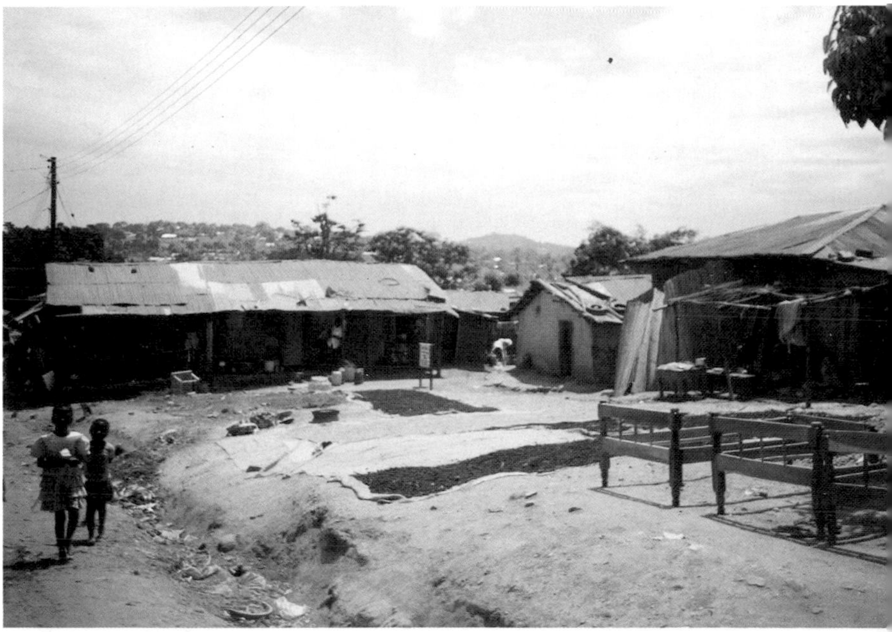

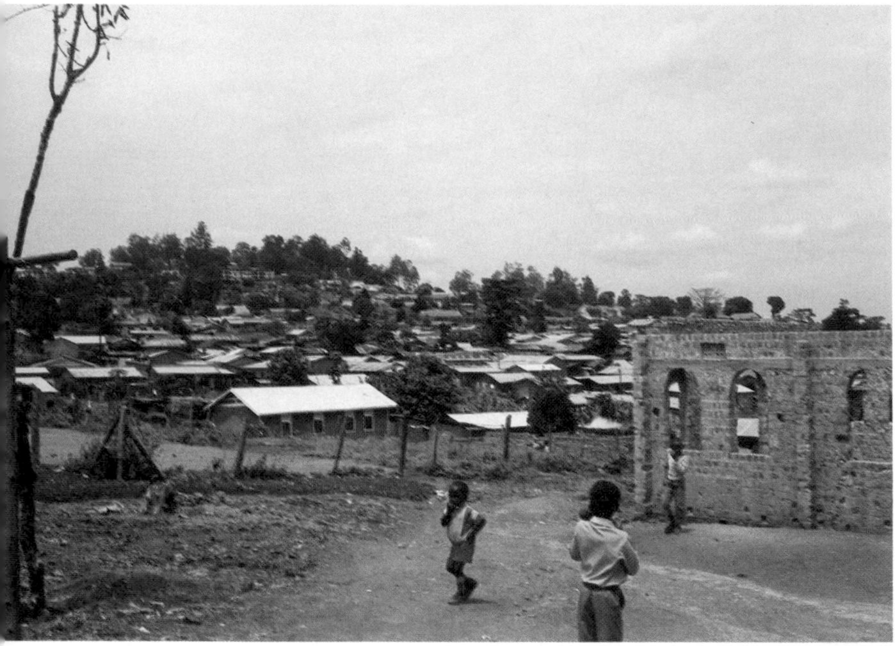

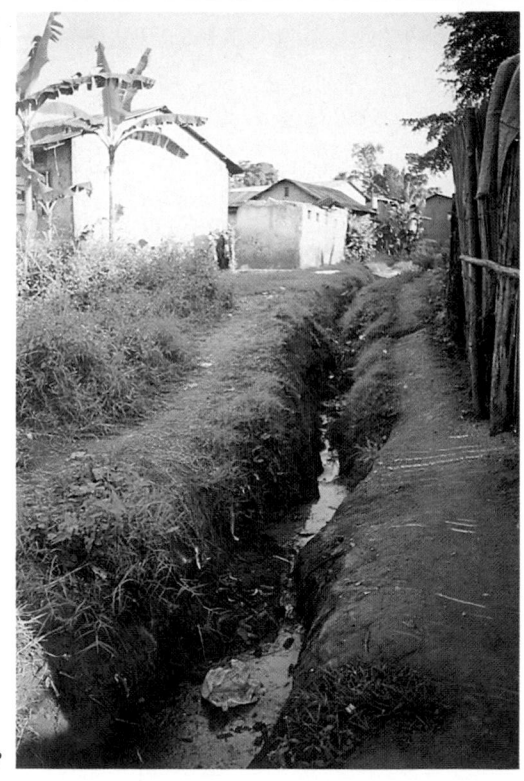

Kamwokya from high ground

Kamwokya drainage

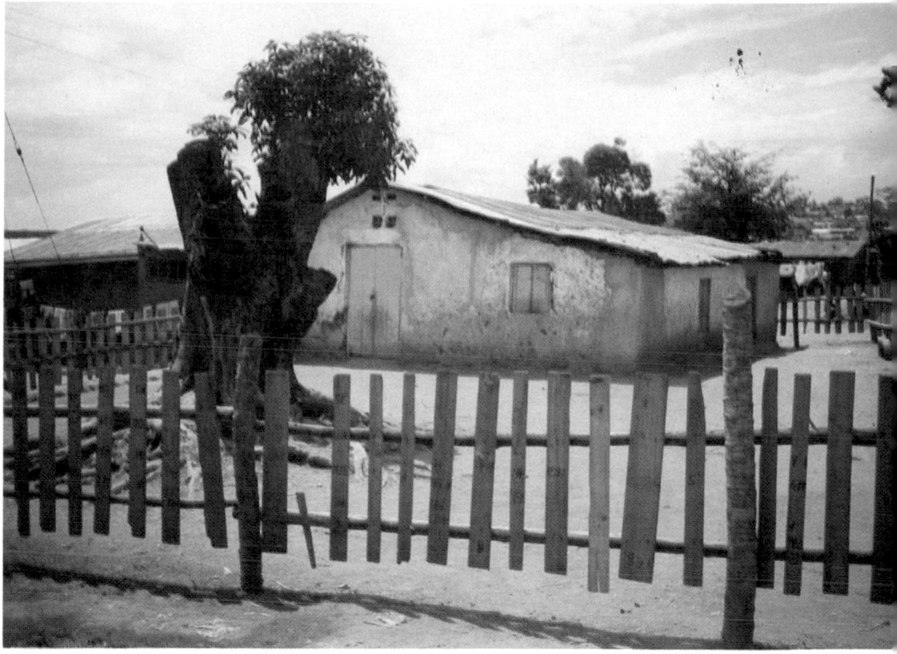

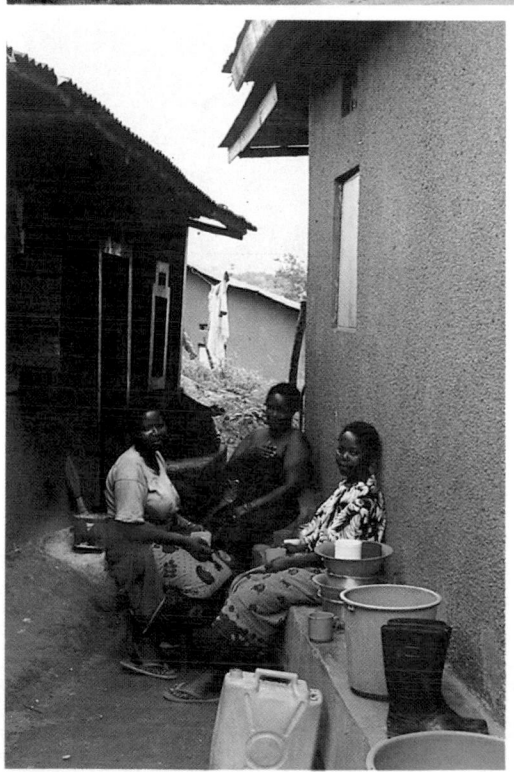

Nursery school doubling as community hall

Tea break

Woman with grandchild

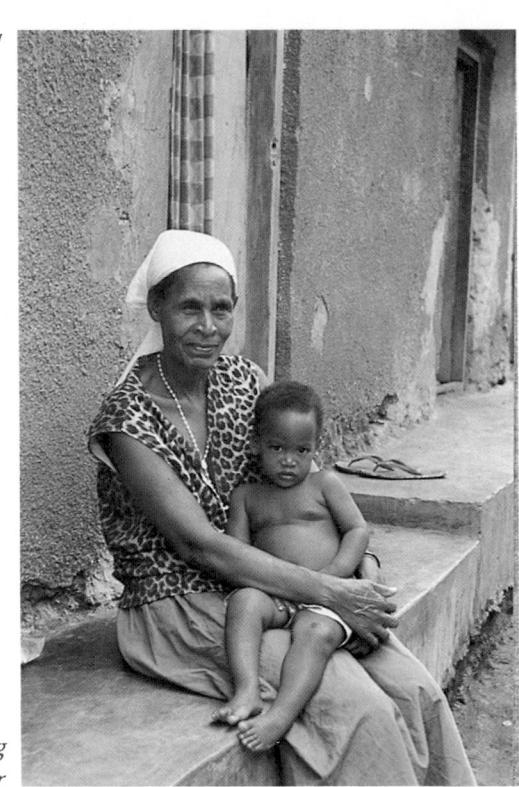

*Traditional bar: drinking
locally brewed beer*

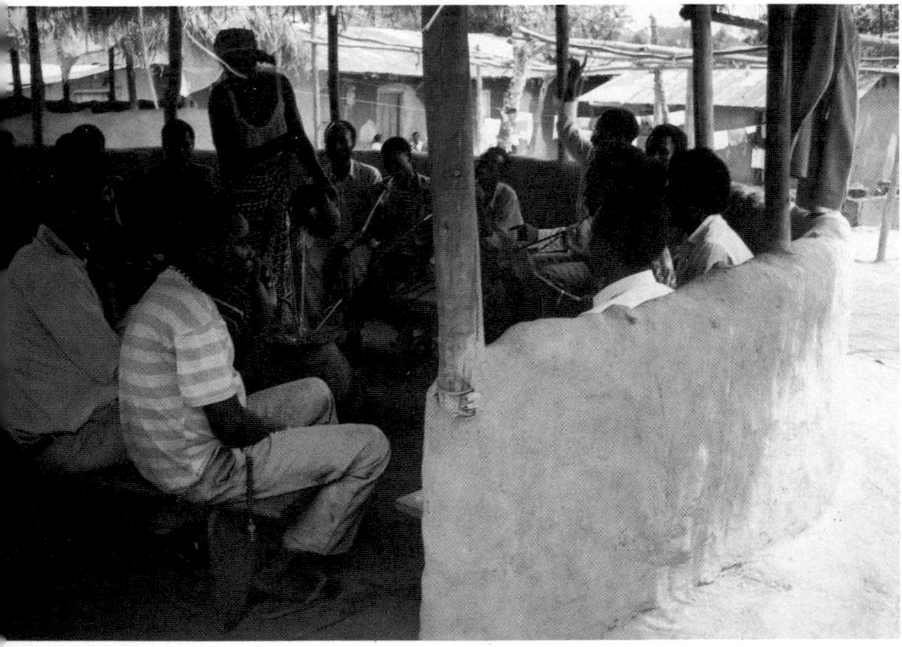

Making a mat

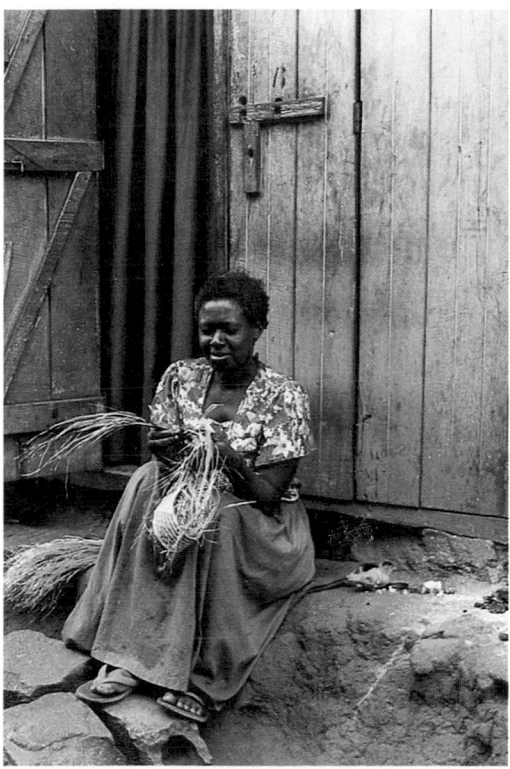

Selling charcoal

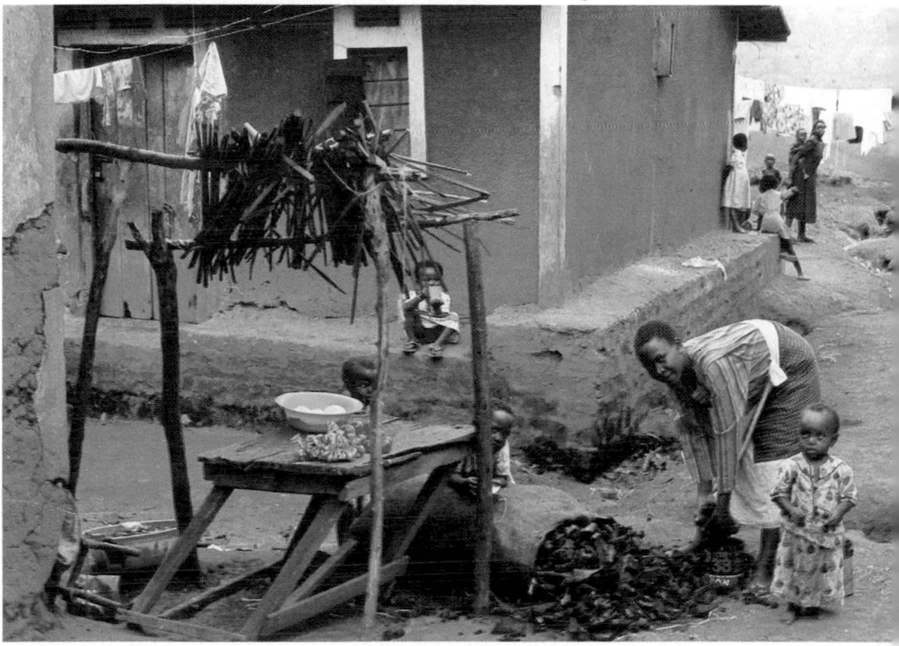

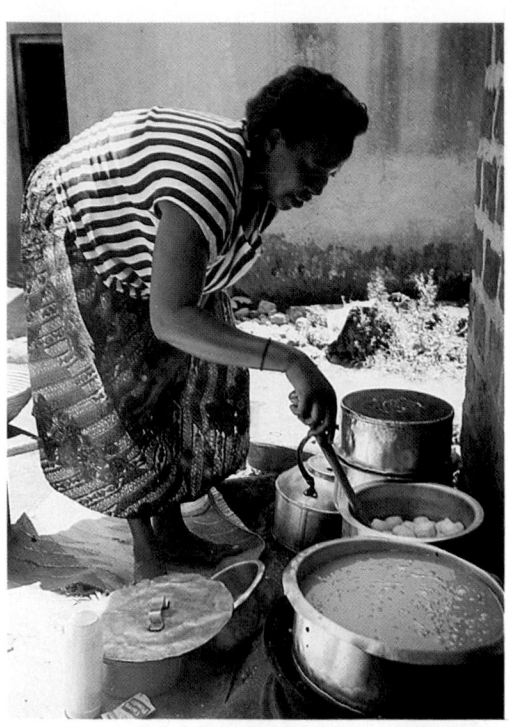

Cooking food for the family and others

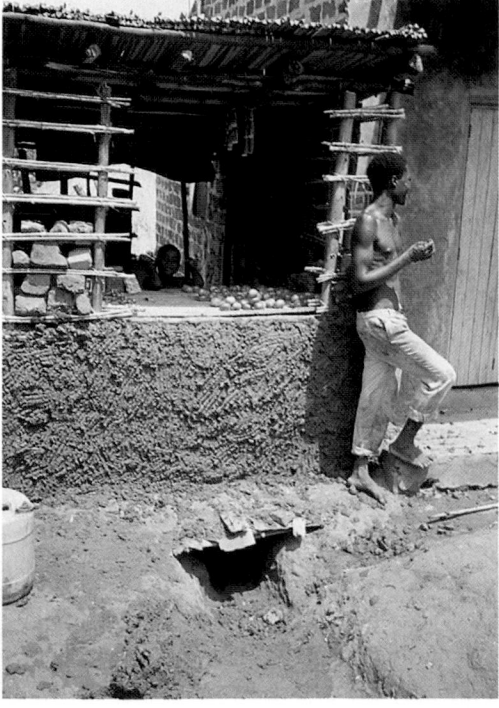

Building a shop

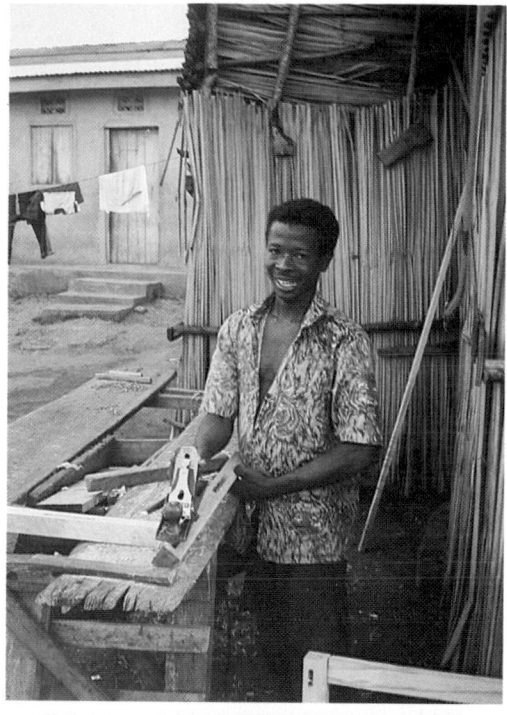

Making furniture

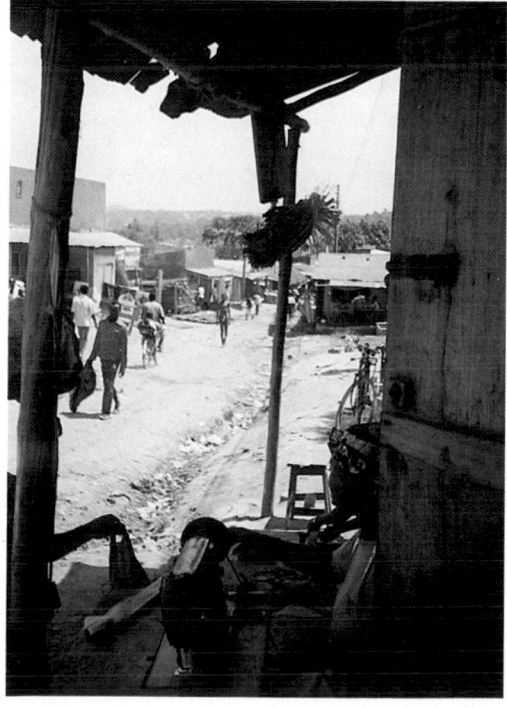

Tailoring with a view

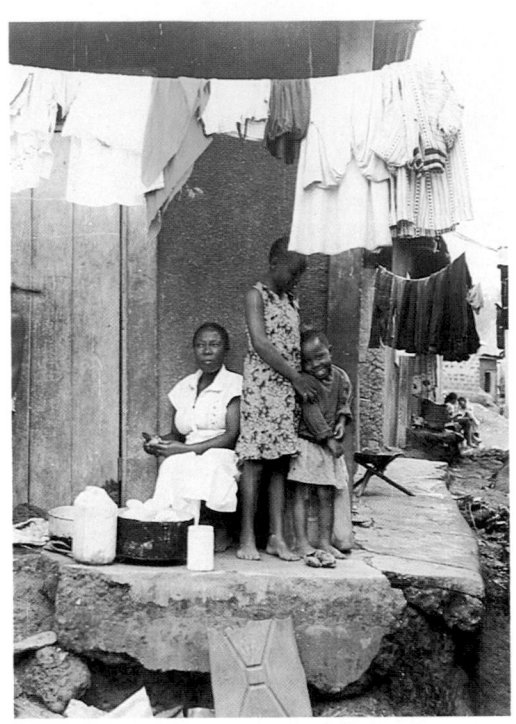

Preparing food to sell

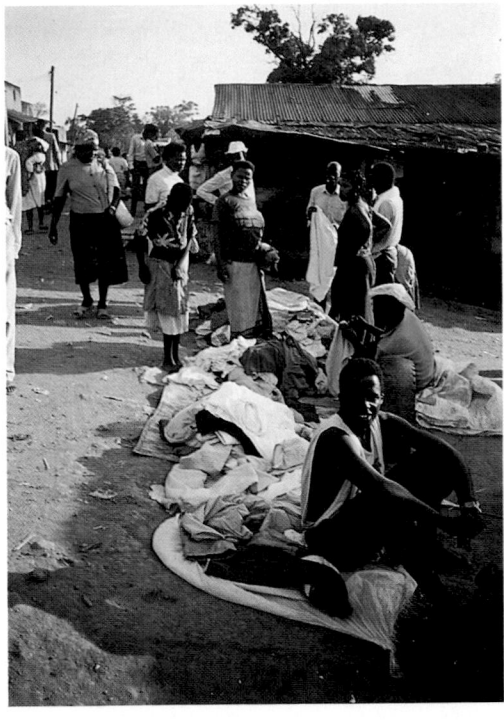

Selling second-hand clothes

vulnerable social groups like women and children (World Bank, 1993c; Barton and Wamai, 1994).

As part of the general crisis, Uganda's health sector largely collapsed during the 1970s. The government hospital infrastructure and many health centres were destroyed, leaving formal health care mostly in the hands of non-governmental organizations, missionary and private practitioners. Funding for the health sector almost disappeared and by 1986 the value of public health budget was only 6.4 per cent of its 1970s levels (Kapoor *et al.*, 1993). Without support, many trained health personnel abandoned government employment. This loss, coupled with poverty-constrained recruiting practices, left a health sector in which half of the staff employed are untrained. Since 1986, most of the health resources have been used to support single-focus vertical programmes, such as control of diarrhoeal diseases, and to rehabilitate hospitals and health centres. These capital expenditures, though essential, have led to a major crisis of financing and donor dependency, with the government unable to raise sufficient recurrent funds to sustain the rehabilitated facilities and vertical programmes (Macrae & Zwi, 1993).

In early 1990 an official inter-ministerial task force on health financing recommended the introduction of a 'cost-sharing' mechanism whereby patients would be required to contribute to the cost of the delivery of health services. The recommendations provoked political controversy and were not implemented. In January 1993, with increased pressure from donor agencies, the Ministry of Health directed health facilities to design and manage their own cost-recovery mechanisms. Most hospitals and other health facilities have subsequently introduced formal user fees. Although policy and guidelines regulating them are not yet in place, their effects are already being felt by the poor and vulnerable, with health conditions progressively deteriorating (Bantebya-Kyomuhendo, 1994). Related to this is the increase and mushrooming of private clinics, drug shops, pharmacies and private individuals operating in their own houses to exploit the need.

A short note on local government and Kamwokya

When, under the leadership of President Museveni, the National Resistance Army (NRA) and the National Resistance Movement (NRM) took over power on 26 January 1986, new structures were introduced to promote participatory democracy and enhance socio-economic development from the grass roots. These are the Resistance Councils (Nsibambi, 1991). The smallest unit of the RC system (RC 1) is the village in rural areas, and the zone in urban areas, of which all residents aged 18 and over are members. In each RC 1 there is an executive RC committee consisting of nine people: a chairman, vice-chairman, general secretary, and secretaries for finance, security, youth, women, information, and mobilization and education. These are elected by the RC members biannually.

Kamwokya II, the focus of this study, is a parish (*muluka*) which constitutes a Resistance Council level 2 (RC 2) made up of ten zones, that is, of ten RC 1s. The ninety people comprising the total of RC 1 committee members elect nine of their number to the executive committee for the RC 2 level. The political system has three more levels above these.

Kamwokya was not selected as a research site on the basis of any rigid demographic socio-economic or cultural criteria: it would not have been possible to recognize such criteria because the results of the 1991 Population and Housing Census for the area were not yet available. It was, however, known as a heterogeneous and densely populated area of Kampala.

The 1991 Census figures later showed its population to be 5,161 in Upper Kamwokya (Ward I: altitude 3450–4025 ft) and 12,079 in Lower Kamwokya (Ward II: altitude 3850–3925 ft) (see Chapter 3). The two wards have always differed appreciably. Upper Kamwokya was in colonial days a 'planned' area within what was then Kampala and Lower Kamwokya lay outside the old municipal boundaries. The latter has developed – mainly since independence – as an entirely unplanned settlement. Its overall population density was and is visibly higher than in Kamwokya I; but (as other chapters will show) there is appreciable variation in density as well as lifestyle within Kamwokya II. This book focuses on the lower ward and any unqualified reference to 'Kamwokya' in the chapters following refer only to Kamwokya II.

Analytical background

This study is about the management of health and illness, and two of its authors are medical doctors. A good proportion of its contents is concerned with the diagnosis of symptoms, the prescription of *materia medica*, and the treatment chosen for particular diseases. Evidence for the match/mismatch of folk and biomedical symptomatology/aetiology has been collected and presented wherever possible. It is, however, the *social* context of these medical matters which decides their meaning for most people, and it is in that context that they can be – need to be – interpreted.

Three dimensions of the context of health/illhealth and treatment-seeking in Kamwokya are sketched out in this section.[5] Each draws on a separate professional literature and is, in the perspective of this book, narrowly focused on a single aspect of a multi-faceted problem. The first (The Development of African Cities) serves to situate Kampala in the context of other African cities and their economies; the second (Healthcare in the Household) reviews women's special responsibility for health and wellbeing, and the constraints on their decision-making in the household sphere; and the third (Varieties of the Urban System) sets out a framework for understanding Kamwokya as an urban system, and the scope for identity and economic activity provided by different kinds of cityscape. They are presented separately as a basis for analysis of the whole in the body of the book.

[5] Notes for the first were prepared by Ogden, the second by Pons and the third by Wallman.

Introduction

The Development of African Cities

Demographics

The image of African cities growing at an historically unprecedented rate through large-scale rural-urban migration is not strictly correct. As in other less developed regions of the world, the rate of change in the urban proportion of the population is not exceptionally high. In the third quarter of this century it grew from 16.7 to 28 per cent, a rate very similar to that pertaining in currently more developed countries in the last quarter of the nineteenth century.

What is unprecedented in today's developing countries is the growth rate of urban populations, particularly in their primate cities. During the 1980s, the urban population of East Africa grew at an average rate of over 7 per cent per annum; those of western Africa at nearly 6 per cent; and those of 'middle' Africa at about 5.5 per cent (UN, 1989). The key difference stems from the fact that natural increase in the cities of the currently developing countries, especially in Africa, remains almost as high as in their rural hinterlands. At the same time, infant mortality in the cities is, if anything, lower than in the rural areas. This combination stands in contrast to the situation which obtained in Europe when its populations had comparably low proportions of urban dwellers.

Africa remains one of the least urbanized regions of the world. In some countries the proportion of urban dwellers is still below 10 per cent (e.g. Uganda and Malawi); in others it reaches about 40 per cent (e.g. Zambia). In a detailed study of 29 developing countries the mean growth rate attributable to natural increase in the 1960s and 1970s was found to be 60.7 per cent. The basic data for such a calculation are not reliable in most African countries; overall the proportion is probably lower – around 50 per cent (Preston, 1988: 14–15).

With young adults making up most of the rural-urban migrants, high urban fertility, and life expectancy around 50 years, the population consists largely of families and households with numerous children and high dependency ratios. In colonial days restrictions placed on rural-urban migration resulted in urban populations with high male/female ratios. Since the 1960s however, this has changed appreciably and has in some cases been reversed. In Kampala, for example, females constituted 51 per cent of the population in 1991. And in some areas they make up an even larger proportion (cf. Nelson, 1979 and 1987, on Mathare Valley in Nairobi).

Urban crisis

In many African countries economic stagnation or decline in the 1970s and 1980s has combined with rapid overall population growth (around 3 per cent per annum in the 1980s) to worsen the situation of ordinary people in both rural and urban areas. African cities are in particular crisis. The real wages of urban workers have fallen sharply, the earlier relative security of formal work has largely gone, and the rural-urban gap has narrowed markedly if not altogether vanished (Jamal and Weeks, 1988).

The net result is not only an urban crisis in the sense of acute problems in providing and maintaining urban services (including health) and municipal administration (Stren and White, 1989) but also that individual and family problems can be met only by recourse to complex sets of survival strategies. Hence the steady growth of the informal economy (Turnham *et al.*, 1990).

The concept of the informal sector has given rise to a voluminous literature (see for example, ILO, 1991 in relation to the studies of the 1980s). But these studies have not, for the most part, embraced the social and cultural aspects of the informal economy as a whole: one important exception is a model distinguishing the characteristics of household, communal, illicit and formal economies. The first three comprise the non-formal (or informal) sphere, generally 'lumped' as a single sector by contrast to the fourth (Gershuny, 1983, and see Harding and Jenkins, 1989). The main focus otherwise has been on work opportunities in small-scale enterprises seen as an alternative to waged or salaried employment and as a means of employing the unemployed. Some of these studies have attempted to assess the proportion of urban dwellers employed in the informal sector. Mettelin (1987), for example, claims that the informal sector absorbs a quarter to one half of the working populations of major African cities, thereby 'surmounting the problem of unemployment'.(!) And in Dar es Salaam, according to Malimyamkono and Bagachwa (1990), virtually every family has one or more – often all – of its members engaged in the informal economy in one or other capacity. Neither government officials nor professionals – let alone workers – can support their families for more than a few days per month on their incomes from formal employment. This position now appears to be general throughout African urban society and not simply among the poor.

The informal economy conceived in this way demands a close analysis of the social texture within and through which it operates – interpersonal relations; social networks; family, kinship and tribal connections; rural-urban linkages; neighbourhood and workplace contexts. Studies on 'getting by' all emphasize that the informal economy is just as much a social, cultural and political phenomenon as an economic one. They call for a holistic if not multi-disciplinary perspective applied, usually on a small scale, in neighbourhoods, households or other fields which lend themselves to intensive investigation by a combination of techniques, including participant observation.[6] This is the approach taken here. The next sections set a background for the household-focused chapters which follow.

---

[6] Among many field-specific studies in urban anthropology/sociology, Southall and Gutkind, 1957; Gutkind, 1973; Stack, 1976; Pons, 1969 and Wallman, 1984 are useful in the discussion of these topics. More generally, Hannerz, 1993, Gregory and Altman, 1989, and Harding and Jenkins, 1989 provide conceptual approaches to economic and/or urban systems.

Health Care in the Household

In the literature generally[7] there is scant mention of the contributions of men to household health provision (but see Maclean, 1966; Janzen, 1978; Jonker, 1988). By contrast, reference to women's role in health-care provision is abundant. 'In general, studies indicate that women play a pivotal role in determining the ... use of health services ... and in providing home nursing for ill children' (Carpenter, 1980: 1210, cited in Graham, 1984: 6). Some studies delineate exactly which decisions women make. Most show them responsible for the day-to-day running of their households, which includes budgeting for major expenditures, up-keep of the physical environment, caring and provision of basic needs (Graham, 1984, 1985; see also Litman, 1974; Blaxter, 1983). From this point of view it might be argued that all a wife-mother's decisions which are related to her household can be understood as health-promoting. House-cleaning, shopping, cooking, bathing and dressing children, washing clothes, saving and budgeting for fuel, rent and transport can all serve to maintain or enhance the health and welfare of the family. This view brings household health very close to the Luganda concept of 'wellbeing' (taken up specifically in Chapter 5). More directly, when a child becomes unwell, its mother is often the first to notice a change, and the first to diagnose the nature and perhaps the cause of the sickness (Graham, 1984; Blaxter, 1983).

Given the health-care responsibilities of mothers, it follows that the raising of standards of 'proper' caretaking and nurture by public health and development campaigns adds to 'the physical and financial burdens of women' (Kellock and Agunda, 1985: 16; see also Smock, 1981). The time and physical labour involved in providing even minimal standards of health for their children is considerable. To collect water for 'adequate' sanitation (no fewer than 50 litres a day according to UNICEF) can require several trips a day to an often distant water source. Fuel must be collected (more if the water is boiled to prevent diarrhoeal disease), food produced and protected from flies and vermin, and cash acquired for clothing, medicines, education, foodstuffs. Visits to the clinic for children's immunization and growth monitoring can involve long queues and (again) a time-consuming return trip.

The amount of time that can be dedicated to childcare is everywhere limited by other responsibilities. In urban areas in particular, the need to concentrate on earning a living outside the home detracts from time for children, even while it provides the income essential for their care (Bantebya-Kyumohendo, 1994 and Chapter 10 below).

There is a paradox of successful caring that can affect a woman in any setting. Graham (1984) calls it the 'responsibility of irresponsible behaviour'.

---

[7] See among many examples, Raikes, 1989; Talle, 1988; Browner, 1989; Kellock and Agunda, 1985; Smock, 1981; Staugard, 1985a and b; Radoki, 1991.

Introduction

In the context of conflicting priorities and a shortage of resources, the pursuit of family welfare may depend on routines 'in which individual health is jettisoned' (*ibid.*: 185). A woman's capacity to care depends in great part on her own wellbeing, so the tendency to sacrifice her own needs for treatment, adequate nutrition or rest may ultimately prevent her looking after her family as she intends.

As well as preventing disease through provision of basic needs in the home, women are likely also to have more or less specialized knowledge of disease symptoms, determining when family members are ill and what kind of care they should be given. 'It is usually women who prescribe remedies, decide at what point in an illness to seek outside attention, and what type of practitioner to consult' (Browner, 1989: 465). Responsibility improves their skills. In one study Latin American wives-mothers were found to be able to identify between 50 and 100 medicinal plants, and to describe the curative properties, preparation and administration of each of them. Children and women without children, by contrast, could only identify 5 to 10 plants and were often misinformed or uninformed about how and when they should be used (*ibid.*). Essentially, most illnesses in Latin America, as in Kampala, are treated neither by Western practitioners nor traditional healers, but by mothers themselves (see also Hogle *et al.*, 1991; and Chapters 6–10 below).

But the ability to implement a treatment decision, like any other, depends on the balance and distribution of authority in the domestic setting. A comparison of evidence from the two continents (Packard *et al.*, 1989) implies that women have more authority over health care in Latin America than in Africa except where men are absent (in which case African women are the more decisive). 'However in both regions women provide care outside the faltering and uneven [*formal*] healthcare system' (*ibid.*: 409). These authors consider the tendency to underestimate women's roles and skills in treatment and caring to be itself a major obstacle to improved health care. Our inference from the Kamwokya study supports their view (see also Hoffman, 1987).

In any event, health-relevant behaviour is governed as much by access to and control over resources as by knowledge of appropriate prevention or treatment. The household resource base includes but is not confined to material items – cash, food, property; time, information, energy and identity are also resources insofar as they are necessary for organizing the material base (Wallman, 1984) and, most crucially in this context, for paying for treatment (Wallman and Baker, 1996). Who has power over which resource is a function both of the type of resource and where it comes from.

Money in cash is obviously essential for providing both basic needs and clinical treatment. Like their control over health-care decisions, the extent to which women as wives and mothers can control money varies with household circumstances, even irrespective of where the money comes from: there is some debate as to whether women even handle the income they have themselves earned (Hakansson, 1988; cf. Ogden, 1991). But it is widely agreed that, where they do, it will be spent on household provision or the needs of children (e.g. Kellock and Agunda, 1985: 29), whereas men tend to spend available cash on business investment or on consumption items such as alcohol and tobacco. The lack of female control over cash is a factor in the management of children's illness in Euro-American as well as Third World settings (see e.g. Litman, 1974; Graham, 1984; Swantz, 1985; Kellock and Agunda, 1985). Women can derive cash from the sale of non-cash resources which are under their own control. For the rural woman this will include surplus food produce, and will have unintended negative effects when she ends up selling food that is needed for the nourishment of her children. Brewing beer (see Nelson, 1978 and Chapter 5), or selling other food items in the market place, is common in rural and urban contexts, as apparently is the commercialization of a woman's own body and sexuality as a means of acquiring cash for the family's needs. (Recall the point above re: responsibility of 'irresponsible' behaviour.)

Varieties of the Urban System

This study deals with combinations of people and place in one densely populated urban area. The perspective taken evolved in the course of the systematic comparison of two inner London areas (Wallman, 1982, 1984, 1985, 1996a). The central questions there were: How do the economic options of the two areas differ? and: What styles or principles of organization do residents in each setting use to manage the options offered by that setting? Adapted to the present purposes, the central question becomes the following: *In the specific matter of coping with illness, in the general business of getting by as an individual, or in the way community resources are managed in Kamwokya, which of the many levels of difference embedded in it makes most difference to what happens?*

A useful analytical focus for understanding both the informal economy of an urban area and its characteristic patterns of group identity is the interrelation of structure and organization in each setting – *structure* being the framework of social, economic or conceptual options, and *organization* the pattern of choices made from amongst those options (Firth, 1951, 1954). This is the first of two angles crucial to the urban perspective of this book. Thus, each city setting provides a framework of options which puts at least an outer limit on how individuals or groups of individuals can make a livelihood within it. They may 'choose', in some sense, among the options offered, but they cannot take up options which are not there. This applies very obviously to the economic aspects of livelihood, but it is less widely recognized that 'getting by' in the city, *especially* in the city, depends also on the skilful management of non-material resources – identity among them. And just as you cannot choose to use job skills in a local system which has no market for them, so a particular form of group identity –

ethnicity, say – is not appropriate, not utilizable, in every city setting, or for every purpose in any one setting. There is no logical limit to the number of identity options available to ordinary individuals. It is because *work* and *locality* so often override or underwrite the identity potential of ethnic origin in urban settings that they are given special notice here. Ethnic difference is regularly observed to coincide with differences in the way work is allocated or organized, and it is normal for people to identify to some extent with the area in which they live. But not even all 'mixed' urban settings are alike. In some, the resource value of local identity clearly outweighs the potential of other options, particularly the ethnic option. It is as though certain kinds of local structure enhance the value of localism over ethnicity, and others have the opposite effect.

The second analytical strut which underpins this analysis of city settings is that they are also social *systems* in which arenas of interaction and opportunity operate as sub-systems of the whole, and which combine to make up its social style. The systems:sub-systems model is directly analogous to anthropological uses of the idea of context. The credo built on them is two-edged; the meaning and/or effect of a thought or action or resource depends on other-things-happening in the context in focus; and (ii) (therefore) its value, effect, etc. is dependent on a particular context and will change when that changes. Thus the salience of difference in any cityscape is determined as much by the urban system as by the original cultures of the people living in it. And it will vary even within that one setting. Who is included amongst 'us' changes with context, and so do the unit and the implications of belonging.

The area described here, for example, strikes the eye as ethnically mixed, but this says nothing about it as an urban system (cf. Wallman, 1996a). Ethnicity as a social or economically salient fact is not about difference as such. It is best understood as the *sense* of difference which can occur when members of a particular cultural, tribal, racial or national group interact with non-members. And to emphasize the urban theme – the facts of migration and compression are such that an encounter with 'not-us' is many times more likely to happen in a city (Hannerz, 1993, Paine, 1992a). The crucial point is that real differences between people are no more (and no less) than *potential* identity markers which will be mobilized, for group identity purposes, only where that particular difference suits the purpose of the encounter at hand.

Each kind of social difference falls into one of three categories: difference which the observer sees (external, manifest, out loud); difference which the actors experience (internal, latent, socially *sotto voce*); and difference of context or situation which makes a difference salient in the first place. Questions of group identity and interaction therefore need to be as much about the city, city-ness, as they are about ethnic affiliation, local belonging or the organization of work.

Analysis of the informal economy of health and treatment-seeking in a particular city setting is primarily the analysis of that setting as an urban system: local organization, infrastructure and socio-economic characteristics provide the conditions of possibility within which day-to-day decisions about treatment, as about everything else, must be made.

The Structure of the Book

Some chapters refer to materials collected by one research method – survey, interview, group discussion, case or situation analysis – and are associated with a single locus of analysis – Kamwokya as a whole, one of the 'cityscapes' within it, the household, individual treatment seekers or providers. Others combine different types of data, or different perspectives on a specified theme or themes.

The sequence of Chapters 2 to 10 in general echoes the broad-and-shallow to narrow-and-deep progression of the enquiry; in Chapter 11 the narrative perspective changes to report a process in which the research subjects look back at the findings. In the same sequence the data become increasingly qualitative, which is to say that the quantitative:qualitative balance shifts towards observations which cannot (and do not need to be) formally enumerated.

The sources of material for the various chapters are also different. Covering the first phase of research in the area, Chapter 3 is based on Uganda census data, and Chapters 2 and 4 on a Broad Brush Survey and other observations of Kamwokya. Chapter 5 draws substantially on responses to Ethnographic and Women's Surveys (ES/WS) carried out in the second phase of the work. Chapters 6 and 7, moving into phase three, are based in combinations of literature, survey, interviews and observation in the field. Chapters 8 and 9 report group discussions convened by Ugandan biomedical colleagues; and Chapter 10 recounts six case studies of individual women, representing the narrowest-deepest analytical focus of phase three. In Chapter 11 the focus again becomes wider and shallower to report the process and procedures involved in making an interactive video which explores perceptions of wellbeing, and of responsibility for disease and infectivity in the community.

To a degree, all of this book is about wellbeing. Some parts of it, however, are more explicit than others. Chapter 5, most importantly, broaches the notion directly, and details the range of elements implied by the concept in Luganda – some of them covered (as we noted earlier) by the anglophone understandings of the word 'health', others quite outside it (see page 11 above). In addition, Chapter 7 spells out the distinction between public and private options for managing the household's health, etc. and underscores the crucial responsibility of women in this domain. And Chapter 10, with a focus on individuals, most plainly demonstrates circumstances in which non-material components of wellbeing – security, self-esteem and reputation among them – can count for more, in treatment-seeking, than the hard facts of livelihood.

These issues could not have been addressed by a single-stranded approach. In the holistic perspective of the book, the interpretation of each set of data is enriched by insights from every other.

A similar mixture of single and multiple perspectives shows in the way authorship is attributed. The main author has been responsible for the overall project and for compiling and editing this volume; others associated in the study are acknowledged on pages ix and x and elsewhere. The aim has been to integrate the perspectives of several disciplines and local interest groups around the health/disease/treatment theme. Parts of the book are so fundamentally team products that it is not possible to discern, let alone to rank, the input of individuals: in those parts authors are not specified. Other chapters (or part chapters), though still constituents of the whole, pertain so directly to the professional expertise and authorship of one or other researcher that their names appear again with the chapter heading.

The contents and source[s] of data, drawings, etc. for each chapter are indicated in every case. Tables and figures are numbered separately for each chapter, maps in a single sequence of capital Roman numerals, and sketches as 1 to 20.

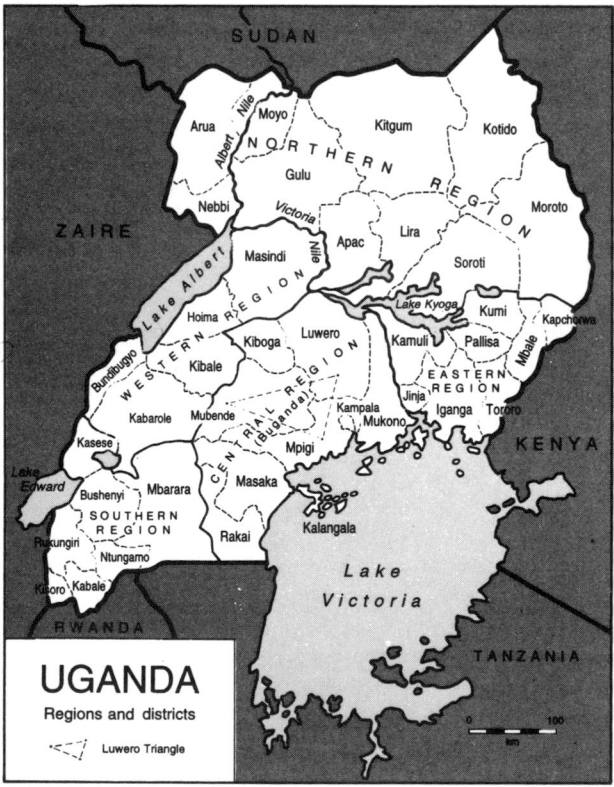

Map I

Two

Kamwokya
(kam-oh-tcha)

The site of our current research in Kampala is the parish called Kamwokya II. The settlement began in about 1960, with the erection of a few mud and wattle dwellings outside the then municipal boundary. Now that the city has grown, Kamwokya lies within it, but it has developed as an entirely unplanned settlement. Uganda's dramatic post-independence history is summarized in Chapter 1, and Kamwokya's relation to it set out in Figure 2.1 (below), but a quick statement of recent demographic and economic events helps to set the scene.

Concerning population: Census data show that between 1969 and 1991 the urban population grew massively, more than doubling both in Kampala as a whole and in the constituent parish. Over the same period, again at both levels, there has been a substantial change in the overall sex ratio and so a decrease in the surplus of adult men over adult women, and a significant excess of girls/young women over boys/young men has developed. These trends are explored in Chapter 3 but are noted here as background to the peculiar gender profile of this city setting. In the foreground of it, two observations from our own research strike the eye: more women than men are 'around' in the daytime; and patterns of livelihood vary with gender: most men come and go, most women stay put. Causes and effects of these differences in the spatial scope of men and women emerge in later chapters of the book.

On the political front: After the National Resistance Army (NRA) and the National Resistance Movement (NRM) took over power in Uganda in 1986, under the leadership of President Museveni, new structures were introduced to promote participatory democracy and enhance socio-economic development from the grass roots. These are the Resistance Councils, popularly known as RCs. The smallest unit of the RC system, the RC I, is the village, or in urban areas the zone. All residents of 18 years of age and over are members of the RC 1. In each RC 1 there is an executive committee of nine people elected by all adult residents every two years. Kamwokya is an RC 2 made up of ten zones (Map VI). The executive committee of these ten RC 1s form the RC 2 constituency,

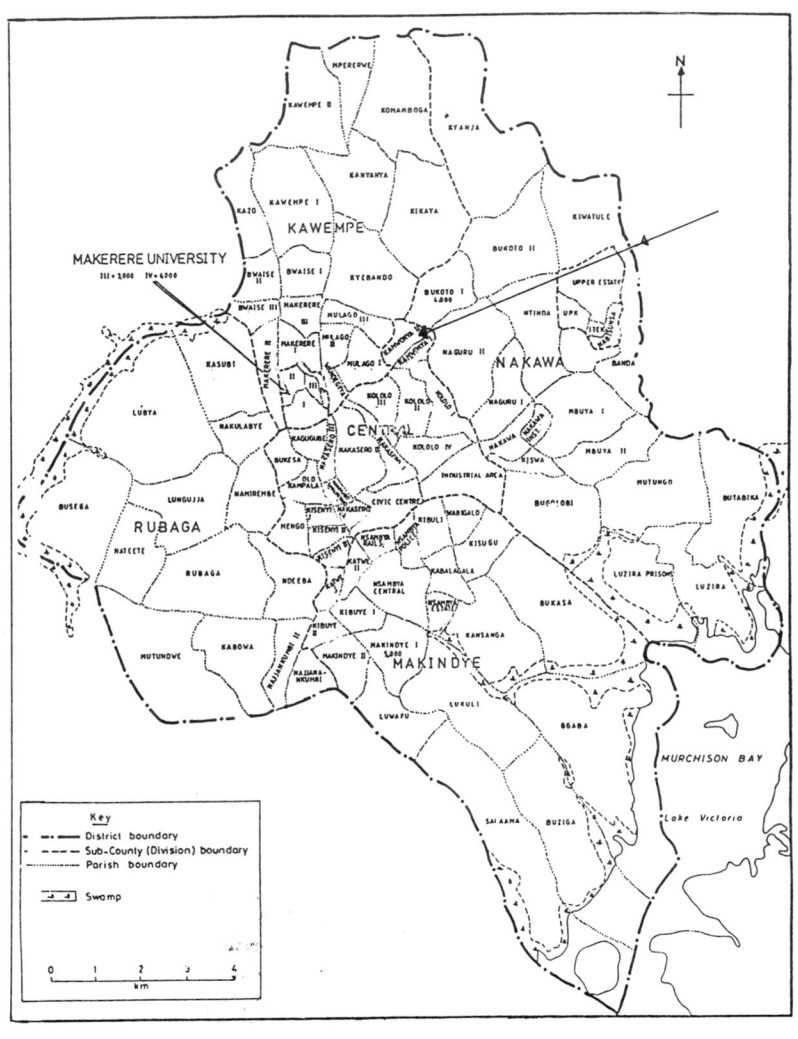

Map II *Kampala, with zones and parishes*

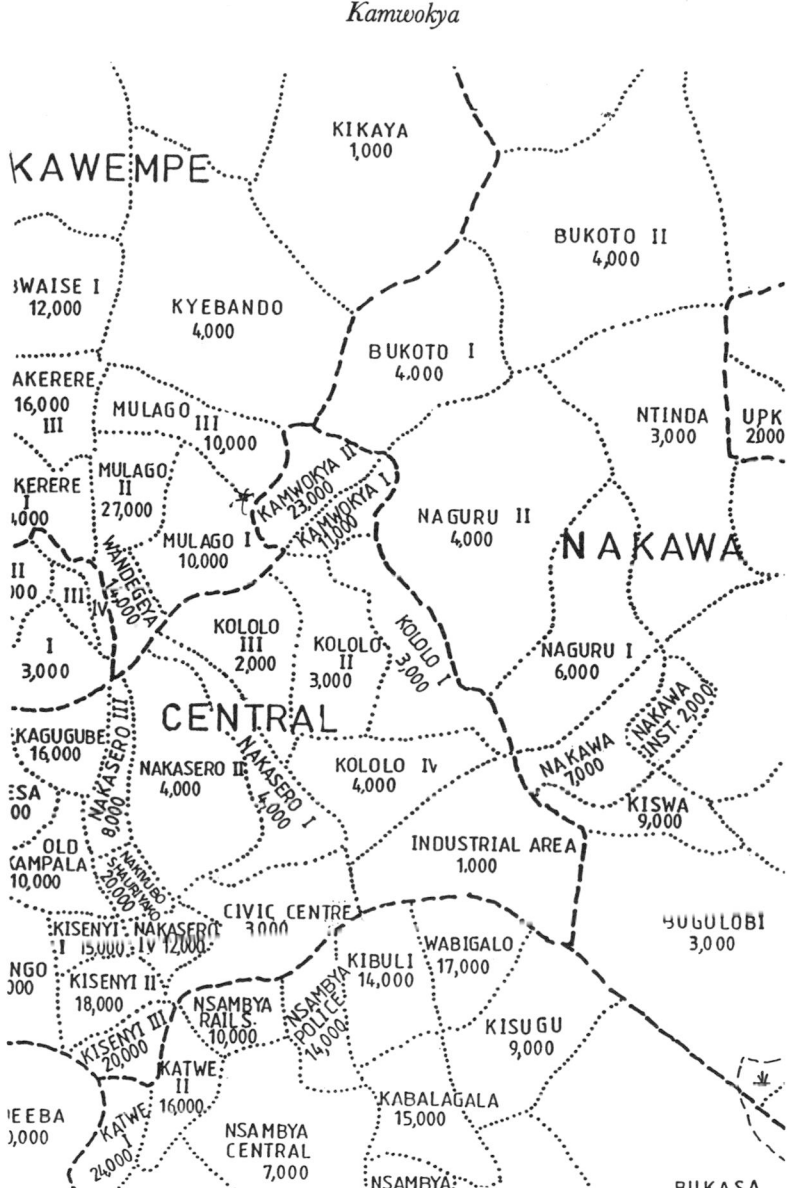

Map III *Kamwokya and surrounding parishes, showing population density to nearest 1,000 per km (1991 census)*

and from these 90 officials, 9 are elected to form the RC 2 committee which governs the parish. The political system has three more levels above these. On the economic front change has directly affected work and the options for livelihood. There has been a near total collapse of the formal economy, and a consequent sharpening of competition to 'get by' in the cracks and niches of informal economic activity. These we might expect to be implicated in definitions of insider:outsider in Kamwokya, and to impinge on the lives of women and men in different ways.

The Physical Setting

(i) Time perspective

Although Kamwokya is a well-established settlement, its expansion as a residential and commercial area is fairly recent, dating from the 1960s and 1970s. It should be stressed that this expansion is on-going; there are many houses under construction and land is still being reclaimed from the swampy edges of the settlement on its northern and eastern boundaries.

Figure 2.1 *Time chart showing highlights in the growth and development of Kamwokya II (1960–94)*

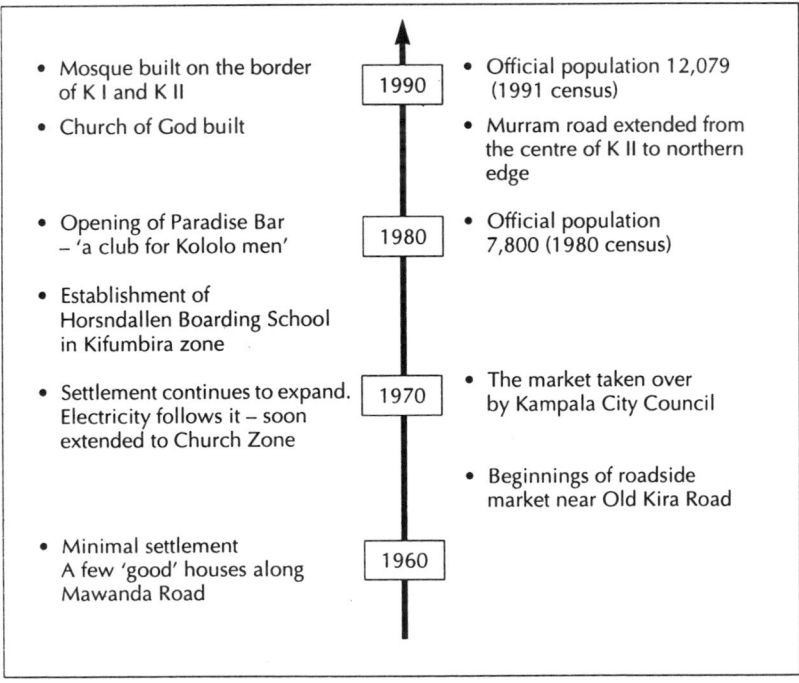

- Mosque built on the border of K I and K II
- Church of God built

1990

- Official population 12,079 (1991 census)
- Murram road extended from the centre of K II to northern edge

- Opening of Paradise Bar – 'a club for Kololo men'

1980

- Official population 7,800 (1980 census)

- Establishment of Horsndallen Boarding School in Kifumbira zone
- Settlement continues to expand. Electricity follows it – soon extended to Church Zone

1970

- The market taken over by Kampala City Council

- Beginnings of roadside market near Old Kira Road

- Minimal settlement A few 'good' houses along Mawanda Road

1960

An elderly man who first settled in the southern (upper) part of Kam-wokya in 1962 claimed that the area was for long known as Kanjokya ('the sun is burning me') and that this later changed to Kamwokya ('it is burning him/her'). The names may have been derived from the fact that walking from one end of the area to the other is a hot, sun-scorching experience. This man also recalled that, when the lower parts of the settlement still consisted of royal plantations, people were afraid to pass through the valley and anyone who had dared to traverse it would say *nsige nsooba* ('I have come tip-toeing'). Today the lower part of the settlement, where drainage channels have since been constructed, is still called *Nsooba*, a name which now refers to both the area and the drainage system.

The name Kamwokya was first used to refer only to 'Upper' Kam-wokya, the present Kamwokya Ward I, located above Kira Road, which was developed before Independence as a residential area primarily for Asians. At that time the present areas of Kamwokya II were sparsely settled if at all, although a roadside market, mainly for passers-by, had begun to develop there by the early 1960s.

Settlement of the area began soon afterwards. There are to our know-ledge no accurate records of the expansion of the settlement in the 1960s and 1970s; but as shown in the Time Chart (Figure 2.1), the population had risen to 7,800 in 1980. It is said that in the troubled years of the 1970s and up to the mid-1980s, Kamwokya had the reputation of being a rough red-light area with several night clubs and a number of bars. Since then, it is claimed, its character has changed appreciably, and Kamwokya has become more respectable. The current population of Kamwokya is estimated to be 14,000 (Chapter 3). It covers an area of roughly half a square kilometre – giving a density of 26,000 per sq. km (Map III) – the second highest in Kampala.[1]

(ii) Land prices, landowners and landlords

Land prices in Kamwokya vary considerably according to whether the land is 'dry' (more expensive) or 'wet', and according to relative distance from the main roads. According to informants the prices range from Ush. 10,000 to Ush. 300,000 per decimal (0.01 of a hectare). These prices are generally higher than those in neighbouring parishes such as Mulago II, Kyebando and Bukoto I, though there is variation in these areas as well.

[1] The population of Kamwokya II, as given in the 1991 Census, was around 13,000. On this basis the official density was calculated at 26,000 per sq. km. However, three caveats: (i) the population is known to have grown since 1991. We asked a number of RC 1 officers to tally recent changes in their separate sub-parishes. The figures showed approximately 10 per cent increase in each. If this is true on average across the parish, it makes a total of 14,500. (ii) On top of this there is a lot of unofficial squatter growth. Kamwokya, after all, is a popular but not an officially recognized settlement (see Chapter 1). (iii) The totals cited vary according to the constituency in mind. A pamphlet describing an AIDS care network in Kamwokya refers to a population of 30,000 (Williams and Tamale, 1991) – presumably the catchment covered by the Catholic Church and its clinic in Kamwokya.

There are several factors in addition to 'dry/wet' land and distance from main roads which reportedly make land in Kamwokya more valuable than these other areas. They include: the good market and commercial area; better security due to the proximity of police stations; good spring water which never dries up and is said to be of better quality than elsewhere; tap water in recent years which the other parishes do not have; and proximity/accessibility to the city centre. The area draws non-residents as an entertainment centre with a good market and lively trades in brewing, tailoring, furniture-making and the like; and it attracts new residents by virtue of its reputation for increasing respectability and desirability as a place to live in Kampala. Relative to some other areas in the city it is central, open and safe. Its population continues to expand almost daily.

The advantages of the Kamwokya commercial and social amenities are said to be factors in the recent spread of well-built houses down into the valley. In these lower-lying 'wet' areas the land costs less but the costs of erecting a house from permanent materials are higher. More has to be spent on laying good foundations of murram (red dirt characteristic of East and Central Africa) and rubble. The erection of houses also takes longer as the foundations should, ideally, be laid three to six months in advance. People who fail to lay good foundations often have problems later on. A good-looking new house in lower Kamwokya already has a large crack of two to three inches down the whole length of the main wall.

RISE IN LAND PRICES OVER RECENT YEARS

Price increases for good 'dry' land have occurred even over the two years of this study:

In 1992 one buyer paid Ush. 1.2 million for ten decimals (1 decimal = 0.1 hectare). In early 1993, another buyer paid Ush. 1.6 million for a similar plot of the same size from the same owner. In mid-1993, a third buyer paid Ush. 1.8 million for land of comparable size and quality again from the same owner.

These examples would indicate an increase of some 50 per cent per year.

In February 1994, a fourth buyer paid Ush. 2.75 million for a plot of the same size but this sale included 7,000 bricks and the plot had an approved building plan. Another case was cited with less precision. A buyer paid 'a million or more' for a plot in late 1992. He did not develop it and sold it in early 1994 for Ush. 3 million, thus making 'one to two million' in 18 months.

Interviews with two old men who came to Kamwokya in its early days revealed that most of the land in the area was then *mailo* land, i.e. land owned by the Kabaka (King) of Buganda. In the early 1960s the Kabaka ceded most of his land to a few of his 'councillors' (members of the Lukiko). At least some paid rent to the Kabaka and others bought land from him. Whatever the precise history, some of these few men acquired titles to the land and, by the late 1960s (after the Obote/Kabaka crisis of 1966), a process of fragmentation set in.

Several informants confirmed that '20–40 years ago' there were only a few landowners while today there are 'hundreds'. But there are said to be only a few large landowners – 'maybe 10 or 20'; others own much smaller pieces of land where they usually have their own houses, but may also let houses or land or both.

The Land Reform Decree of 1975 passed by the Amin regime abolished all land rent, but 'letting and renting went on officially as before'. This is apparently still the position today, though there is talk that the present government intends to change the law.

Landlords fall into two categories: those who let houses, and those who let land and allow people to build their own houses. There are large as well as small landlords in both categories. A few examples demonstrate the range:

The Chairman (RC 1) of Central zone said that 'most of the Central Zone is owned by one person "who collects rent from squatters" '. This is, he said, 'underground rent'. The area is very congested with temporary structures. Each 'squatter' pays about Ush. 2000 per month and it is estimated that there are 40 such units bringing the owner some Ush. 80,000 per month in addition to rent from shops and better buildings which he owns. It was unclear how or when this landlord acquired his land...

There is one landlord who owns land and buildings in Kamwokya as well as in Bukoto and Kyebando. His property in Kamwokya belonged to twin brothers whose father had acquired it from the Kabaka. When the father died, the twin sons inherited the property. They were unable or uninterested in maintaining the property and they sold it to the present owner who was a resident of Bukoto '...before or just after independence'. At the time the new landlord was not wealthy but he established himself as a brewer, bought a juke box for one of his drinking places, and 'gradually built himself up', erecting houses, trading, etc. The houses are of poor quality, mainly of mud and wattle, but he is said to collect well over a million shillings per month in rents and is considered a wealthy man...

Another wealthy landlord lives in a flat in the Market Area where he owns many commercial premises as well as better quality residential houses. He is a businessman as well as a landlord. He built the mosque and the school next to it, and also owns the Cuntafrica Theatre...

The number of small landlords is said to have grown especially fast since the early 1980s. Many owners are increasingly willing to sell land. People who settled as 'squatters' paying rent unofficially are now buying the land on which they built their houses from the landowners. In many cases, the landowners no longer live locally.

(iii) Roads, tracks and pathways

There are no tarmacked roads inside Kamwokya's boundary. On its southern border it is separated from Kamwokya I by the Kira Road, part of which is a two-way road with considerable motor and other traffic. The other part, Old Kira Road, which runs on the inside of the boundary, is still in a reasonable state of repair. Mawanda Road, which forms the boundary between Kamwokya II and Mulago I, is also a good road but with much less traffic than Kira Road (see Map IV, p. 30).

Within Kamwokya II there are three murram tracks which can be used by vehicles. The first bisects the settlement from south to north. The lower northern section has been made usable by vehicles only in the last year or two, and it ends at a small foot bridge over the drainage channel. The second murram track runs roughly parallel to Kira Road from Mawanda Road to the 'centre' of Kamwokya II where it meets the south–north road. A third track runs inside the settlement's border with Mulago III.

There are also many partial tracks (Map IV); some can be negotiated by vehicles driven very cautiously. Most lead on to innumerable foot-paths that crisscross the entire area, in some cases through open spaces, in others through narrow passages between houses built only a few feet apart.

(iv) Dwellings and other buildings

For the first (Broad Brush Survey) mapping of houses, shops and other structures, a two-fold classification of 'permanent buildings' and 'semi-permanent and temporaries structures' was set up. The criteria for the first were walls of hard-baked bricks or durable blocks; roofing of corrugated iron sheets, tiles, asbestos or concrete; and doors and windows of wood and glass. The criteria for the second category were walls of soft or unbaked bricks or of reeds plastered with mud; roofing of tins, old iron sheets, reeds, grasses or polythene; doors and windows of make-shift materials including wood but usually without glass panes. However, when attempting to classify buildings by these measures, the observers found variations and combinations which led them to use less specific criteria such as the apparent durability and general appearance of individual houses.

There are two main areas of permanent buildings. The first stretches along Kira Road from a section of Mawanda Road zone through the Market Area and into the Contafrica zone. It runs through the trading centre where the permanent buildings consist partly of residential houses and partly of shops, bars, and other commercial premises. There are also several public buildings such as the main market, the Catholic Church and the Drama Hall (theatre). The second stretches along Mawanda Road in the western part of the settlement. Here the buildings are mainly houses.

Map IV shows that there are also pockets of permanent buildings along some stretches of the murram road bisecting Kamwokya II from south to north, and on the northern and north-eastern sides where land has in recent years been reclaimed from the swampy areas along the *nsooba* drainage channels. But in these areas, as in some others lying in the inner parts of the settlement, permanent houses are scattered, seemingly at random, between semi-permanent and temporary structures.

Variation in the quality of houses can be seen from outside by differences in size, in amenities and facilities, in apparent security and in their respective surroundings. Most of the permanent houses have electricity, piped water, water closets, nearby soak-pits, hedges and/or security fences, and many have burglar-proof windows and doors. Few of the semi-permanent houses and virtually none of the temporary structures have any of these. There is, nevertheless, great variation in outside appearance within both categories, especially in the semi-permanent/ temporary categories (Sketches 1–9).[2]

Most of the permanent buildings give the impression of having been built according to plans, except in the centre of the trading areas (around the market) where, in the words of one observer, 'competition and corruption have ruled out proper planning'. Here there is much congestion, with houses adjoining each other or being separated only by narrow passages.

Permanent houses in other areas are usually placed well apart from each other. Except in one section of the Mwanda Road zone, they do not appear to form part of planned areas, but they have clearly been planned as individual residences. Most of them are located in the upper part of the settlement facing the good roads that run along the southern and western boundaries. With internal piped water, toilets and electricity, and with fences, hedges and other demarcations, the houses are seldom surrounded by cluttered shacks. They are relatively free from rubbish and usually stand on plots which are recognizably their own. There are few loiterers around them and few roadside vendors.

In contrast to most permanent houses, the semi-permanent and temporary structures are much smaller, often consisting of only one or two rooms and commonly adjoining each other. Few have clearly demarcated areas, uncluttered surroundings or burglar proofing of any kind. The unplanned or, at best, partially planned nature of the houses is noticeable. Many have small additional rooms or lean-to structures, either under construction or already in use. The areas around the dwellings are usually congested with poorly constructed latrines and 'bathrooms' and the daily clutter of charcoal stoves, old plastic bags and piles of rubbish.

Privacy, cleanliness and hygienic conditions decline rapidly as one moves from the surroundings of some of the better semi-permanent homes into the areas of temporary structures. There are sharp contrasts between the better areas and the 'slum areas in the valley', and the differences occur over extremely short distances. The mixture of housing types and living conditions is a salient feature of Kamwokya II, setting it off sharply from Kamwokya I where all the houses are permanent, and are built in regular rows facing on to wide open tarmac roads.

(v) Water and sanitation[3]

The main contrasts between the 'good' and 'bad' areas of Kamwokya are highlighted by their respective water and sanitation facilities. In

---

[2] These sketches were made by Abraham Kafeero, a Makerere University student observer on the Broad Brush Survey (BBS).

[3] Because these facilities, or the lack of them, are fundamental to the perception and reality of wellbeing in Kamwokya, they reappear as the focus of discussion several times in the course of the book.

general, most of the population living in the areas of semi-permanent and temporary houses rely for their water supplies on two springs in the lower valley area and some half dozen water tap sites. These sites have a total of 28 taps located in different parts of the settlement and in some cases at appreciable distances from each other.

The main sites occupied by the water sellers indicate areas in which water is a major daily problem; these all lie toward the lower end of the valley. People in this area either buy water from the sellers or collect it themselves from the two springs or from water taps. One of the springs is in a poor state of repair and water from it is available free of charge. The other spring is supervised by an RC caretaker who is required to charge Ush. 10 per jerry can. The demand is so great, however, that there is also a 'special line' for express services at a rate of Ush. 50 per jerry can.

There are innumerable rubbish dumping sites scattered throughout Kamwokya. The Kampala City Council supervises only three sites. These have skips which are supposed to be emptied regularly, but are in fact usually overflowing with refuse (Sketch 10). All the formal dumping sites are located in the upper part of Kamwokya, close to the Kira Road.

Sanitation and the provision of adequate toilet/latrine facilities is a major problem for most Kamwokya residents. In the upper market area there is a block of latrines erected and maintained by the Kampala City Council. It is built out of cement blocks and has a caretaker who charges Ush. 50 for their use. The observers noted, however, that these facilities were nevertheless ill-kept and dirty (Sketch 11). Apart from a new RC toilet block under construction (in 1993) (Sketch 12), virtually all visible external latrines in the settlement are made of semi-permanent or temporary materials, and their cleanliness and adequacy decline steadily the further one moves into the poorer areas.

The observers noted only three large soak pits, although there are many smaller ones scattered throughout the settlement. They serve the purpose of draining dirty water that is thrown into them or that drains into them from intended or unintended sewers and streams. In many cases, however, the soak pits are themselves clogged and overflowing (Sketch 15).

In the centre of Kamwokya there is a brewers' area. There latrines are usually erected on the premises of traditional drinking places by the owners and are used by their families as well as by their numerous customers. They are usually kept locked and their use is strictly controlled by the brewers (Sketch 13).

Away from the brewers' zone, and especially in the lower parts of the valley, the condition of toilets and bathrooms is far worse. This is partly due to the poverty of the population, but also on account of the high level of the water table in the valley. Where there is a high water table, the pit latrines cannot be dug much deeper than one metre and the inhabitants compensate for this by erecting platforms (Sketch 14).

These platform latrines like others in the areas of semi-permanent and temporary housing, are usually erected by groups of neighbours who attempt to restrict their use by keeping them padlocked and passing the keys around as required. Not surprisingly, much inconvenience is caused by these practices. Moreover, children are not normally permitted to use the adult latrines. Instead, they either use potties and polythene bags or smaller latrines are constructed for them. The latter are usually exposed pits, about one metre in depth, and covered with logs on which the children squat. They are at times also used by adults but because they are exposed, adults tend to use them only under cover of darkness.

Bathrooms, like toilets, are usually constructed out of poor quality materials, often even more flimsy than the toilets. Their quality also deteriorates progressively as one moves down the valley towards the swamps. Here they are normally made of sacks, rags or papyrus reeds and seldom have roofs or doors (see Sketches 15 and 16). Old towels or 'Kanga' cloths are commonly used to curtain the entrance.

Both in the poorest areas and in the 'better' areas of semi-permanent houses, the bathrooms are habitually used only in the very early morning or the evenings in order to avoid the embarrassments they cause. And when they are used during the day, adults use them partially clothed. They seldom have adequate drainage, and often none at all, so that the overflow – sometimes smelling of urine – runs into open sewers. Few have properly constructed soak pits, and such soak pits as there may be are usually clogged. As in the case of toilets, bathrooms are often 'communal' and groups of neighbours attempt to restrict their use. People can be seen waiting outside 'their' bathroom for others to complete their ablutions.

Open sewers run throughout the greater part of Kamwokya, but, again, mainly in the poorer areas where they form a fairly dense network. The flow of dirty water is highest in the early morning and the evening. It commonly passes by the very front of houses where small bridges are built to allow the inhabitants access to their front doors (Sketch 8). In the worst areas water sellers and food vendors will at times be seated on the ground a foot or two away from these sewers.

(vi) Communal, commercial and service premises

Kamwokya is an important centre of communal life and commercial activity not only for its own residents but also, in varying degrees, for the inhabitants of neighbouring parishes and for other passers-by, especially along the Kira Road.

Unlike many other parishes in Kampala, Kamwokya has no government school, which means that many of its children have to leave the settlement daily to attend schools elsewhere. Kamwokya does have several private nurseries and primary schools, however, one of which is a boarding school. It is also an important centre of religious life. The Catholic Church, the local Church of Uganda (Anglican), and a mosque all have catchment areas extending well beyond their own boundaries. This is also true of three Protestant sectarian churches.

Kamwokya

Map V (p. 31) shows that most of the communal establishments stretch across the southern (upper) end of Kamwokya. This area has the main market at its centre, but also includes many small dry goods shops, the 'special hire' (taxi) park, and the main point of entry for vehicles. The range of goods and services available in this part of Kamwokya exceeds the day-to-day needs of the poorer local residents, but caters well for outsiders, giving Kamwokya its distinctive character and value as a commercial centre. Other parts of the settlement contain commercial and service points which are used more by the local people. There is a smaller market located in Kifumbira I/Mulago III, for example, which operates at night, selling smaller quantities at lower prices than the main market. Local residents also buy food and other necessities (such as charcoal, soap, salt, matches, etc.) from small kiosks and roadside vendors located throughout the settlement.

These observations contribute appreciably to a definition of Kamwokya. In addition to being a settlement with 'good', 'poor' and 'mixed' residential areas, it is a centre of communal activities and of a variety of commercial and entertainment services which attract adherents, customers and clients from outside its own boundaries. There are thus two intertwining elements in the life of Kamwokya. The first consists of highly localized, almost village-like, activities and routines; the second lies in its less parochial and more 'urban' life which calls for assessment and analysis in the context of its wider setting.

The Urban System

(i) The distribution of difference

Kamwokya Parish is mixed in every sense, and its heterogeneity shows in variation from one part of the parish to another. Pursuing the analysis of it as an urban system (outlined in Chapter 1), the first and most straightforward question to address is: How closely do all these kinds of difference overlap?

Figure 2.2 shows the ethnic origins of our survey population. The Baganda are numerically dominant and, not by coincidence, the original 'locals' in this part of Uganda. They have usefully been called the 'host' group, all the others being 'migrants' by contrast (Parkin, 1969), and Luganda, along with English, is the *lingua franca* in Kampala. Traditionally the Baganda differed from the rest by family culture as well as status in the region. In the early days of migration, these differences showed in styles of organization in town – notably in what looked like 'ethnic clustering' among migrants (*ibid.*: 92–4; McGee, 1973).

Next in size are smaller but still substantial proportions of Batoro and Banyankole – technically 'migrants' but some of many years, even generations, residence in the city. Each of the remaining (seventeen) ethnic groups is locally represented by quite small numbers. Because the number

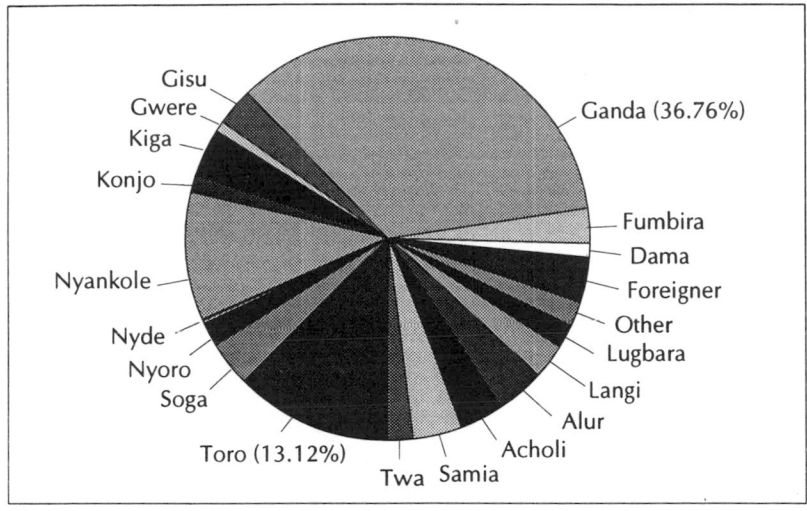

Fig. 2.2 *Ethnic distribution, Kamwokya, 1993*
(data from Ethnographic Survey 1993)

of respondents resident in each zone is in any case tiny, and the Census office has been reluctant to specify ethnic origin as such, we followed the official lead and cumulated the figures by region of origin (Figure 2.3). In the Uganda context, region is a reasonable proxy for ethnicity since the home area of each tribe is concentrated in one or other part of the country.

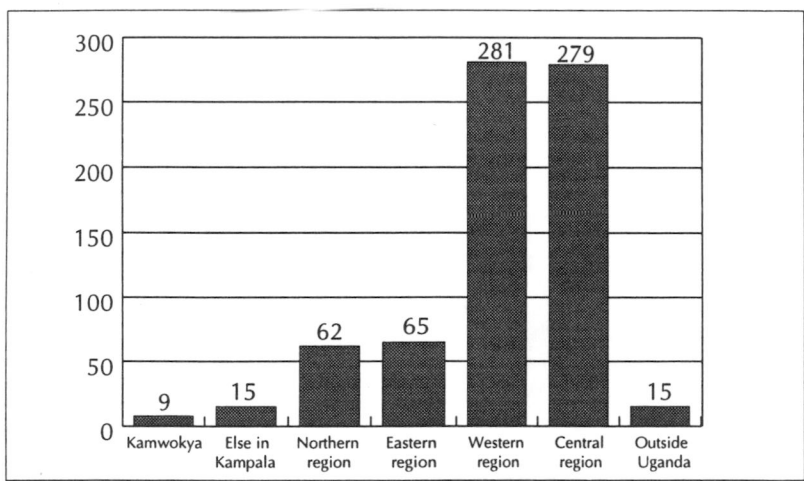

Fig. 2.3 *Place of other origin: 'home area'*

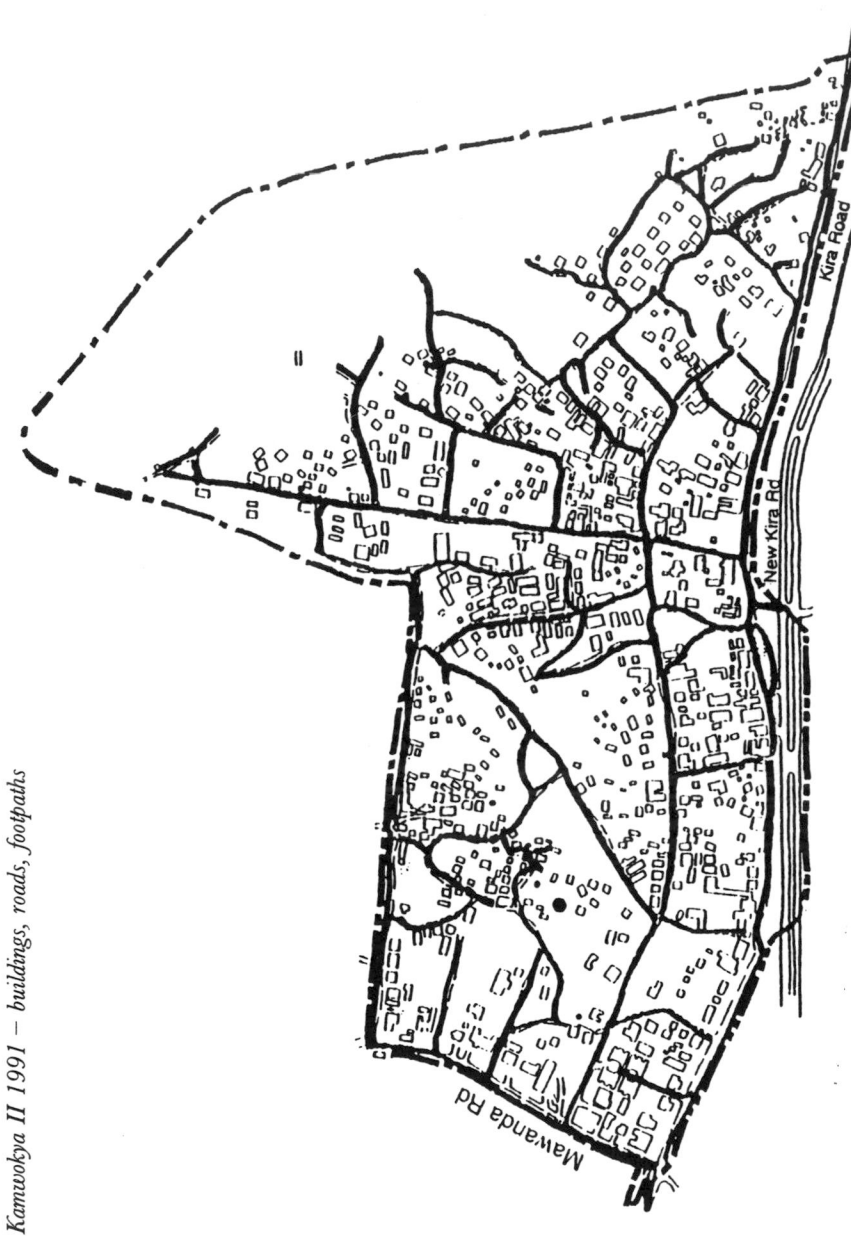

Map IV *Kamwokya II 1991 – buildings, roads, footpaths*

Map V *Communal, commercial and service premises*

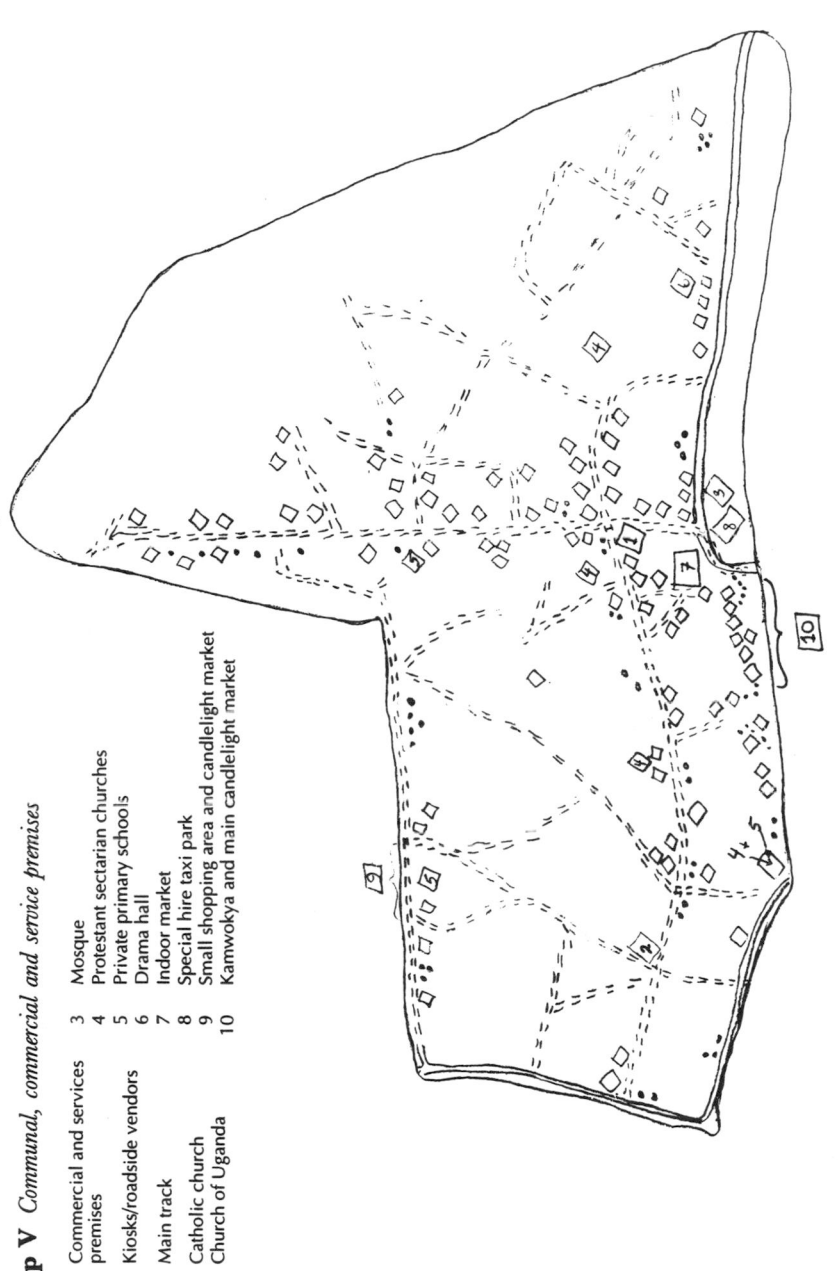

□ Commercial and services premises
∴ Kiosks/roadside vendors
// Main track
1 Catholic church
2 Church of Uganda
3 Mosque
4 Protestant sectarian churches
5 Private primary schools
6 Drama hall
7 Indoor market
8 Special hire taxi park
9 Small shopping area and candlelight market
10 Kamwokya and main candlelight market

Map VI *Population densities in each enumeration area and land contours*

- densities in 000s per sq. km.
- overall density 23,000

Census zones and enumeration zones

Kisenyi II Zone	01–04	Kifumbira II Zone	20–21
Church Zone	05–10	Mawanda Road Zone	23–24
Green Valley Zone	11–13	Market Area	25–26
Central Zone	14–15	Contafrica Zone	27–29
Kifumbira I Zone	16–19	Kisenyi I Zone	30

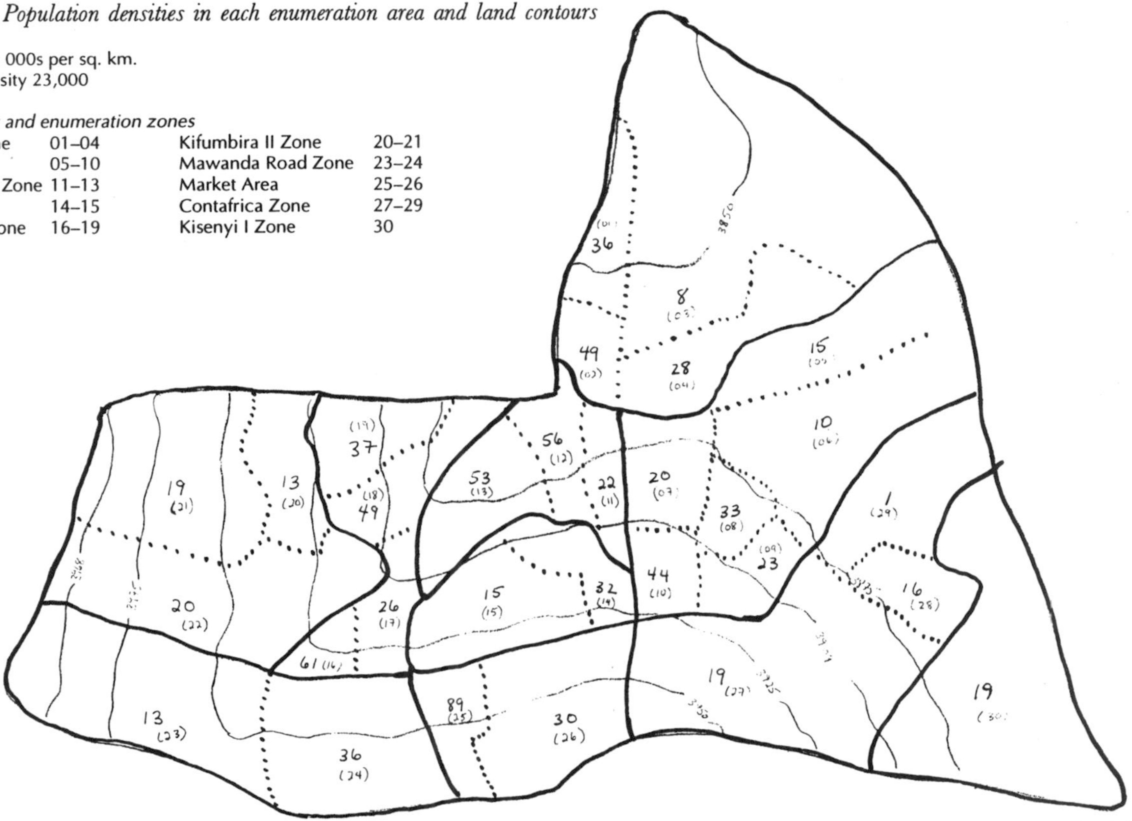

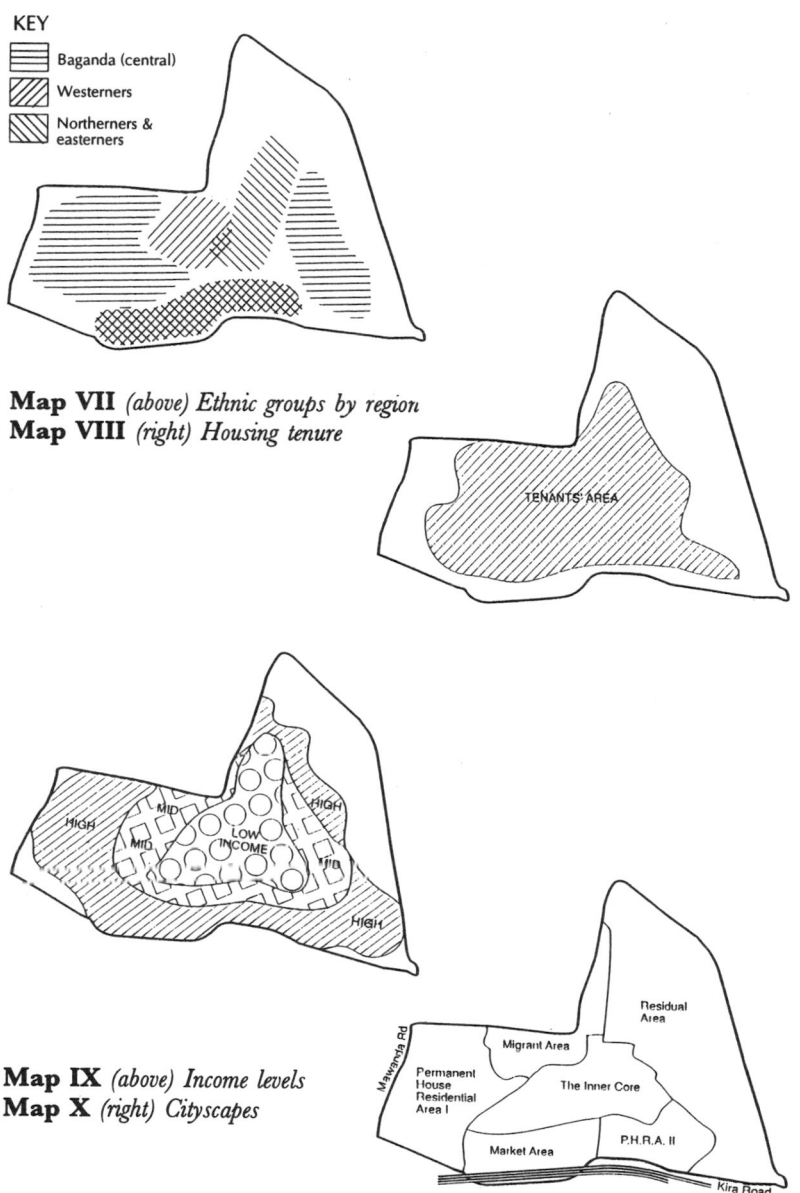

Map VII *(above) Ethnic groups by region*
Map VIII *(right) Housing tenure*

Map IX *(above) Income levels*
Map X *(right) Cityscapes*

[4] Maps VII, VIII and IX are effectively sketch maps, produced on the combined basis of observers' impressions and insiders' knowledge. Map X was constructed by matching small area statistics from the 1991 census with evidence of physical difference across Kamwokya (Pons, 1993/4b).

On this basis, Map VII shows that there is still ethnic clustering but other evidence shows this confounded by economic and structural factors which challenge the assumption that the clustering is ethnically led. The various levels of difference are unpicked in a sequence of maps showing tenure, income levels and cityscapes across Kamwokya (Maps VIII, IX, X).[4] If the four maps are notionally superimposed, it immediately becomes clear that the four dimensions vary together, each ethnic/regional group being consistently over-represented in one or other tenure, income and cityscape category. But to observe that things vary together is not to know that one causes the other: there may be yet another factor driving the system. In any case the clustering may be sustained by forces different from the original impetus to get together.

Work could be crucial on both fronts. Particularly persuasive is the likelihood that opportunities for 'getting by' are different in the five cityscapes and that they match the aspirations and skills of some categories in the population more than others.

(ii) The movement of people

Initially we had assumed Kamwokya to be a relative self-contained community: many people appear to live their lives almost exclusively within the settlement. That assumption is sustained by the homogeneous look of the map sequence in the previous section. Accumulated the maps suggest a central, low-income ethnically homogeneous core, with the boundaries of the various sub-systems overlaid so tightly that the local system is hard to enter and not easy to leave (cf. Wallman, 1985, 1996a).

But it was also clear from the outset that many residents leave Kamwokya every day, for work, school or social purposes, and that many non-residents come there to use its commercial and other services. The analytical point is that the distribution of difference across the parish is a feature of the urban system different *in kind* from the movement of people in and out of it. Any contradiction between the two sets of evidence becomes instructive as soon as they are visualized as analytically separate sub-systems of the whole. Ultimately the question *What kind of an urban system is this?* demands their recombination (attempted in later chapters). More immediately, in-flows and out-flows of people (also) demonstrate the rhythm of daily life. Aware that complete coverage was impossible, we concentrated on three observation points along Kira Road. Observers counted passengers coming in or leaving on wheeled transport only: cars, lorries, buses, *matatus* (minibus taxis), bicycles and motorcycles; and the vast majority were *matatu* passengers. Hundreds of *matatus* (locally known as taxis) pass in both directions along New Kira Road. Some terminate their journeys from Kampala city centre at Kamwokya but most proceed further and stop only if they have passengers who want to get off there or if they see people at the *matatu* stages wanting to get on.

[4] See foot of page 33.

Counting people getting on and off was relatively easy. It was more difficult to know, especially with those getting on, whether they were Kamwokya residents. Some enter and then leave again, while others move in and out on foot from other entry points. We know too, for example, that there is pedestrian traffic *through* Kamwokya along the south/north murram road leading to the Mulago III/Kyebando border. And so on.

All in all, a precise count cannot be possible. But there is interest in the proportions of the sexes on the move and in the evidence that more people appear to enter Kamwokya than leave it during daylight hours. Throughout the day there are appreciably more men than women leaving from the main exit point near the market. In the late afternoon/early evening men outnumber women by more than 2 to 1. Presumably many of the incomers at this time leave again during the evening but we were not able to attempt any assessment of numbers.

On the basis of observations made for the Broad Brush Survey (Pons, 1993/4a), we calculated that from 7.00 to 9.00 a.m. 367 people per hour were visiting or passing by the shops. This rose to 430 between 9.00 and 10.00 before falling back to 314 between 10.00 and 11.00 and to 244 from 11.00 to 12 noon. There was little change over the lunch period but the figures began to rise again later: to 279 per hour from 3.00 to 5.00 p.m. and to 579 between 5.00 and 6.30 p.m.

Children made up approximately a third of the total in the early morning (7.00–9.00 a.m.) but their proportion fell back to a quarter during the day, rising again to about a third in the late afternoon. These changes presumably reflect the impact of school attendance, but it is of interest to note that children form a significant proportion of people in this type of public place at all times.

The proportions of men and women on the move did not vary much: 67 per cent were men from 7.00 to 10.00 a.m. with little variation; 71 and 68 per cent from 10.00 to 11.00 and 11.00 to 12 noon respectively, and similarly up to the late afternoon when the proportion of men fell slightly to 60 per cent. The variations are slight and probably have little significance, especially when we consider the element of estimation they contain. But the general preponderance of men is important when viewed in conjunction with other figures (see below). Throughout the day, 64 per cent of adults on the move were men and 36 per cent women.

The intersection of two paths on the edge of the market area is always busy but many of the shoppers are leisurely (mainly women and children), whereas most men walk past hurriedly. The composition of the passers-by and the directions in which they moved varied a great deal at different times of the day. A few of the shoppers, especially young children, appeared to be from nearby homes, but the majority of all who traversed the intersection were clearly moving with other than shopping purposes in mind.

Throughout the day food and goods are sold, invariably in small quantities and, in the case of cooked foods and cigarettes, usually for immediate consumption. But there is variation in the numbers, age and sex of the people in view, and in the direction of traffic flow throughout the day. For example, between 7.00 and 9.00 a.m. 576 people passed through (288 per hour). Of these, 331 were moving towards Kira Road and 127 towards Mawanda Road. It is thus a fair assumption that over 80 per cent were heading for Kamwokya's central trading area or for transport along Kira Road. Although children were prominent as shoppers, they constituted only 7 per cent of the population enumerated. Towards midday the number of passers-by had fallen to 106 per hour and the flow of people towards Kira Road had reduced to a third of the total. The proportion of children was still only one in twenty. After 1.00 p.m., however, the proportion of children rose to 40 per cent. It was even higher between 4.00 and 5.00 p.m. by which time the number of passers-by had risen to 374 per hour, many now moving back towards the residential areas.

Taking adults only, the sex composition of those on the move through this intersection varied according to the time of day. From 7.00 to 9.00 a.m. three-quarters were men and from 9.00 to 10.00 am 83 per cent were men, after which the proportion of men fell fairly steadily to below half in the early afternoon, rising sharply again in the late afternoon, up to nearly 80 per cent between 6.00 and 6.30 p.m. Taking figures throughout the day as a whole, about three-quarters of the adults on the move were men and just over one quarter were women. Both the overall movement and the more local focus of women are important characteristics of the Kamwokya urban system. Implications and explanations of the latter are taken up in the discussions of population (Chapter 3) and livelihood (Chapters 5 and 10).

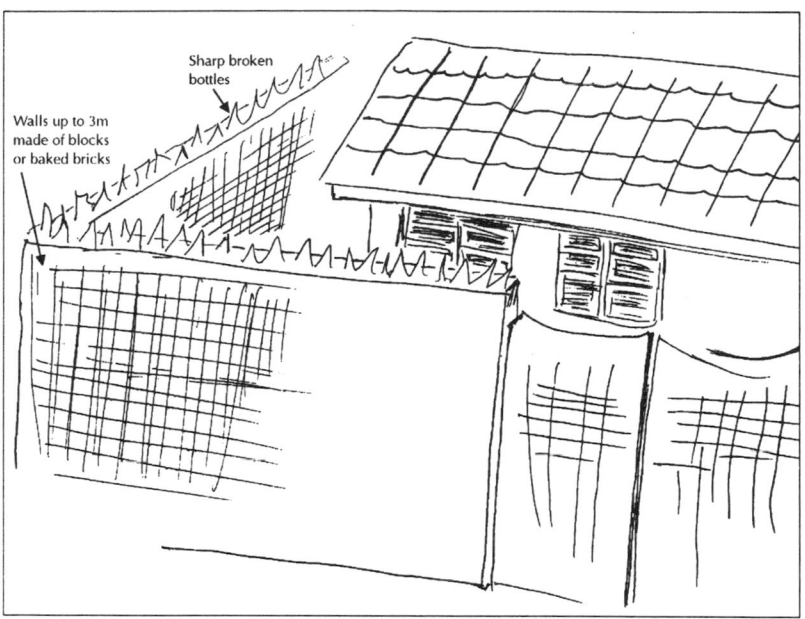

Sketch 1 *Permanent house with well-built protective wall*

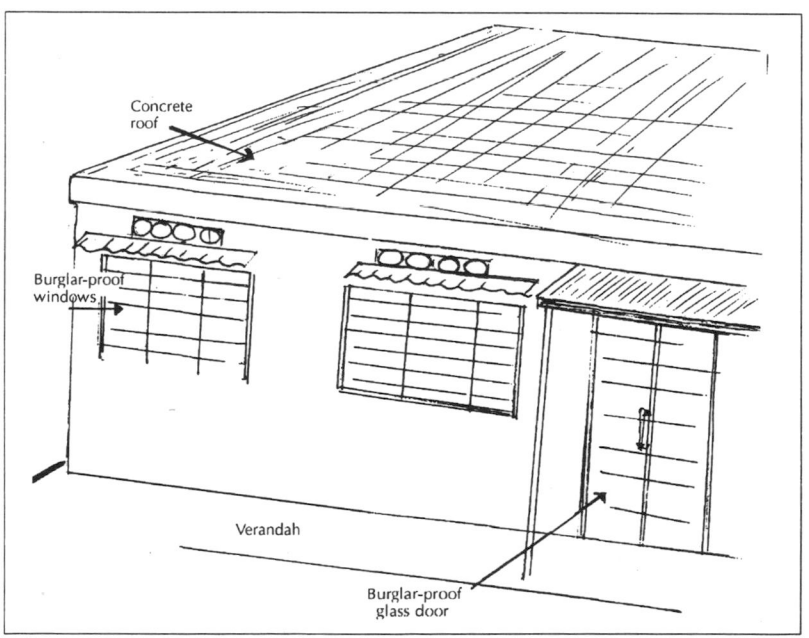

Sketch 2 *Permanent residential house with concrete roof and burglar-proof windows and door*

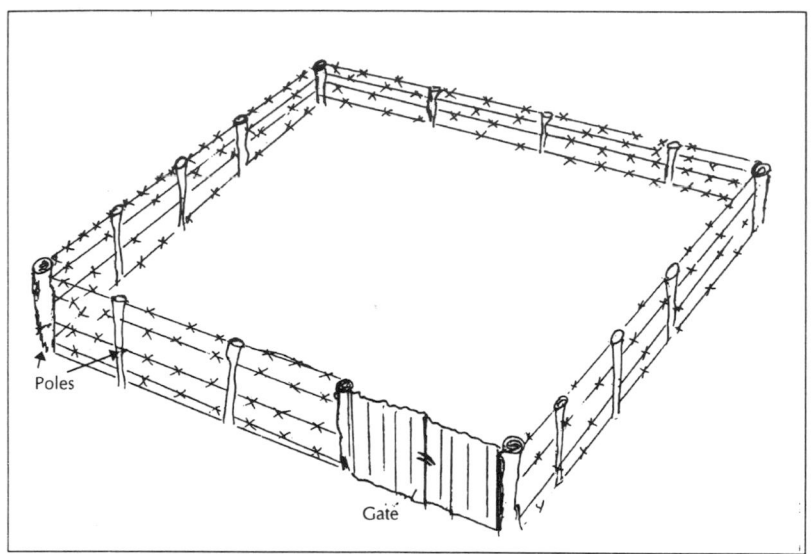

Sketch 3 *Barbed wire fence for a good residential house*

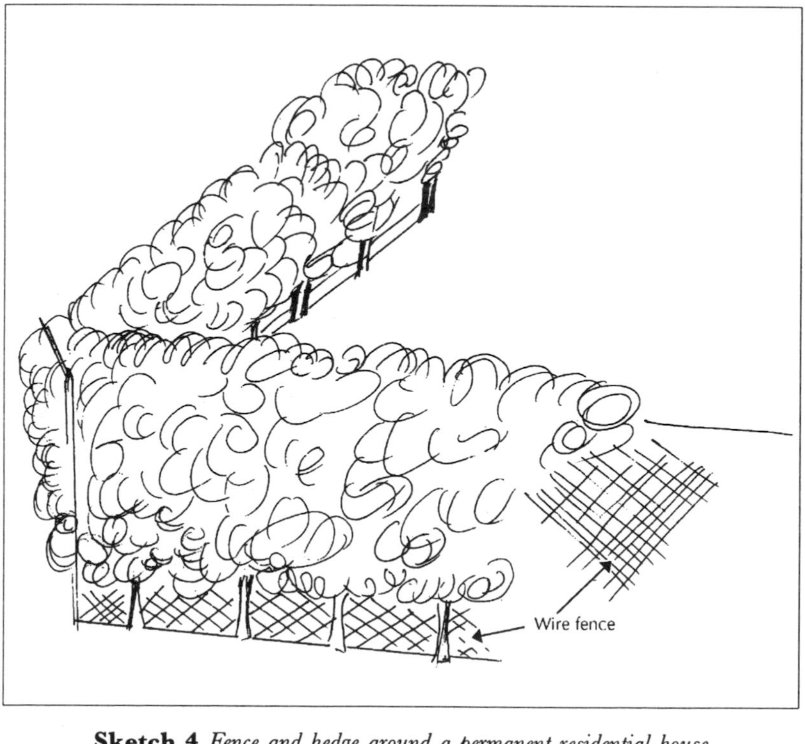

Sketch 4 *Fence and hedge around a permanent residential house*

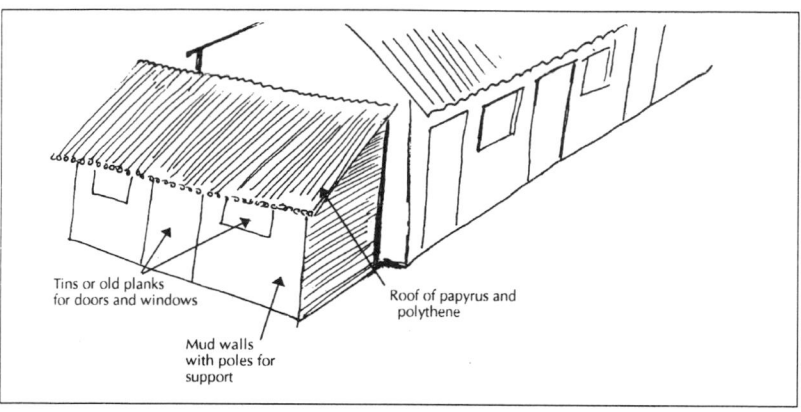

Sketch 5 *Semi-permanent papyrus-roofed house. (Houses of this kind are usually attached to other semi-permanent dwellings or shops)*

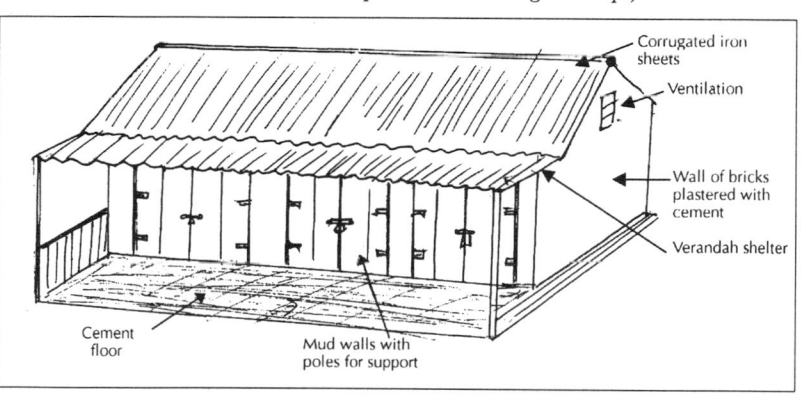

Sketch 6 *Well-built shops with residential premises at back*

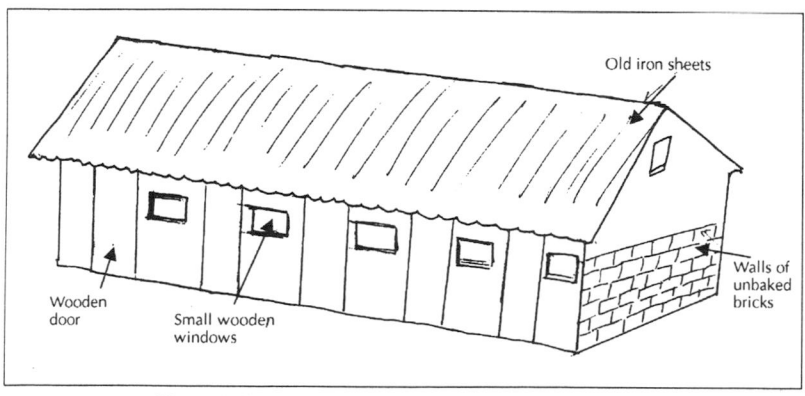

Sketch 7 *Newly built semi-permanent houses to let. (This type of house often has only one or two rooms)*

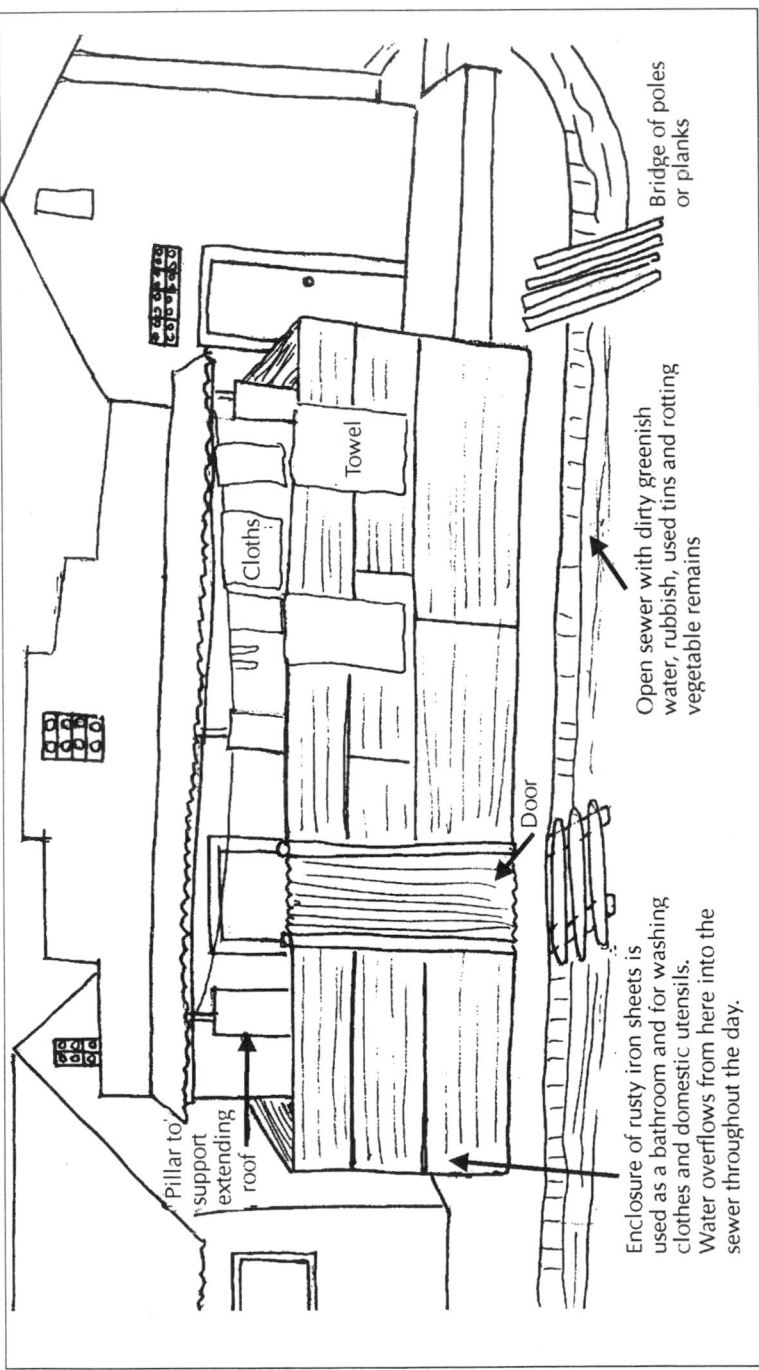

Sketch 8 *Adjoining houses in a slum tenant area*

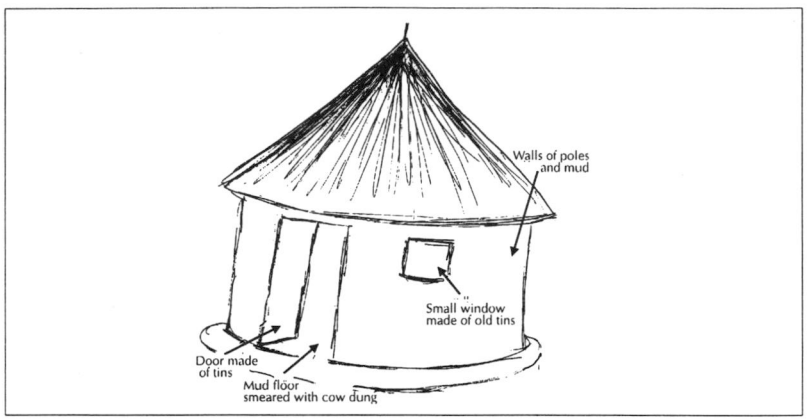

Sketch 9 *Temporary grass-thatched hut*

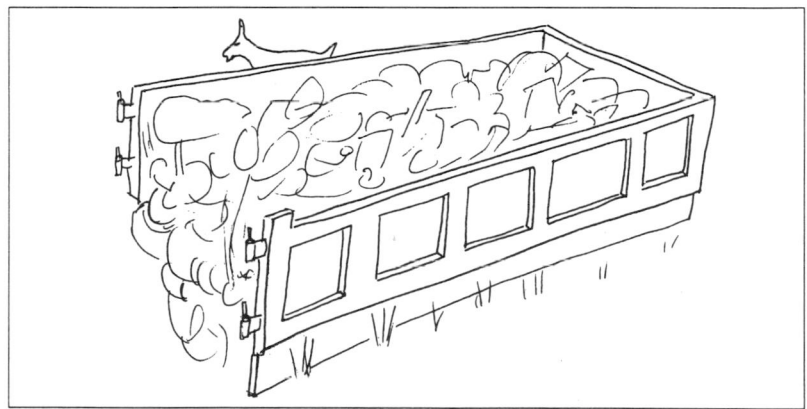

Sketch 10 *Kampala City Council rubbish skip*

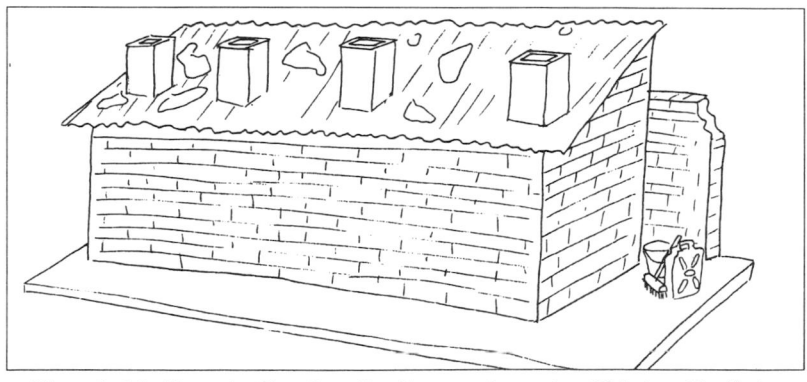

Sketch 11 *Kampala City Council toilet near the market. This is a Ventilation Improved Pit Latrine (VIP toilet).*

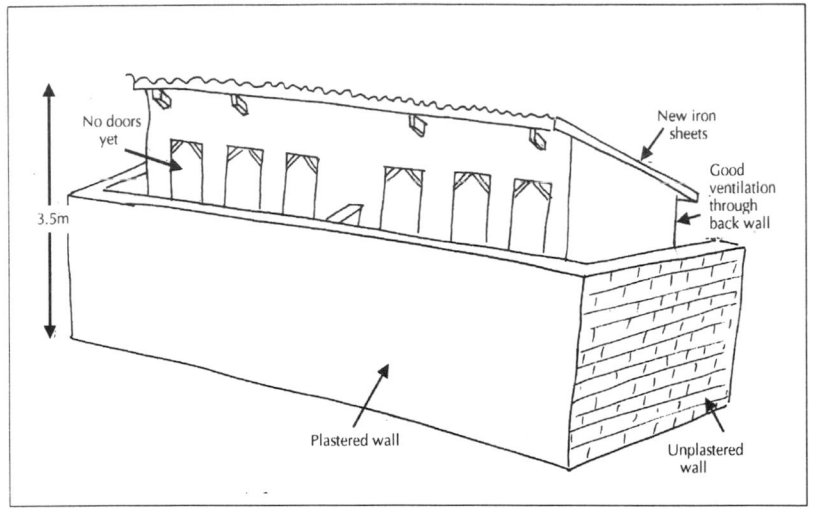

Sketch 12 *RC Toilets under construction in February 1993*

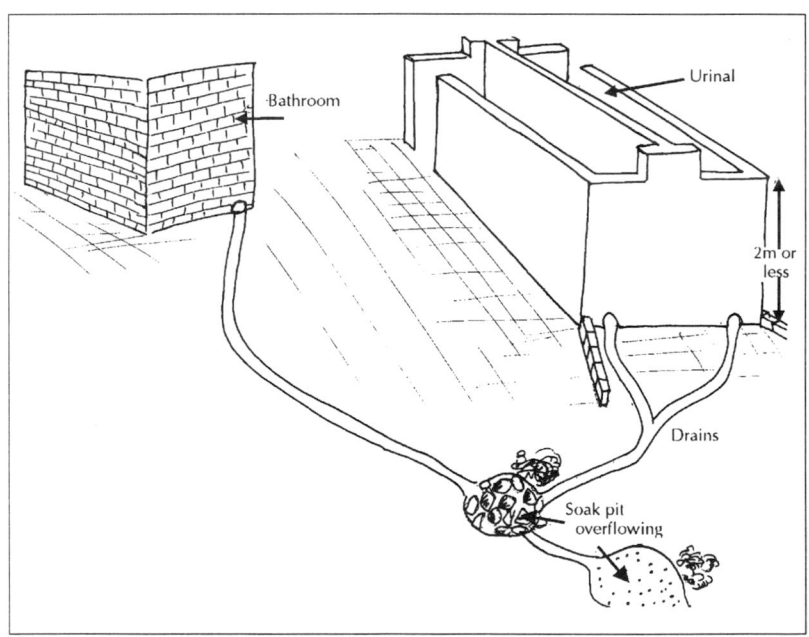

Sketch 13 *Urinal and bathroom in Brewers' Zone*

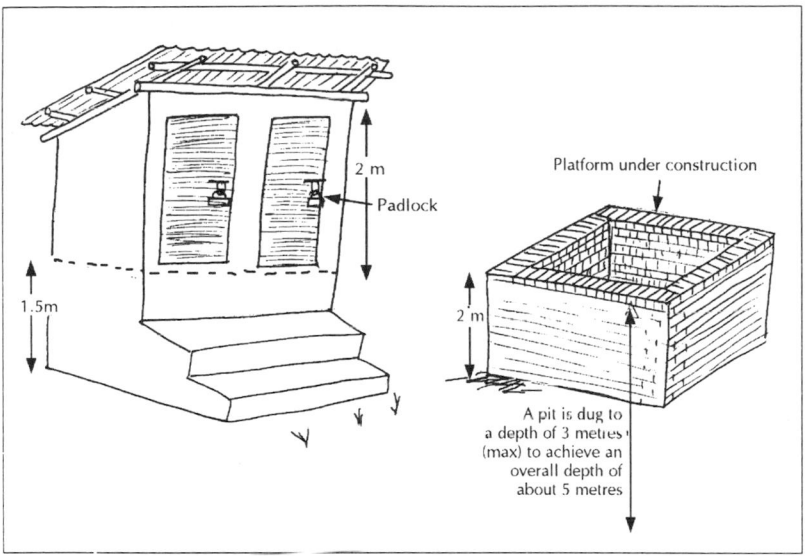

Sketch 14 *Platform toilet. This type of platform toilet is found in swampy areas with a low water table. Children do not use these toilets. They use potties or polythene bags which are then thrown away by older ones.*

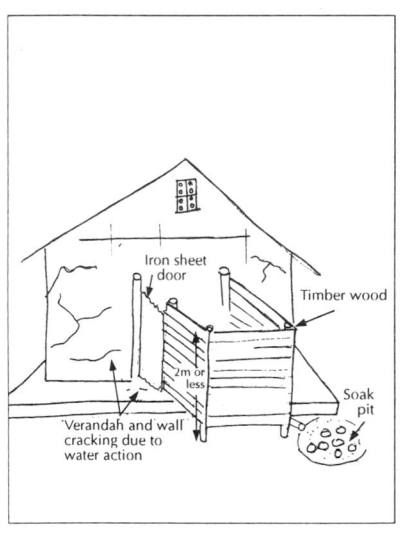

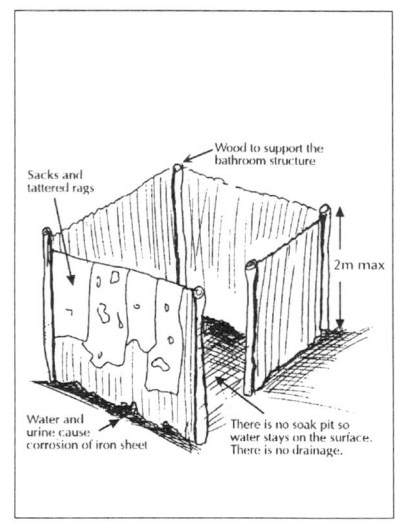

Sketch 15 *Bathroom in a tenant's house*

Sketch 16 *A bathroom structure in a swamp slum area*

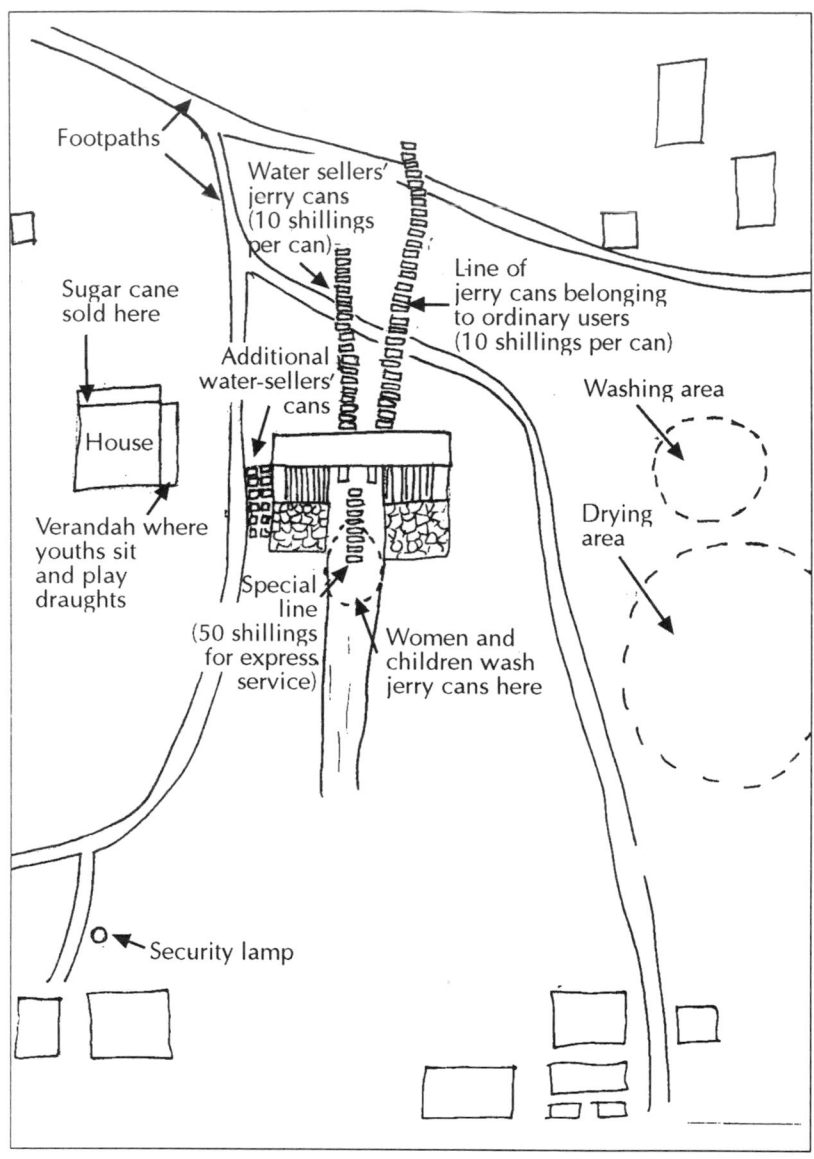

Sketch 17 *Organizational lay-out of Spring 'A'
(supervised and recently renovated). (Not to scale)*

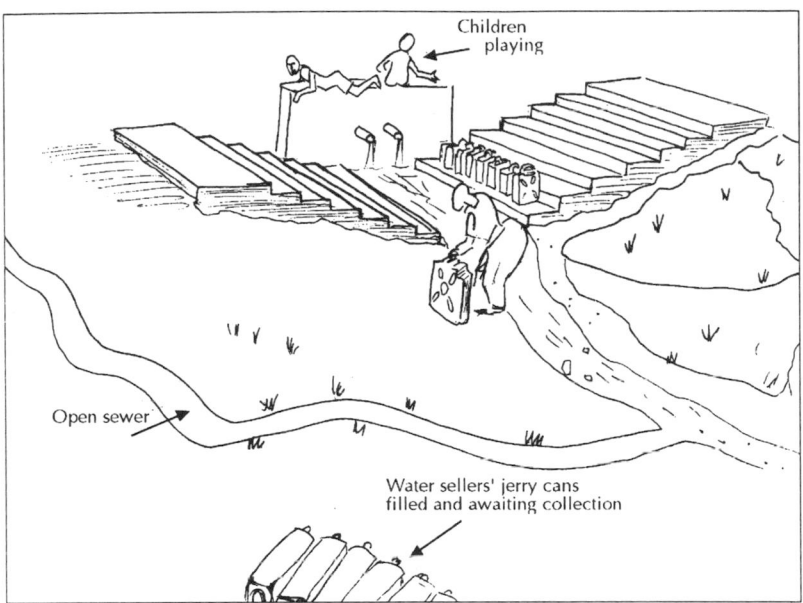

Sketch 18 *Spring 'B' (unsupervised and due for renovation). Spring next to open sewer. There is a toilet 15m away. The drain has dirty water and stones. The dirty water is used by locals to wash their jerry cans. Water from the spring is free.*

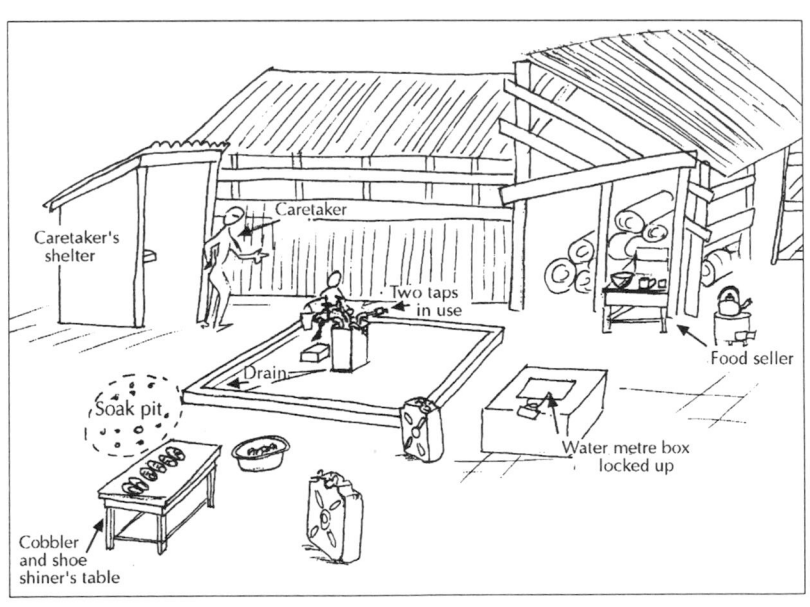

Sketch 19 *An RC water selling tap*

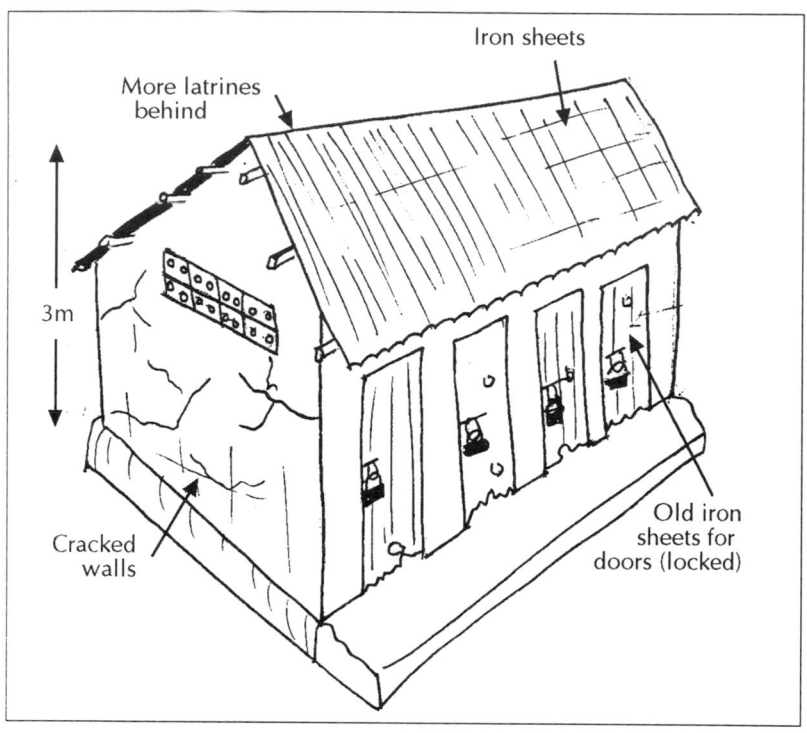

Iron sheets

More latrines
behind

3m

Cracked
walls

Old iron
sheets for
doors (locked)

Sketch 20 *Pit latrines in the Brewer's Zone*

Three

People in Place

VALDO PONS

This chapter reviews socio-demographic data drawn from the Uganda Censuses for 1969, 1980 and 1991. While its general purpose is to begin to fill out the picture of Kamwokya sketched in Chapter 2, it also has three specific aims:

- *to place the population of Kamwokya within the context of Kampala as a whole;*
- *to map and account for socio-demographic variations within the parish; and*
- *to highlight and try to explain imbalances in the age/sex composition of the parish and the city, most importantly the excess of girls/young women over boys/young men which has arisen since 1969.*

With these aims in view, the chapter depends most heavily on data drawn from the 1991 Census. We also use age/sex data drawn from the 1969 Census, and sex ratios from the 1980 Census (which unfortunately did not publish any information on age). The Census materials are supplemented by observations made in the field, and by some results of the Ethnographic Survey conducted in 1993. That survey had other than census objectives, being more concerned to see households and local people in the round, embedded in systems of relationships rather than as units of population (see Leach, 1967). It covered a non-random sample of contiguous households cutting a broad swathe through the parish. Its data are not (and did not set out to be) statistically representative, but reasonably close correspondence on a few salient characteristics – age, sex, ethnicity, etc. – gives us the confidence to cite certain items not covered by or not available from the Census Office. And as is indicated below, we have grouped the component Census Enumeration Areas into five sub-sets, 'cityscapes', so that the uneven distribution of social and demographic characteristics across the parish can be shown in relation to – perhaps even explained by – some very marked variations in its economic geography.

Introduction: Kampala and Kamwokya

In January 1991 Kamwokya II had a population of 12,071. This had increased from 7,800 in 1980 and 5,658 in 1969. There are no earlier figures for the parish, but we known from elderly local informants that the area was sparsely settled before Independence in 1962 when it probably had no more than 500 inhabitants, if that.

At the time of our study the population was still rising rapidly. An estimate based on the records of seven of the parish's ten RC zones puts the number of inhabitants in mid-1994 at between 15,000 and 16,000, an increase of some 3,500 in the two and a half years which had elapsed since the census was conducted in January 1991 (see Chapter 2, Note 1).

Our access to the 1991 Census Data and our use of them call for brief explanation. The ten RC zones in Kamwokya were for census purposes sub-divided into a total of 30 Enumeration Areas (EAs). The RC zones ranged in population from 560 to 1,835 with a mean of 1,271, and the 30 EAs ranged from 24 to 992 with a mean population of 402. The Census Office was willing to provide us with certain bivariate data for the RC zones but not for the EAs as some resultant cells would have been so small that individuals might have been identified. The Office was, however, willing to supply us with single-variable data for the EAs and certain bivariate tabulations for any reasonably large populations made up by EA combinations of our choice.

In the first instance we requested single-variable tabulations for the EAs. We plotted the data on maps which we then compared with our fieldwork knowledge of the parish. On this basis, we judged that limited bivariate data for five social areas or 'cityscapes', established through our own combination of EAs, would provide a better basis for a profile of the parish than similar data for the RC zones (Chapter 2). We then returned to the Office with our requests, most of which were granted.

The first areas we delineated were as follows: (Maps VI and X)

The Migrant Area (EAs 1, 2, 12, 13, 18 and 19) with a population of 2,355 and a density of approx. 48,000 persons per sq.km.

The Market Area (EAs 24, 25 and 26) with a population of 1,829 and a density of approx. 39,000.

The Permanent House Area (in two parts covering EAs 20, 21, 22, 23 and 27) with a population of 2,650 and a density of approx. 17,000.

The Inner Core (EAs 7, 8, 9, 10, 11, 14, 15, 16 and 17) with a population of 2,873 and a density of approx. 28,000.

The Residual Area (EAs 3, 4, 5, 6, 28, 29, 30) with a population of 2,274 and a density of approx. 13,000.

The parish as a whole had a density of about 23,000 per sq.km. (By mid-1995 this must have been nearer 30,000). It is the third most congested parish in Kampala where the highest densities tend to be found in low-lying areas at the bottom of the city's numerous hills.

The differences in density between areas within Kamwokya II reflect this tendency. The Migrant Area is close to the swamp on the lower slopes of Kololo Hill. The Market and Permanent House Areas are on higher ground, but the Market Area was the first part of the parish to be settled and it has a longer history of the sub-division and intensive use of plots lying immediately behind its commercial premises. This accounts for its density being higher than in the Permanent House Area. The Inner Core Area lies below the Market Area and occupies an intermediate position with regard to both altitude and density.

In our analysis we make most use of the data for the Migrant, Market and Permanent House Areas. The main socio-demographic characteristics of the Inner Core tend, as in the case of its density, to be intermediate to extremes in the first three areas. The Residual Area, as the name we have given it implies, is of little importance in outlining variations in the features of the parish population.

(i) Population growth and declining sex ratios

In 1969 Kampala had a population of 329,497. By 1980 this had risen to 458,503 at an average annual rate of 3.1 per cent. This period included the turbulent years of the Amin regime and there is evidence that the rate of growth, modest for an African capital of the times, was inhibited by insecurity in the city (O'Connor, 1988: 92: Jamal, 1991: 96). But between 1980 and 1991, the population rose from 458,503 to 774,241 at the substantially higher rate of 4.8 per cent per annum.

Table 3.1 compares the increases by sex for Kampala and Kamwokya II. During the intercensal period 1969–80 the percentage increases in the two populations were similar. In the intercensal period 1980–91 the increases for both the city and the parish were substantially higher than

Table 3.1 *Population by sex for Kampala and Kamwokya II, 1969, 1980 and 1991*

Year	Males	Intercensal increase	Females	Intercensal increase	Total	Intercensal increase	Sex ratio
Kampala							
1969	182,294		147,837		330,770		123 (126[a])
		27%		53%		39%	
1980	232,215		226,288		458,503		103
		62%		75%		70%	
1991	377,225		397,016		774,241		95
Kamwokya II							
1969	3,281		2,377		5,658		138
		25%		56%		38%	
1980	4,085		3,715		7,800		110
		45%		65%		55%	
1991	5,942		6,131		12,073		97

Note: a) The 1969 Census published separate data for Africans and others. The ratio of 123 was for the total population and 126 for Africans only (cf. footnote to Table 3.2)

for 1969–80, but Kamwokya's percentage rise was somewhat lower than that of Kampala.

Over both periods and for both localities the increases in the female population were significantly higher than in the male population. As a result, Kampala's sex ratio fell from 123 males per 100 females in 1969 to 103 in 1980 and 95 in 1991, while that of Kamwokya fell from 138 to 110 in 1980 and 97 in 1991. This fall in sex ratios is no doubt in part a continuation of a longer-term trend. In colonial days the sex ratio in Kampala was much higher, even if it was not known precisely (Southall and Gutkind, 1957), and the post-independence influx of females has been a significant aspect of the changes which took place in many African cities following on decolonization. There clearly were other factors also at work which we refer to later.

That the sex ratios of the city and the parish are now virtually the same should not be taken to imply that there is relative uniformity in either. There are appreciable variations in the parishes immediately surrounding Kamwokya II: Kamwokya I has a ratio of 87; Mulago I a ratio of 77; Mulago III and Kyebando ratios of 103 and 106 respectively; and Bukoto I a ratio of 96.

Within Kamwokya II the ratios range from a high of 110 in the Migrant Area to 81 in the Market Area and 93 in the Permanent House Area, with intermediate ratios of 97 and 100 in the Inner Core and Residual Areas respectively. Such variations assume significance as we examine other socio-demographic differences between the Areas.

(ii) Composition by age and sex

The 1991 age and sex distributions (including age-specific sex ratios) for Kampala and Kamwokya II are shown in Tables 3.2 and 3.3 and the resultant population pyramids are depicted in Fig. 3.1. The pyramids for the two populations are remarkably similar, though the parish has slightly lower proportions of children/young people and correspondingly higher proportions of adults. On the whole, it also has slightly greater imbalances between the sexes of the same age.

The first point of major interest common to both populations is the excess of girls/young women over boys/young men. Not having age distributions for 1980, we turned to the 1969 Census for comparison. The relevant data for both the city and the parish in 1969 are set out, in a form as comparable to the 1991 data as the census sources allow, in Tables 3.4 and 3.5, and to facilitate comparison age-specific sex ratios for both areas and both years are set out side by side in Table 3.6. In addition, Fig. 3.2 presents population pyramids for Kampala in 1969 and 1991 and Fig. 3.3 for Kamwokya II for both years.

It is clear that declines in sex ratios have been accompanied by important changes in age composition and in age-specific sex ratios. In both populations there are now appreciably larger proportions of children aged 5–15 years, especially girls. And the imbalance persists up to the age

Table 3.2 *The African[a] population of Kampala by age and sex 1991*

Age	Males No.	%	Females No.	%	Both Sexes No.	%	Sex Ratio
0-4	66,076	8.6	68,099	8.9	134,175	17.5	97
5-9	42,006	5.5	47,750	6.2	89,756	11.7	88
10-14	36,352	4.7	50,130	6.5	86,482	11.3	73
15-19	40,228	5.2	58,994	7.7	99,222	12.9	68
20-24	53,080	6.9	56,881	7.4	109,961	14.3	93 ⎤
25-29	47,938	6.2	42,611	5.5	90,549	11.8	113 ⎬ 107[b]
30-34	32,438	4.2	25,293	3.3	57,731	7.5	128 ⎦
35-39	19,995	2.6	14,720	1.9	34,715	4.5	136 ⎤
40-44	12,616	1.6	8,820	1.1	21,436	2.8	143 ⎬ 140
45-49	8,315	1.1	5,732	0.7	14,047	1.8	145 ⎦
50-54	6,021	0.8	5,163	0.7	11,184	1.5	171 ⎤
55-59	2,951	0.4	2,392	0.3	5,343	0.7	123 ⎬ 107
60-64	2,209	0.3	2,944	0.4	5,153	0.7	75 ⎦
65-69	1,222	0.2	1,384	0.2	2,606	0.3	88 ⎤
70-74	859	0.1	1,517	0.2	2,376	0.3	57 ⎬ 66
75-79	494	0.1	698	0.1	1,192	0.2	71 ⎥
80+	681	0.1	1,351	0.2	2,032	0.3	50 ⎦
Total	373,481	48.6	394,479	51.4	767,960	100	95

Notes: Italic figures here and in subsequent tables show the ratio average for the age range indicated.
a) The 1969 Census gave separate figures for the different races. In tabulations of the 1969 data we have used the figures for Africans only. In order to maximize comparability, we have in this table used citizenship data given in the 1991 Census and counted as *African* the citizens of Uganda and all its neighbouring countries.

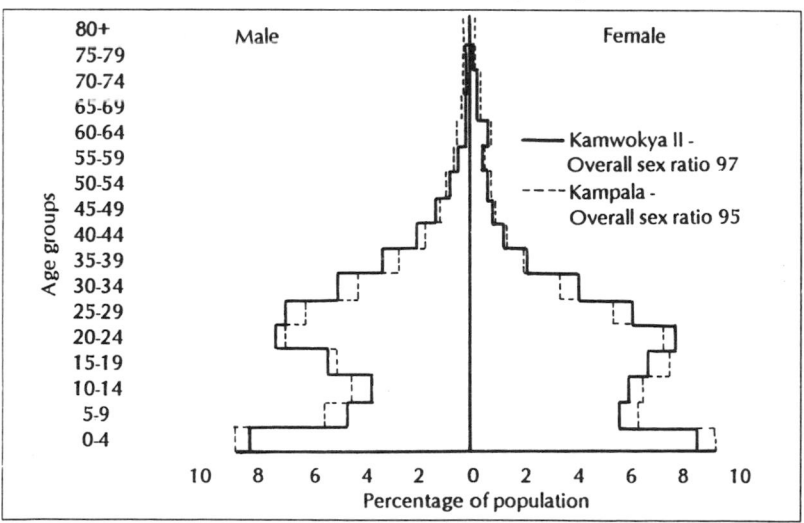

Figure 3.1 *Population pyramids for Kamwokya II and Kampala in 1991*

Table 3.3 *Kamwokya II: Population by age and sex in 1991*

Age	Males No.	%	Females No.	%	Both Sexes No.	%	Sex Ratio	
0-4	982	8.1	1,067	8.8	2,049	17.0	92	
5-9	566	4.7	690	5.7	1,256	10.4	82	
10-14	476	3.9	729	6.0	1,205	10.0	65	
15-19	651	5.4	827	6.8	1,478	12.2	79	
20-24	872	7.2	950	7.9	1,822	15.1	92	
25-29	831	6.9	752	6.2	1,583	13.1	111	*106*
30-34	610	5.1	479	4.0	1,089	9.0	127	
35-39	382	3.2	242	2.0	624	5.2	158	
40-44	237	2.0	123	1.0	360	3.0	193	*167*
45-49	139	1.2	89	0.7	228	1.9	156	
50-54	95	0.8	68	0.6	163	1.3	140	
55-59	42	0.3	25	0.2	67	0.6	168	*129*
60-64	26	0.2	33	0.3	59	0.5	78	
65-69	12	0.1	15	0.1	27	0.2	80	
70-74	7	0.1	13	0.1	20	0.2	54	
75-79	4	0.03	9	0.1	13	0.1	44	*58*
80+	10	0.1	20	0.2	30	0.2	50	
Total	5,942	49.2	6,131	50.8	12,073	100	97	

Table 3.4 *The African population of Kampala city by age and sex in 1969*

Age	Males No.	%	Females No.	%	Total No.	%	Sex Ratio	
0-4	24,844	8.5	25,786	8.8	50,630	17.3	96	
5-9	15,013	5.1	17,157	5.9	32,170	11	88	
10-14	10,556	3.6	11,288	3.9	21,844	7.5	94	
15-19	17,357	5.9	17,139	5.9	34,496	11.8	101	
20-24	25,981	8.9	17,583	6.0	43,564	14.9	148	
25-29	23,770	8.1	13,819	4.7	37,589	12.9	172	*163*
30-34	16,040	5.5	8,873	3.0	24,913	8.5	181	
35-39	10,762	3.7	5,362	1.8	16,124	5.5	201	
40-44	6,155	2.1	4,029	1.4	10,184	3.5	153	*185*
45-49	4,428	1.5	2,177	0.7	6,605	2.3	203	
50-54	2,830	1.0	2,136	0.7	4,966	1.7	132	
55-59	1,549	0.5	740	0.3	2,289	0.8	209	*139*
60-64	1,409	0.5	1,303	0.4	2,712	0.9	108	
65-69	663	0.2	528	0.2	1,191	0.4	126	
70-74	615	0.2	659	0.2	1,274	0.4	93	*106*
75+	832	0.3	807	03	1,639	0.6	103	
TOTAL	162,804	55.7	129,386	44.3	292,190	100	126	

Table 3.5 *Kamwokya II: Population by age and sex in 1969[a]*

Age	Males No.	%	Females No.	%	Total No.	%	Sex Ratio
0-4	438	7.7	527	9.3	965	17.1	83
5-9	227	4 0	276	4.9	503	8.9	82
10-14	172	3.0	174	3.1	346	6.1	99
15-19	369	6.5	370	6.5	739	13.1	100
20-34	1,564	27.6	779	13.8	2,343	41.4	201
35-49	416	7.4	184	3.3	600	10.6	226
50-64	70	1.2	48	0.8	118	2.1	146
65+	25	0.4	19	0.3	44	0.8	132
TOTAL	3,281	58.0	2,377	42.0	5,658	100	138

Note: a) Data for 1969 are available only in 15-year age groups above the age of 20.

Table 3.6 *Age-specific sex ratios for Africans in Kampala City and for Kamwokya II 1969 and 1991*

Age	1969 Kamwokya	Kampala	1991 Kamwokya II	Kampala
0-4	83	96	92	97
5-9	82 ⎫	88 ⎫	82 ⎫	88 ⎫
10-14	99 ⎬ 94	94 ⎬ 94	65 ⎬ 75	73 ⎬ 76
15-19	100 ⎭	101 ⎭	79 ⎭	68 ⎭
20-24	⎫	148 ⎫	92 ⎫	93 ⎫
25-29	⎬ 201	172 ⎬ 163	111 ⎬ 106	113 ⎬ 107
30-34	⎭	181 ⎭	127 ⎭	128 ⎭
35-39	⎫	201 ⎫	158 ⎫	136 ⎫
40-44	⎬ 226	153 ⎬ 185	193 ⎬ 167	143 ⎬ 140
45-49	⎭	203 ⎭	156 ⎭	145 ⎭
50-54	⎫	132 ⎫	140 ⎫	117 ⎫
55-59	⎬ 146	209 ⎬ 139	168 ⎬ 129	123 ⎬ 107
60-64	⎭	108 ⎭	78 ⎭	75 ⎭
65-69	⎫	126 ⎫	80 ⎫	88 ⎫
70-74	⎬ 132	93 ⎬ 106	54 ⎬ 58	57 ⎬ 66
75+	⎭	103 ⎭	50 ⎭	57 ⎭
TOTAL	138	126	97	95

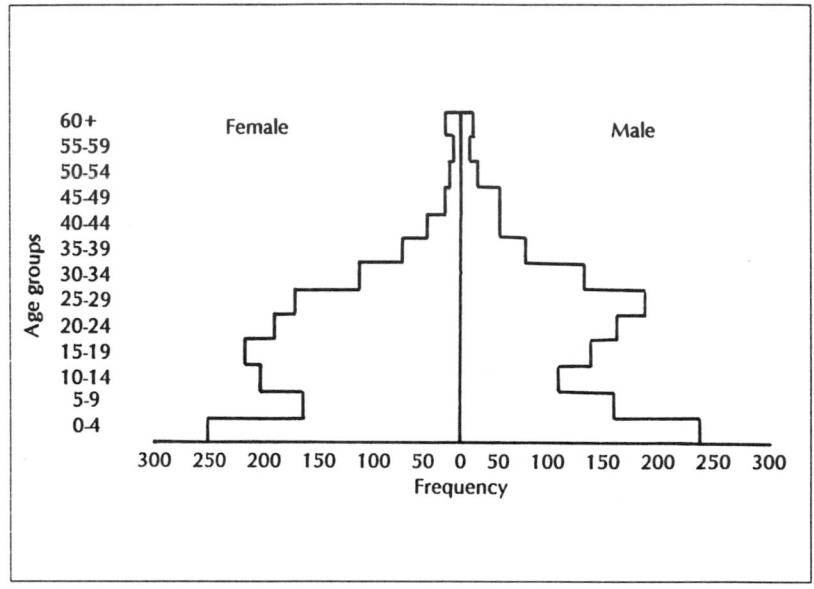

Figure 3.2 *Population pyramid, Kamwokya 1993*

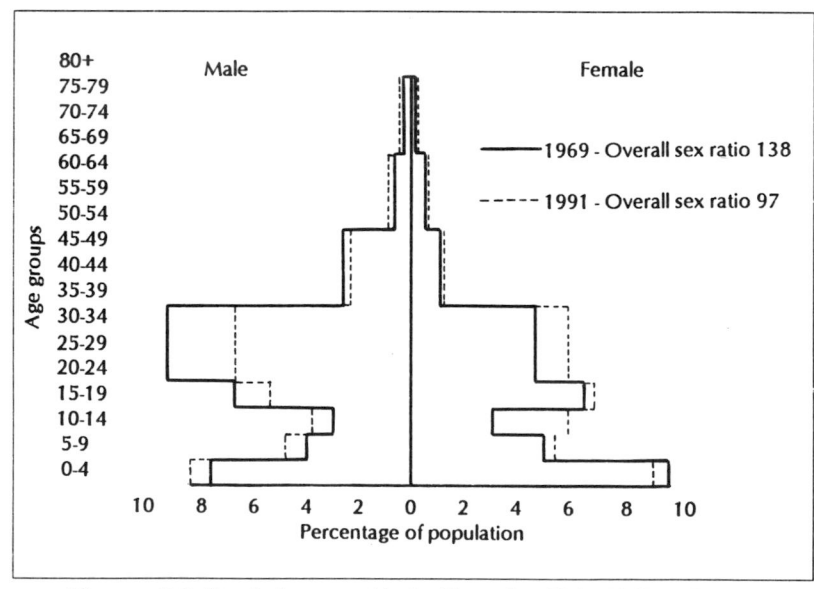

Figure 3.3 *Population pyramids for Kamwokya II in 1969 and 1991*

Table 3.7 *Population by age and sex in the Migrant Area of Kamwokya II, 1991*

Age	Male No.	Male %	Female No.	Female %	Total No.	Total %	Sex ratio
0–4	158	6.7	203	8.6	361	15.3	78
5–9	101	4.3	113	4.8	214	9.1	89
10–14	79	3.4	112	4.8	191	8.1	71
15–19	128	5.4	155	6.6	283	12.0	83
20–24	198	8.4	174	7.4	372	15.8	114
25–29	211	9.0	142	6.0	353	15.0	149
30–34	147	6.2	91	3.9	238	10.1	162
35–39	85	3.6	49	2.1	134	5.7	173
40–44	65	2.8	21	0.9	86	3.7	⎫
45–49	30	1.3	22	0.9	52	2.2	⎬ 207
50–54	19	0.8	15	0.6	34	1.4	⎭
55–59	8	0.3	1	0.04	9	0.4	
60–64	6	0.3	7	0.3	13	0.6	⎫
65–69	2	0.1	3	0.1	5	0.2	⎪
70–74	0	0.0	2	0.1	2	0.1	⎬ 56
75–79	0	0.0	1	0.04	1	0.04	⎪
80+	2	0.1	5	0.2	7	0.3	⎭
Total	1,239	52.6	1,116	47.4	2,355	100	110

Table 3.8 *Population by age and sex in the Market Area of Kamwokya II, 1991*

Age	Male No.	Male %	Female No.	Female %	Total No.	Total %	Sex ratio
0–4	155	8.5	170	9.3	325	17.8	91
5–9	83	4.5	118	6.5	201	11.0	70
10–14	89	4.9	132	7.2	221	12.1	67
15–19	103	5.6	127	7.0	230	12.6	81
20–24	127	7.0	140	7.7	267	14.6	91
25–29	95	5.2	113	6.2	208	11.4	84
30–34	59	3.2	76	4.2	135	7.4	77
35–39	39	2.1	46	2.5	85	4.6	85
40–44	29	1.6	23	1.3	52	2.8	⎫
45–49	21	1.1	13	0.7	34	1.9	⎬ 108
50–54	10	0.5	21	1.1	31	1.7	⎭
55–59	6	0.3	4	0.2	10	0.5	
60–64	1	0.1	9	0.5	10	0.5	⎫
65–69	1	0.1	6	0.3	7	0.4	⎪
70–74	1	0.1	6	0.3	7	0.4	⎬ 11
75–79	0	0.0	3	0.2	3	0.2	⎪
80+	0	0.0	3	0.2	3	0.2	⎭
Total	819	44.8	1,010	55.2	1,829	100	81

Table 3.9 *Population by age and sex in the Permanent House Area in Kamwokya II, 1991*

Age	Male No.	%	Female No.	%	Total No.	%	Sex ratio
0–4	212	7.9	225	8.4	437	16.3	94
5–9	154	5.7	154	5.7	308	11.5	100
10–14	121	4.5	207	7.7	328	12.2	58
15–19	145	5.4	196	7.3	341	12.7	74
20–24	177	6.6	203	7.6	380	14.2	87
25–29	149	5.6	167	6.2	316	11.8	89
30–34	121	4.5	102	3.8	223	8.3	119
35–39	90	3.4	55	2.1	148	5.4	164
40–44	45	1.7	21	0.8	66	2.5	⎫
45–49	34	1.3	21	0.8	55	2.1	⎪
50–54	23	0.9	17	0.6	40	1.5	⎬ 173
55–59	7	0.3	4	0.1	11	0.4	⎪
60–64	7	0.3	6	0.2	13	0.5	⎭
65–69	3	0.1	2	0.1	5	0.2	⎫
70–74	2	0.1	0	0.0	2	0.1	⎪ 114
75–79	1	0.03	3	0.1	4	0.1	⎬
80+	3	0.1	3	0.1	6	0.2	⎭
Total	1,294	48.3	1,386	51.7	2,680	100	93

group 20–24. This is markedly different from 1969 when sex ratios in the 10–14 and 15–19 age groups were at or near parity, and when men aged 20–24 heavily outnumbered women of the same age. (A more detailed year-by-year analysis of the Kampala data, which cannot be set out in full here, showed that it is at age 23 that parity between the sexes is reached, but only at 25 that there is an appreciable excess of men – a ratio of 111.) We may also note (a) that the excess of men over women in the adult age groups up to 55–59 is less in both populations than it was in 1969, and (b) that today's appreciable excess of old women over old men is also new. This doubtless has more significance in the context of concerns other than ours.

Turning to the situation within Kamwokya in 1991, the excess of girls/young women over boys/young men was marked in all areas. The data for the Migrant, Market and Permanent House Areas are given in Tables 3.7–3.9 respectively, and the population pyramid for the Migrant Area is plotted against that for the Market Area in Figure 3.4 and of the Permanent House Area in Figure 3.5.

With the single exception of parity in the age group 5–9 in the Permanent House Area, girls/young women outnumber boys/young men in all age groups in all areas (including the two areas for which the evidence is not represented here). But the rate and extent to which the imbalance changes as we go up the age ladder varied appreciably. In the

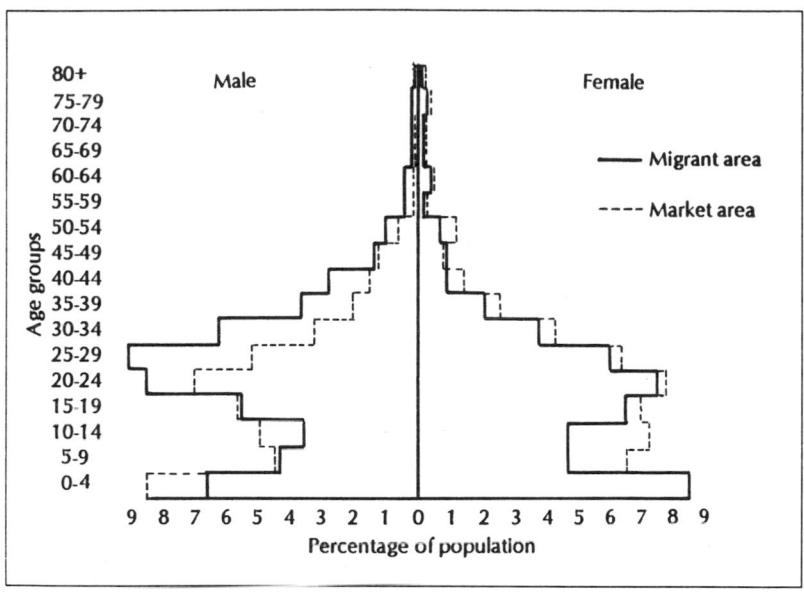

Figure 3.4 *Population pyramids for the Migrant and Market Areas of Kamwokya II, 1991*

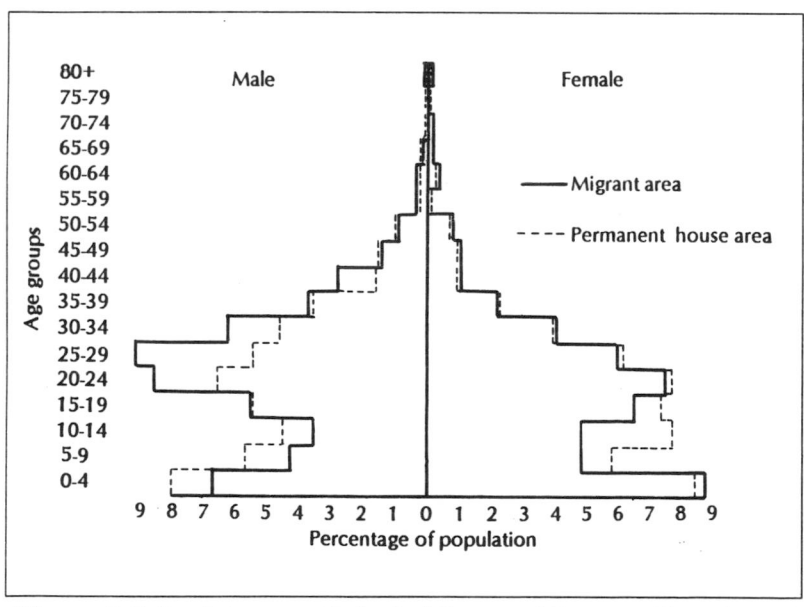

Figure 3.5 *Population pyramids for the Migrant and Permanent House Areas of Kamwokya II, 1991*

People in Place

Migrant Area, with the highest overall sex ratio, the imbalance is reversed in the age group 20–24; in the Market Area, with the lowest overall ratio, it persists into the mature adult age groups; and in the Permanent House Area it is reversed in the 30–34 age group. (In the two areas for which the figures are not given, the reversal was in the age group 25–29, intermediate to the Migrant and Permanent Home Areas.) It can also be seen that the Migrant Area has high sex ratios in the middle adult age groups, in sharp contrast to the Market Area, while the Permanent House Area falls between these extremes.

We later comment on this pattern of variations in the light of our review of other differences between the areas.

(iii) Household size

The mean household size in Kampala was 4.0. Households with male heads (69 per cent) had a mean of 4.1 and those with female heads (31 per cent) a mean of 3.8.

In Kamwokya II the mean size of all households was 3.4, ranging from a low of 2.9 in the Migrant Area to 3.6 in the Market Area and 4.2 in the Permanent House Area. The Inner Core and Residual Areas each had means of 3.3. We do not have census data on the sex of the heads of households but the ethnographic survey gave a return of 73 per cent males and 37 per cent females.

(iv) Places of birth and the migrant nature of the population as a whole

The regions of birth of the population of Kamwokya and its five areas are shown in Table 3.11. At the time of writing, comparable data for the city have not yet been published, but we know that 42.6 per cent of the Kampala population were born in the city as against 38.5 per cent for Kamwokya. (According to our ethnographic survey, most of those born in Kampala were born in Kamwokya itself.) Within Kamwokya this figure ranges from 31.3 per cent for the Migrant Area to 46.6 per cent in the Market Area. These two areas also have the highest and lowest

Table 3.10. *Places of birth of the Ugandan population of Kamwokya II by area[a] (%)*

Place of birth	Migrant Area	Market Area	Permanent House Area	Inner Core Area	Residual Area	All Areas
Kampala	31.3	46.6	39.1	38.4	41.1	38.5
Central Region	22.8	29.0	23.3	28.7	16.4	24.1
(Kampala + Central subtotal)	54.1	75.6	62.4	67.1	57.5	62.6
Western Region	32.3	16.5	19.6	23.4	17.4	22.0
Eastern Region	5.0	6.1	11.2	5.3	15.6	8.4
Northern Region	8.6	1.8	6.7	4.2	9.5	7.0

Note: a) Persons born outside Uganda constituted 1.8 per cent and are excluded from this table.

proportions of Westerners, but with the higher proportion in the Migrant Area.

In general, the differences between other areas are relatively small. The table does not, however, reveal either the full extent to which there are local concentrations of people from the same region, or the essentially migrant nature of the populations, since most of the locally-born are children.

On the first point, although all but three EAs in the parish had majorities from the Central Region (including Kampala), a number had well above average representations of Westerners and Northerners: for example, one EA in the Migrant Area had 46 per cent Northerners and two had 41 and 45 per cent Westerners. Moreover, from our field observations we gained the impression that the arbitrary boundaries of EAs had the effect of masking some concentrations (cf. our remarks on ethnic affiliations below and in Chapter 2). On the second point, the extent to which the birthplaces of children tend to distort overall migrant profiles may be gauged from Tables 3.11 and 3.12 for the Migrant and

Table 3.11 *Age and sex in the Migrant Area by place of birth (Kampala or elsewhere)*

Age	Born in Kampala				Born elsewhere				Total	% born in Kampala	Sex ratio among immigrant pop.
	Males		Females		Males		Females				
	No.	%	No.	%	No.	%	No.	%			
0–4	126	5.4	171	7.3	32	1.4	32	1.4	361	82.2	100
5–9	60	2.5	63	2.7	41	1.7	50	2.1	214	57.5	82
10–14	38	1.6	55	2.3	41	1.7	57	2.4	191	48.7	72
15–19	39	1.7	36	1.5	89	3.8	119	5.1	283	26.5	75
20–24	26	1.1	28	1.2	172	7.3	146	6.2	372	14.3	118
25–29	15	0.6	15	0.6	196	8.3	127	5.4	353	8.5	154
30–34	8	0.3	10	0.4	139	5.9	81	3.4	238	7.6	172
35–39	2	0.1	10	0.4	83	3.5	39	1.7	134	9.0	213
40–44	4	0.2	3	0.1	61	2.6	18	0.8	86		
45–49	0	0.0	0	0.0	30	1.3	22	0.8	52		
50–54	3	0.1	2	0.1	16	0.7	13	0.6	34		
55–59	2	0.1			6	0.3	1	0.04	9		
60–64					6	0.3	7	0.3	13	7.7	176
65–69					2	0.1	3	0.11	5		
70–74					0	0.0	2	0.11	2		
75–79					0	0.0	1	0.04	1		
80+			2	0.1	2	0.1	3	0.11	7		
Total	323	13.7	395	16.7	916	39.0	721	30.6	2,355	30.5	127

Males born in Kampala: 13.7 }
Females born in Kampala: 16.7 } 30.4%
Males born elsewhere 39.0 }
Females born elsewhere 30.6 } 69.6%

[a] All these are percentages of the total population (2,355)

59

Table 3.12 *Age and sex in the Market Area by place of birth (Kampala or elsewhere)*

Age	Born in Kampala				Born elsewhere				Total	% born in Kam-pala	Sex ratio among immigrant pop.
	Males		Females		Males		Females				
	No.	%	No.	%	No.	%	No.	%			
0–4	141	7.7	148	8.1	14	0.8	22	1.2	325	88.9	60
5–9	67	3.7	89	4.9	16	0.9	29	1.6	201	77.6	55
10–14	59	3.2	72	3.9	30	1.6	60	3.3	221	59.3	50
15–19	51	2.8	47	2.6	52	2.8	80	4.4	230	42.6	65
20–24	35	1.9	32	1.8	92	5.0	108	5.9	267	25.1	85
25–29	21	1.1	22	1.2	74	4.1	91	5.0	208	20.7	81
30–34	11	0.6	16	0.9	48	2.6	60	3.3	135	20.0	80
35–39	9	0.5	9	0.5	30	1.6	37	2.0	85	21.2	81
40–44	3	0.2	1	0.1	26	1.4	22	1.2	52		
45–49	3	0.2	6	0.3	18	1.0	7	0.4	34		
50–54	0	0.0	3	0.2	10	0.5	18	1.0	31		
55–59	1	0.1	1	0.1	5	0.3	3	0.2	10		
60–64			2	0.1	1	0.1	7	0.4	10	15.2	87
65–69			1	0.1	1	0.1	5	0.3	7		
70–74			2	0.1	1	0.1	4	0.2	7		
75–79			1	0.1	0	0.0	2	0.1	3		
80+			0	0.0	0	0.0	3	0.2	3		
Total	401	21.9	452	24.7	418	22.9	558	30.5	1,829	46.6	71

Males born in Kampala	21.9	46.6%
Females born in Kampala	24.7	
Males born elsewhere	22.9	53.4%
Females born elsewhere	30.5	

Market Areas when the Kampala-born are classified by age and sex. See also the population pyramids of the local and non-local by birth in Figures 3.6 and 3.7.

In all areas there are large majorities of adults born outside Kampala. But there are again consistent differences between areas. In the Migrant Area the proportion born in Kampala falls to 14.3 per cent in the 20–24 age group, whereas in the Market Area it remains at a level of about 20 per cent up to age 40. In the Permanent House Area it fell to 17.9 per cent in the age group 20–24 and in the Inner Core Area to 15.3 per cent in this same age group. (The distributions for these latter areas are not shown here.)

Another point of central interest to us is that the age-specific ratios of immigrants in both the polar cases of the Migrant and Market Areas tend to fall in line with those examined for all residents in the previous section. This was equally the case in the other three areas and thus in Kamwokya II as a whole, which clearly indicates the sex-selective tendencies in the migration of young people.

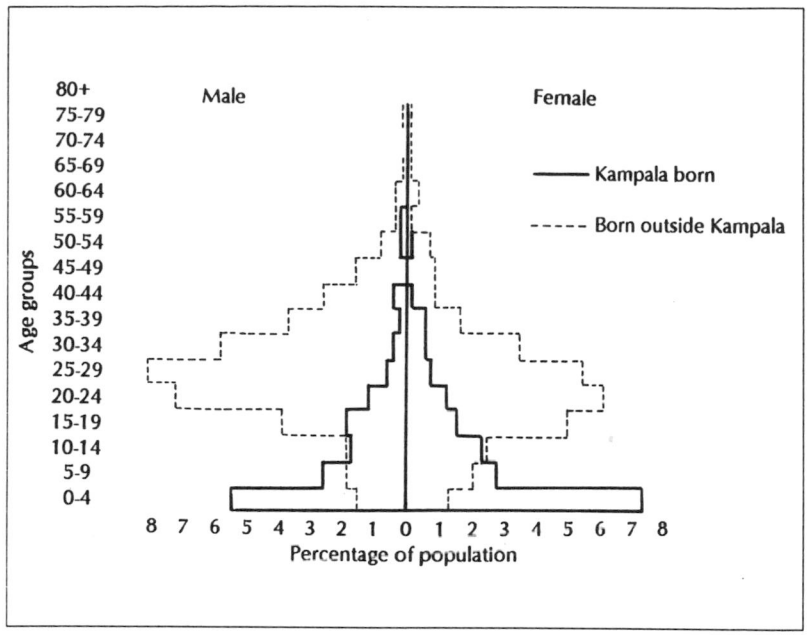

Figure 3.6 *Population pyramids for residents of the Migrant Area born in Kampala and elsewhere*

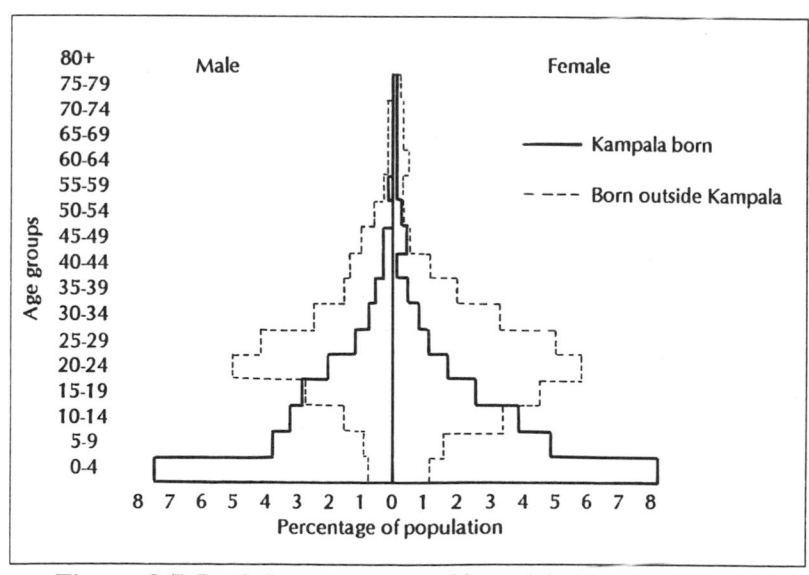

Figure 3.7 *Population pyramids for residents of the Market Area born in Kampala and elsewhere*

People in Place

(v) Religious and ethnic affiliations

Tables 3.13 and 3.14 set out the religious and ethnic affiliations of the populations of Kampala and of Kamwokya II and its five areas. The main differences between them in religion are that the parish had a larger proportion of Catholics and a lower proportion of Muslims. Within Kamwokya II there were more marked differences. The Migrant Area was over 50 per cent Catholic (and up to 70 per cent in one of its EAs), but it had the lowest proportion of Muslims (10.5 per cent). In contrast the Market Area had the lowest proportion of Catholics (34.4 per cent) and the highest of Muslims (36.2 per cent), making it the most diverse area in this respect. (In one of its EAs, there were about one-third Catholics, one-third Church of Uganda and one-third Muslims.)

Table 3.13 *Religious affiliation of people in Kampala and of Kamwokya II by area (%)*

Religion	Kampala	Kamwokya II Total	Migrant Area	Market Area	Permanent House Area	Inner Core	Residual Area
Roman Catholic	39.4	46.2	53.3	34.4	46.3	51.3	47.3
Church of Uganda	38.5	36.9	34.4	39.0	42.8	33.3	35.4
Muslim	19.8	15.4	10.5	26.2	13.3	13.8	16.4
Minor Christian Churches	1.5	0.9	0.9	0.2	1.5	1.3	0.4
Others	0.8	0.6	1.0	0.2	1.1	0.3	0.4

Table 3.14 *Ethnic groups of the populations of Kampala and Kamwokya II by area (%)*

Ethnic Group	Kampala	Kamwokya II Total	Migrant Area	Market Area	Permanent House Area	Inner Core	Residual Area
Baganda	60.6	39.8	27.3	59.3	39.0	38.2	40.1
Banyankole/ Bahima	5.0	7.6	5.8	7.1	7.6	8.3	8.3
Batoro/ Batuku/ Basongora	3.6	11.1	17.4	7.3	11.2	11.2	7.4
Ifeso	3.3	3.7	2.0	2.1	4.5	3.2	6.5
Basoga	3.2	2.9	1.2	2.9	3.3	1.7	3.0
Bakiga	2.8	4.1	4.6	2.4	5.0	5.0	10.6
Acholi/Labwor	2.6	3.1	4.6	1.0	2.9	1.2	5.1
Bafumbira	1.2	6.0	13.0	2.6	2.9	8.2	2.3
Others	17.6	21.7	24.1	15.3	23.6	23.0	16.7

Note: a) The percentages refer to all groups constituting at least 3% of either the Kampala or the Kamwokya populations.

62

In ethnic composition, the city and the parish differed very appreciably, with a far lower proportion of Baganda in the Parish (39.8 per cent) than in the city (60.6 per cent). The Baganda were, however, the single largest group in all Areas, but the main difference was again between the Migrant Area (27.3 per cent) and the Market Area (59.3 per cent), where the proportion of Baganda was much the same as in the city as a whole. In general, the Market Area was the most homogeneous, and the Migrant Area the most mixed, with significant proportions of Batoro/Batuku/Basongora (17.4 per cent) and Bafumbira (13 per cent).

As in the case of regional origins, however, ethnic clustering cannot be adequately judged from the arbitrarily drawn EA divisions which underlie our areas. Looking at the figures for individual EAs as well as for neighbouring parishes, it is clear that some groups are much more clustered than others. For example, the Bafumbira, although dispersed throughout Kampala, are markedly concentrated in and around Kamwokya's Migrant Area, with 42 per cent in one EA and 22 per cent in another, and also making up 10 per cent of the adjoining parish of Mulago III where they are mainly settled along the border with Kamwokya II. Similarly, there is a neighbourhood in the Migrant Area, popularly known as 'the Acholi quarter', where the Acholi make up 29.4 per cent of one EA and 13.2 per cent in an adjacent one.

According to local informants, such concentrations have historical roots and were more marked in the past. The proportion of Acholi in 'the Acholi quarter' was, we were told, higher in the days of the Amin regime but declined towards the end of the Obote II period. It is also said that ethnic concentrations in general are declining with the current increasing pressure of demand for accommodation in parishes like Kamwokya II, which have relatively easy access to the city centre. In addition, some informants reported that in the past landlords were more inclined to give preference to tenants of their own group, whereas now it is 'money that counts'.

(vi) 'Activity status' and occupations

The Uganda Census classifies the population aged 10 years and over by 'activity status' as shown by sex in Table 3.15 for Kamwokya and Kampala and, in a slightly simplied form, in Table 3.16 for the Migrant, Market and Permanent House Areas within Kamwokya.

The main difference between Kamwokya and Kampala is that Kamwokya had a larger proportion of economically active (54.5 per cent as against 47.9 per cent) with a correspondingly lower proportion of students (21 per cent as against 25.9 per cent), but this differential was approximately the same for both sexes in the two populations. The differences in the proportions of men and women who were economically active were also similar (71 per cent males and 37.9 per cent females in Kamwokya as against 65.2 per cent males and 32 per cent females in Kampala).

Table 3.15 'Activity status' by sex of all aged 10 years and over in Kampala and Kamwokya II (%)

Activity status	Male	Kamwokya Female	Total	Male	Kampala Female	Total
Employee	42.0 ⎫	18.5 ⎫	30.3 ⎫	41.2 ⎫	17.5 ⎫	28.9 ⎫
Self-employed	29.0 ⎬ 71.0	19.4 ⎬ 37.9	24.2 ⎬ 54.5	24.0 ⎬ 65.2	14.5 ⎬ 32.0	19.0 ⎬ 47.9
Household worker	2.0	34.1	18.0	2.6	35.8	19.8
Student	21.7	20.4	21.0	27.0	24.8	25.9
Unpaid family worker	1.1	3.8	2.4	0.9	2.7	1.8
Looking for work	3.3	2.4	2.8	2.8	2.1	2.5
Disabled/too old to work/ others	0.9	1.5	1.2	1.5	2.5	2.0
Total no.	4,370	4,346	8,716	244,962	264,342	509,304

Local differences within Kamwokya were again more marked. We may note the following in particular: the proportion of economically active was higher in the Migrant Area (58.9 per cent) than in the Market Area (50.8 per cent) and the Permanent House Area (49 per cent); and the proportion of students in the Migrant Area was correspondingly lower (14.1 per cent) than in the Market Area (27.4 per cent) and the Permanent House Area (29.6 per cent). As school attendance is a major indication of socio-economic status, we return to this in more detail in the following section.

The most marked differences by sex in classification as 'economically active' were between the Market Area and all other areas, including the Inner Core and Residual Areas not shown here. The Market Area was the only one in which the proportion of economically active men (43.1 per cent) was lower than the corresponding proportion for women (62.2 per cent).

Table 3.17 sets out occupational categories by sex for Kamwokya and Kampala and Table 3.18 for the Migrant, Market and Permanent House Areas. These tables are based on all who were returned by the Census as *having an occupation*. They therefore exclude household workers, students and categories such as disabled or 'too old to work'. (There were various

Table 3.16 *'Activity status' by sex of all aged 10 years and over in the Migrant, Market and Permanent House Area of Kamwokya II (%)*

Activity status	Migrant Area Male	Female	Total	Market Area Male	Female	Total	Permanent House Area Male	Female	Total
Employee	44.2 }77.7	15.6 }36.0	31.4 }58.9	33.0 }60.3	20.0 }43.1	25.8 }50.8	40.1 }62.2	22.6 }36.8	31.0 }49.0
Self-employed	33.4	20.4	27.5	27.3	23.1	25.0	22.1	14.2	18.0
Household worker	2.0	40.8	19.4	2.1	24.3	14.4	1.9	25.8	14.5
Student	13.9	14.3	14.1	31.6	24.1	27.4	30.4	28.8	29.6
All others	6.4	9.0	7.6	6.0	8.5	7.4	5.5	8.6	6.9
Total numbers	986	800	1,786	579	715	1,294	928	1,008	1,936

People in Place

discrepancies in the census data between the absolute numbers returned as having occupations and the 'economically active' in the 'activity status' figures, but we judged that these were not such as to distort the general analyses given here.)

The main differences to note from Table 3.17 are between the proportions in 'higher occupations' (managers down to clerks) of 21.4 per cent for Kampala and 16.3 per cent for Kamwokya, and the higher proportion of service workers in Kamwokya (38.7 per cent) than in Kampala (33.1 per cent). The latter no doubt reflects Kamwokya's importance as a commercial centre serving a population drawn from beyond its own borders. But service work was nonetheless the single largest category in both populations and most markedly for women.

Table 3.17 *Occupations by sex of all aged 10 years and over returned by the Census as 'economically active' in Kampala and Kamwokya II (%)*

Occupation	Kampala			Kamwokya		
	Male	Female	Total	Male	Female	Total
Managers	1.8 ⎫	0.6 ⎫	1.4 ⎫	1.0 ⎫	0.2 ⎫	0.7 ⎫
Professionals	3.9	2.2	3.3	1.8	1.0	1.5
Associate professionals (technicians)	10.4 ⎬ 20.3	10.8 ⎬ 23.4	10.5 ⎬ 21.4	8.5 ⎬ 16.5	6.4 ⎬ 15.2	7.8 ⎬ 16.3
Clerks	4.2 ⎭	9.8 ⎭	6.2 ⎭	5.6 ⎭	7.6 ⎭	6.3 ⎭
Service workers	27.1	43.8	33.1	30.0	53.9	38.7
Machine operators and craftsmen	31.1	7.9	22.8	26.4	9.3	20.1
Elementary occupations (labourers, etc) and agricultural workers	21.5	24.9	22.7	26.8	21.6	24.9
Total numbers	159,011	89,486	248,497	3,152	1,810	4,962

Table 3.18 shows that there were only 11.1 per cent in 'higher occupations' in the Migrant Area as against 28.1 per cent in the Permanent House Area (one EA in this area had 50.8 per cent). The Market Area differed in another respect, namely that almost a half of its economically active population was engaged in service work.

(vi) School attendance

The school attendance figures from the Census are of interest in confirming and underlining socio-economic differences. School fees are one of the most pressing financial demands on family budgets and a constant source of anxiety at all social levels. In general, if children/young people do not attend school it is because they or their families cannot afford the fees.

Table 3.18 *Occupations by sex of all aged 10 years and over returned by the Census as 'economically active' in the Migrant, Market and Permanent House Areas of Kamwokya II (%)*

Occupation	Migrant area Male	Migrant area Female	Migrant area Total	Market area Male	Market area Female	Market area Total	Permanent House Area Male	Permanent House Area Female	Permanent House Area Total
Managers	0.3 ⎫	0.3 ⎫	0.3 ⎫	1.6 ⎫	0.0 ⎫	0.8 ⎫	1.7 ⎫	0.5 ⎫	1.2 ⎫
Professionals	0.8 ⎪	0.0 ⎪	0.6 ⎪	1.4 ⎪	0.9 ⎪	1.1 ⎪	5.3 ⎪	3.3 ⎪	4.4 ⎪
Associate prof.	⎬10.9	⎬11.7	⎬11.1	⎬15.7	⎬13.3	⎬14.5	⎬28.2	⎬28.1	⎬28.1
(technicians)	5.6 ⎪	7.5 ⎪	6.1 ⎪	7.3 ⎪	5.6 ⎪	6.5 ⎪	13.8 ⎪	11.1 ⎪	12.6 ⎪
Clerks	4.2 ⎭	3.9 ⎭	4.1 ⎭	5.4 ⎭	6.8 ⎭	6.1 ⎭	7.4 ⎭	13.2 ⎭	9.9 ⎭
Service workers	28.8	54.7	36.2	37.4	61.1	48.6	24.9	38.1	30.4
Machine operators and craft workers	22.9	9.4	19.0	31.2	9.5	21.2	23.3	9.9	17.6
Elementary occupations (labourers, etc.) and agricultural workers	37.4	24.1	33.6	15.5	16.1	15.6	23.5	24.0	23.8
Total numbers	770	307	1,077	369	338	707	587	425	1,012

Table 3.19 *School attendance in the Migrant, Market and Permanent House Areas of Kamwokya by age and sex (%)*

| | | Males | | | |
Age	Area	At school	Left school	Never attended	No.
5–9	A	49.0	1.0	50.0	102
	B	48.2	0.0	51.8	83
	C	59.4	0.0	40.6	155
10–14	A	78.5	11.4	10.1	79
	B	80.9	14.6	4.5	89
	C	90.1	8.3	1.7	121
15–19	A	36.2	49.6	14.2	127
	B	59.2	38.8	1.9	103
	C	63.2	31.3	5.6	144

| | | Females | | | |
Age	Area	At school	Left school	Never attended	No.
5–9	A	49.6	0.0	50.4	115
	B	53.4	0.0	46.6	118
	C	59.7	1.3	39.0	154
10–14	A	69.9	16.8	13.3	113
	B	76.5	18.2	5.3	132
	C	76.0	13.5	10.5	208
15–19	A	15.0	73.2	11.8	153
	B	41.7	52.8	5.5	127
	C	43.1	50.3	6.7	195

A = Migrant Area; B = Market Area; C = Permanent House Area

Table 3.19 shows the differences in school attendance by age and sex for the city and the parish. In both, the differences between the sexes in the total population at school are relatively small, though they tend to increase from the 5–9 age groups to the 15–19. For both sexes and throughout the age scale, however, there is a consistent tendency for the proportions at school in Kamwokya to be lower than in Kampala.

We may also note in passing (a) that for both sexes in both populations the proportions at school in the age groups 10–14 are appreciably higher than in the 5–9 age group, reflecting the relatively late age at which children go to school; and (b) that in both populations the proportion of girls aged 15–19 falls more steeply than that of boys, with the net result that there are many more girls (especially given their excess over boys at this age) who have either left school or never attended (70.7 per cent in Kamwokya as compared with 51.9 per cent for boys).

Table 3.20 gives comparable figures for the Migrant, Market and Permanent House Areas of Kamwokya. The difference between the Migrant and Permanent House Areas is particularly marked. Between the ages of 5 and 9 there is a difference of about 10 per cent for both boys

Table 3.20 *School attendance in Kampala and Kamwokya by age and sex 15–19 years (%)*

Age		At School	Left School	Never Attended	Total No.
			Males		
5–9	Kampala	56.4	0.6	43.0	42,219
	Kamwokya	54.9	0.2	44.9	566
10–14	Kampala	88.5	6.9	4.6	36,550
	Kamwokya	82.1	10.1	7.8	476
15–19	Kampala	52.1	43.4	4.5	40,024
	Kamwokya	48.1	44.5	7.4	647

Age		At School	Left School	Never Attended	Total No.
			Females		
5–9	Kampala	58.6	1.1	40.3	47,918
	Kamwokya	54.8	0.9	44.3	690
10–14	Kampala	76.9	4.7	8.4	50,292
	Kamwokya	73.9	15.8	10.3	729
15–19	Kampala	34.9	58.8	6.3	58,873
	Kamwokya	29.4	62.0	8.7	820

and girls, and this increases in the higher age groups. Only 15 per cent of girls aged 15–19 in the Migrant Area were at school, against 43.1 per cent in the Permanent House Area. Thus 85 per cent of girls of this age in the Migrant Area have either left or never attended school, as against 57 per cent in the Permanent House Area. The proportions in the Market Area approximate to those in the Permanent House Area, and those in the Inner Core and Residual Areas (not given here) tend to approximate to those for the parish as a whole.

Conclusions and Comments

We saw that the age/sex composition of Kamwokya is similar to that of Kampala as a whole. Most of the parish's socio-demographic characteristics (with the main exception of ethnic composition) also resemble those of the city, though there is a slight but consistent tendency for the parish population to be less 'advantaged' (fewer people in higher occupations, greater congestion, lower school attendance rates, etc.)

Local differences within the parish are more appreciable, with the Migrant Area having a very different set of characteristics from those of the Market and Permanent House Areas. The Inner Core Area tends to fall between these extremes and is, in that sense, most 'typical' of Kam-wokya. We do, however, know that none of these areas is homogeneous or 'pure': there is considerable variation in all respects in each of the areas.

Against this summary view, we return to the issue of sex ratios set out in Sections (i) and (ii) and especially to the excess of girls/young women over boys/young men. Two observations have been made: one is that in the past two decades the pattern of age/sex ratios has changed in much the same way as in the total Kampala population; the other is that the pattern on the ground is complex and variable and it is evident that micro-local factors affect the distribution of people by age and sex. And two very different levels of explanation can be applied to these observations: one is *what people say*: the other *what the historical record and the comparison of areas suggest.*

First level of explanation: what local people say
(a) Girls/young women, sometimes as young as 8 or 9 years, are sent to town to do housework in the homes of their kin or of other families.
(b) Some girls/young women who drop out of village school go to town to trade (more so than boys).
(c) Young boys are more likely to be sent back to their villages – i.e. their father's villages – than are young girls.
(d) Orphan girls are more readily assimilated into town homes than are orphan boys: the girls are more useful.
(e) Some girls working in town are paid very poor wages, if any, and are commonly 'abused by the bosses', i.e. by the adult men in the house. So it is not unusual for them to break away, but to stay in town rather than to venture back to their villages.
(f) Boys (and their parents) often consider education to be more important for them than for girls. But, as town schools are more expensive than village schools, they may be sent back to the less expensive village schools for their education even if the education is of poorer quality.
(g) School fees in town are high and girls are often in a better position to make a little money on the side than are boys. Schoolgirl prostitution exists, though some informants claimed that it is not as widespread now as it was some years ago.
(h) Young men complain that life in town is harder for them than for girls. There are various elaborations on this: parents at times treat their girls better than their boys (giving them more money) in order to 'keep them', to dissuade them from accepting money from men; and while schoolboys do have relationships with schoolgirls they have difficulty in maintaining a steady relationship because the girls are tempted away by approaches from older men with more money.
(i) Many people return to their villages after some years in town. Some informants consider that a woman is likely to return earlier than her husband in order to produce crops to feed the family.

(j) The assumption that the two wars and AIDS may be factors affecting sex ratios in town is widespread but not substantiated. With frequent movement back and forth between Kampala and the countryside it is difficult to see a direct connection, or to envisage which way any cause/effect links would operate. In any case the young men 'missing' in the urban demographic pyramid are largely not of the age groups most vulnerable to either disaster.

(k) AIDS may, however, have a different and indirect connection. It is 'common knowledge' that adult men search out and value young girls as sexual partners on the grounds that the risk of STD/HIV infection is lower with them than with older girls and adult women. This explanation implies, in effect, a particular demand niche for young girls in the urban economy which may allow disproportionate numbers of them to survive in town.

(l) Finally, it was also suggested to us that the proportions of men and women in town may be skewed by their different involvement with 'dual residence'. People living partly in town may see advantages in declaring themselves rural rather than urban or *vice versa*. Informants seemed to think that men would be more likely to see advantages in claiming residence in their 'home area' outside Kampala. The reverse, they say, is likely to be true for women.

All these explanations are plausible, but no more than partial, and we cannot possibly know what weight should be attached to any of them. Whatever the case, however, the change in Kamwokya's and Kampala's population structures between 1969 and 1991 must in some way reflect, or be a response to, the quite fundamental changes in Ugandan society and its economy over the same period.

Second level of explanation: recent history and comparison between areas
It is plainly unlikely that the years of social, economic and political turmoil did not have far-reaching effects on the way Ugandans manage their livelihoods. In fact, we know they did – from relative prosperity in the 1960s, through the years of *magendo* and the *mafuta mingi* (lit. much fat) economy, to the relative economic and social stability that has come about in recent years.

This relative stability has been achieved with, and partly through, an informal economy which requires and allows individuals to use all their personal and family assets to achieve a 'living wage' (Obbo, 1980, 1991). Whatever the true balance of cause and effect, the present economic system is some kind of outcome of the past two decades. And given the structures of opportunity and constraint that typify it, girls and young women are now more viable in the urban setting than boys and young men. Patterns of migration appear to have adapted to match this situation.

Our hypothesis therefore is that the proliferation of alternative means of making a living engendered by the collapse of the formal economy draws more girls/young women than boys/young men into town and encourages them to stay there once they have arrived. To the extent that this broad hypothesis is valid, we should expect different types of 'social areas' in town to develop different age/sex ratios. Opportunities to achieve a living wage, including opportunities to find cheap accommodation, clearly vary considerably according to local circumstances, as do the chances of many rural migrants to stay in town at all. Those of different age, sex and ethnic group inevitably find their niches in different types of areas according to their personal and family resources. In the case of Kamwokya this is abundantly illustrated by the differences we have noted between different areas.

As a general conclusion, we would stress that Kamwokya's relative similarity to Kampala in its socio-demographic characteristics is an accident of history (i.e. of its particular mix of areas), as is its difference in ethnic composition. Some of the parishes adjacent to it have quite different profiles, as we noted with regard to overall sex ratios alone.

Four

Community Life
I
Observers' Views

First impressions from a colleague's diary begin to bring the rather dry facts of place and population to life:[1]...

Kamwokya II Parish is situated four miles or so from the centre of Kampala on the slopes of Kololo Hill. A busy tarmac road takes you to the upper end and from there you can enter the area by walking (or driving) down the slope on one of the dirt roads. Kamwokya is a very busy place, with many women, men and children moving around on its roads and narrow passages. Officially there are close to 14,000 people in its half square kilometre, but one hears figures quoted as high as 30,000. Certainly the centre part is very crowded. Since the settlement is unplanned, with houses being built over night, it is impossible to know exactly how many people live in the area.

The energy of the settlement is immediately striking. Few people just sit or hang around. Everybody is active: women washing clothes, cooking, carrying water, dealing with their children, selling vegetables at the market or brewing the local beer; men repairing houses, bicycles, radios, shoes, anything indeed that might conceivably be repaired. They wash cars and make furniture and charcoal stoves. There are tailors and barbers and hawkers and people advertising their wares. It is noisy – pleasantly noisy on the whole: lots of laughter, music coming from radios and cassette recorders; children everywhere.

There is a big indoor market at the upper part of the settlement, close to the tarmac road, and people come from all over Kampala to shop there. The market building is a large square hall with straight rows of numbered stalls and a few small rooms built to serve as eating rooms or 'restaurants'. Here too there are people milling around. A large number of women seem to be preparing food, green bananas (matoke), onions, tomatoes, pineapples, potatoes, beans, dried fish, fresh meat, etc. The market is open from 7 in the morning to 7 at night and then a candlelight market continues outside in the open

[1] Solveig Freudenthal. See also Chapter 11.

space by the road. Some leftovers from the stalls inside are sold there, but also other goods are bought by women who come to the evening market from their homes or other places of work.

Along the track leading into the centre of Kamwokya there are many bars and shops: grocery shops, butchers, drug shops, second-hand clothes shops and so on. There are several video clubs, where young men watch action films like Karate Kid *and* Rambo. *The better areas contrast sharply with the poorer ones down in the valley. In the poor areas, which local people call the slums, there are garbage heaps and rubbish everywhere, smelly latrines, filthy gutters and greenish water flowing in front of every house as well as open sewers. Anyone going on foot through the settlement must jump over puddles or ditches of dirty water in many places. Most of the better looking houses are located in the upper part of the settlement facing the good roads, but their drainage system looks no better than anywhere else. The dirty water from the richer people's houses in the upper part of the slope runs directly down to the people living at the bottom of the valley.*

Kamwokya people that say they are religious but they don't mean one religion. There are a number of churches and one mosque in the Parish. The mosque is at the top of the road as you enter Kamwokya. A bit further down is the large Catholic Church, then St John's Anglican Church, Church of Uganda, Church of God, Born Again, Seventh Day Adventists and some which the people call 'mushroom' churches, because they grow up over night...

Each of the vignettes which form the body of this chapter focuses on one aspect of community life in Kamwokya. Inevitably the effect is to simplify a very complex picture. And just as inevitably the selection of items worthy of focus is guided by the interests of the observers rather than the priorities of the actors (which are the particular subject of Chapter 11).

It is also appropriate to note that these seven snapshots are the result of different kinds of observation. The first three ('The Market and Shopping'. 'Activity around a Protected Spring' and 'Sunday Morning') are drawn from BBS files – whether as transcripts of field notes, summaries of reports written by various observers, or sketches drawn by one of them. The contents of 'Football' and 'Drinking' emerged from combinations of conversations and walkabout; and the 'RC Court Case' and 'Neighbouring' situations are based on shorter or longer periods of participatory fieldwork.

In terms of their significance to the wider theme of this book, they fall into yet other groups: 'The Market and Shopping' illustrates the bustle of economic activity, and the 'Protected Spring' example carries forward the story of water (begun in Chapter 2). 'Sunday Morning' shows the religious fervour of Kamwokya residents, and 'Football' and 'Drinking' (some of) the leisure pursuits and friendship patterns of men. The RC court case demonstrates the authority of Resistance Councils at the local level, as well as the clash of attitudes with regard to the social and sexual lives of young adults. Finally, 'Neighbouring' brings the focus back to the constraints and resources affecting the lives of women, and adds another strand to the discussion of support systems and the idioms of belonging which continue throughout the book.

(i) The Market and Shopping

The main market is owned and administered by the Kampala City Council. The produce sold is of good quality and the prices are said to be lower than in the central Kampala market, but higher than in smaller markets around the Kamwokya area. In this respect it is an intermediary market catering for many of Kamwokya's residents as well as for visiting shoppers and passers-by.

The market hall is built of wood and corrugated iron sheets. Its floor appears to have been cemented in the past, but over time it has been damaged and broken so that it gives the impression of stones laid in what is usually muddy earth.

The market supervisor and his assistants are responsible for opening the market at 7.00 a.m. and closing it at 7.00 p.m. They also collect fees from the stall holders and restaurant owners and are expected to maintain law and order and to settle disputes between customers and attendants or between stall holders in the market. On one day, many people are gathered around the office to watch young boys being punished. According to bystanders they are bastards who are commonly known to steal. The chief market supervisor reprimands them and orders that they be taken to the police. One old woman is heard saying that the increase in the number of children on the street is the fault of mothers who do not leave the children with their parents (presumably with their fathers). She also blames the authorities who release the children on payment of a fine.

At dawn there is little activity around the market. A few night guards are still walking around and there are always lorries, stacked with *matoke* to be unloaded. When the market opens, kiosk holders and roadside vendors are already beginning to operate.

At 7.00 a.m. a market assistant opens the doors and the stall holders or their employees begin to arrive, set out their stalls, clear things up and generally prepare for the day ahead. By 8.00 a.m. there are 40 or more attendants around the stalls and intense activity – clearing up, cooking and serving early customers in the restaurants. By 9.00 a.m. the number of stall attendants has risen to 100 or more. A good half are Baganda and most of them are women. But there are quite marked differences in the sex and ethnic composition of attendants at the different stalls.

Children play a significant role. Both boys and girls are used by adults to carry goods around, to fetch goods from other stalls, to throw away refuse and the like, in addition to sometimes serving customers. On the whole, they are most frequently seen serving customers early in the morning before their parents/employers have arrived and on Sundays when business is slacker. Older children who serve on Sundays have been at school during the week.

The level of activity in the market has two peaks: the first between 9.00 and 11.00 a.m. and the second from 5.00 p.m. to closing time. When business is slack there is a good deal of leisurely activity among the stall attendants. Some women turn to mat-making, knitting and weaving, while they chat with neighbours. Others, especially boys, play cards and other games.

Competition between attendants to attract customers is most marked at the fresh produce stalls. Attendants are usually able to speak a few words in two or more languages and they compete for attention by addressing customers in whichever they judge most appropriate. Or they use 'cool words' like: 'Hullo Auntie, Uncle, Son…' in Lugunda, English or other languages.

Throughout the day, but especially in the early mornings, there are many Kamwokya customers. Some were house-girls (and sometimes house-boys) sent to the market to buy food for their parents or other adults. Others, mainly women, were taken to be locals because of their untidy dress (wearing slippers, etc.) or because they had small children with them. Most local shoppers went direct to stallholders whom they clearly knew well; they did not look around for cheaper prices and they bought in small quantities.

Towards the mid-morning and late afternoon peaks of activity, the shoppers were more varied and included middle- and higher-income earners. Some arrived and left by car, others had walked from the Kira Road where the *matatus* put down and pick up passengers. They were usually better dressed and conducted themselves differently. They move around the stalls, and inspect the quality, quantity and prices before buying. Some also went to stalls where it was evident from the greetings, smiles and conversations that customer and attendant knew each other well enough to have established credit arrangements. Such customers usually buy in larger quantities than the poorer locals.

Between 6.00 and 7.00 p.m. there is much movement in and around the market. Some customers are still coming in for hurried shopping but attendants are beginning to pack up their stalls to go home or to transfer the produce to the open space outside the market which then becomes even livelier than it is during the day. The open space outside is where the candlelight market operates, with people selling goods off tables or even from the ground. The prices here are lower than in the official daytime market. Much of the produce consists of leftovers from the stalls inside. But the vendors are not all stall holders. Some have been outside since morning, and others (mainly women) come to the evening market straight from their homes or from other work.

The market lies within an area which is busy from early morning to about 10.00 p.m. Above a row of shops which front on to the market there are open spaces which provide parking both for lorries, pick-up vans and cars and for 'special-hire' cars (taxis). Further up still, on the Kira Road, are the *matatu* bus stages from which there is a constant stream of comings and goings. There are two repair garages and innumerable kiosks, roadside vendors, tailors, car washers, shoe-shiners and the like, especially along the pavements and other spaces in front of the line of larger shops which face on to the Kira Road.

As in the market, the busiest shopping times are mid-morning and mid-to-late afternoon. But the general liveliness of the scene in front of the shops is affected by the large numbers of passers-by, some hurrying without stopping and others lingering to chat to the shopkeepers or to friends along the way.

(ii) Activity around a Protected Spring

A description of available water sources and their distribution was given in Chapter 2. These observations were made over a full day around a spring located in the lower part of Kamwokya II close to the swamp.

Sketches of three different water sources appear as Sketches 17–19. The waterspring observed 'in action' is shown in Sketch 17. It is a 'protected' spring which has recently been renovated. It has a cement 'pavement' and two large pipes through which the water gushes. On both sides of the pipes there are cement steps used by people to reach the water supply. Below the spring there is a well-constructed drainage channel of stones which allows excess water to drain away without creating stagnant pools. An RC attendant supervises the use of the spring and was seen to collect payments from the users.[2]

By 8 a.m. 12 men, 14 women and 33 children (18 boys and 15 girls) were gathered around the spring. The male attendant was already busy supervising operations. A few people near the head of the householders' queue seemed to have come very early as the men wore jackets and the women and children were wearing warm clothes to protect them from the early morning cold. There were three lines of large 20-litre jerry cans spread around the spring as shown in Sketch 17. The first line was made up of cans belonging to local householders, the second had cans belonging to water sellers, and the third was a special line for people in a hurry. The first two lines were much longer than the third and the owners of the cans, whether households or water sellers, were charged Ush.10 per can. Owners of cans in the special express line were charged Ush.50. The number of cans in the first two lines was much larger than the number of people: many users leave their cans under the supervision of the attendant and only return when they expect them to be near the filling point.

---

[2] Local informants, both RC officials, later insisted that no payment is required. People use protected as well as unprotected springs when they do not have money to pay for tap water. But they conceded that if someone helps you get the water because you do not want to walk in the mud, you may 'give them something'. Alternatively, perhaps, the payments observed were 'unofficial' in contrast to payments for tap water which are officially sanctioned.

Between 8.00 and 9.00 a.m. the scene around the spring became livelier, with some people taking away full cans and larger numbers joining the queues. On one occasion two women began to quarrel and ended up fighting until the spring attendant separated them. One stayed on to get water and the other went home without it. The number of children increased. Most of them placed their cans in the householders' line, then ran around and played while keeping an eye on their cans and periodically breaking away from their groups to move the cans forward. When their cans had been filled, they struggled to take them away or to move them to one side until an older member of the family came to fetch them. At this time the general atmosphere was noisy and lively. People chatted in a way which indicated that they knew each other well. The languages most frequently heard were Luganda, Lunyankole, Ateso and Lugbara.

At this time the water sellers were mainly young adults, well-built and strong. Many appeared to be Northerners. Taking the water away they carried one jerry can in each hand and 'walked away majestically', then returned to the spring with 10–15 empty cans roped together on their backs.

One water seller was seen stacking his filled cans a little distance from the spring. No one interfered with them. He then returned at 10-minute intervals to carry away two at a time. Another was seen bringing 20 empty cans to the spring but placing only one in the line. Apparently by agreement with the spring attendant, the one can in the line reserved the right to fill the other 19 at the appropriate time. By 9.45 a.m. several other carriers were doing the same, and this had the effect of shortening the water sellers' line of cans. The householders' line continued to extend, while the special line had disappeared altogether. Between 10 a.m. and 12 noon the line of householders' cans gradually diminished but the water sellers were, if anything, busier than before. It takes about 40 seconds to fill one large can and so with two pipes delivering water, approximately 180 cans per hour are carried away.

The sun was getting hot and most of the women and children were retiring to the shade of nearby trees, only coming forward either to move their cans or to fill them. Some people awaiting their turn played cards or drafts or simply chatted. The smaller children continued to run around, in the sun or in the shade.

Between 12 noon and 2.00 p.m. the water sellers were as busy as ever, but the line of householders' cans had decreased to about a quarter of its morning length. Between 2.00 and 3.00 p.m. the scene was much quieter. Very few householders were fetching water and most of the water sellers took a lunch-time rest. Soon after 3.00 p.m., however, there was a general increase in activity, with householders and water sellers starting to come back to the spring. And by 4.00 p.m. the scene was 'back to normal' with the first two lines lengthening and the special line re-appearing. There was also a noticeable increase in the number of children, some of them carrying smaller 5-litre cans. The attendant separated the children with small cans from the rest and gave them water free of charge. A few elderly people began to arrive and were also allowed to by-pass the queues.

By 5.00 p.m. more and more people of all categories were coming to the spring and the overall scene was getting livelier by the minute. This surge of activity continued into the peak hour of 5.30 to 6.30 p.m. Men, women and children from local households now exceeded the water sellers and there were large numbers of full jerry cans stacked on the side waiting to be carried away in all directions.

Towards nightfall two members of the local defence unit arrived to take over supervision of the spring from the attendant. The fetching of water began to decrease between 6.30 and 7.00 p.m., but this was the time when the proportion of women at the spring reached its peak. It was also the time when there were many people hanging around casually. The general scene appeared even livelier after a bright security light lit up the whole area at 7.30 p.m.

(iii) Sunday Morning

The Catholic and Anglican Churches in Kamwokya II have by far the largest followings but the smaller sectarian churches are also lively. All the churches have catchment areas extending well beyond Kamwokya II, and between them provide very active programmes of mission work, Bible study, welfare programmes (notably for AIDS victims and their families), leisure activity groups for children, and sewing and tailoring classes for women. Observations made in three churches on one Sunday in January convey the liveliness of religious life in Kamwokya.

a. *The Catholic church* is a large modern building with a seating capacity of approximately 300 and with several rooms attached as well as outbuildings in a secure enclosure.

Mass began promptly at 7.00 a.m. The church was filled to capacity and there were a number of people outside in the entrance. The church is divided into three sections. The area on the far right of the altar was mainly occupied by children, about 60 in number with more girls than boys. About 200 adults were present, women sitting on the right-hand side of the church and men on the left. There were more women than men. Some of the women sat on mats in the entrance to the church, while most of the men were inside.

At the beginning of the mass all made the sign of the cross. Hymns were sung and most members of the congregation uttered words of praise after each hymn. The first readings were taken from the Books of Corinthians and Revelations. The priest then read from St Luke's Gospel and preached for about 15 minutes.

At 7.30 Holy Communion was served by two priests. Most of the adults and some of the children took communion, filing past the altar before returning to kneel at their seats. Those sitting outside followed as did late-comers who looked for empty spaces on the men's side of the church after taking communion.

At 7.50 the priest blessed the congregation and sat down. A man in the front row then got up to give out special announcements. These included the names of couples to be married and a statement of the offerings collected: Ush.755 from the children, 5,500 from the men and 7,000 from the women.

The priests left the church at 7.55 a.m. followed by the congregation, many of whom lingered outside to greet friends. The entire mass had been conducted in Luganda, though a few people were overheard conversing in Lukiga and Lunyankole outside.

By 8.20 a.m. most people had left and the church yard was clear.

b. *St. John's Church of Uganda* is also a large modern building with a seating capacity of approximately 350. It has two services on Sunday mornings, the first in English and the second in Luganda. At 8.35 a.m. a group of six 'saved' men are setting up the microphone and loudspeaker system to be heard outside the church. They are joined by six young women wearing nice tidy uniforms. Each tests the microphone in turn.

At 8.45 a.m. a visiting choir stands up to sing to the congregation. After three songs they resume their seats on a bench in front. The congregation then stands up and begins to sing from English hymn books provided by the church. After singing a few hymns, the choir faces the congregation and begins to sing songs that are not in the hymn book, inviting the members of the congregation to join in. The atmosphere becomes lively with singing and clapping. From time to time the choir leader pauses to read short quotations from the Bible.

About 9.15 a.m. the service becomes more formal. The Canon of the Church welcomes the visiting clergy and choir and then announces the first reading by a male member of the congregation who leaves his seat to walk to the front of the church. The first reading is followed by more singing by the choir and a second reading by a female member of the congregation.

By 9.40 am. the church is full to capacity and late-comers gather outside in the entrance. A sermon by the first visiting preacher begins at 9.45 and ends at 10.10 am. It is delivered with great conviction and regular exhortations for members of the congregation to repeat aloud some of his principal statements. Another sermon by the second visiting preacher follows up to 10.30 a.m. and is even more animated than the first.

The sermons are followed by prayers and invitations for those who want to be 'saved' to come to the front of the altar and be blessed. Four young women, a boy of about 16 and a man of about 25 go forward. The whole congregation claps and one of the preachers prays aloud for them.

The choir now sings while members of the Church Council stand in the nave of the church to collect offerings. The preacher receives the offerings, raising them above his head. He turns to face the altar and prays for some two minutes with his arms held high. More offerings are then made by members of different residential zones, the leaders from various zones taking it in turn to move forward followed by the residents of the zones they represent. During this time, the choir leads the congregation in lively singing accompanied by constant clapping which continues until all the people from the different zones have returned to their seats. One of the preachers then leads the congregation in a closing prayer and all members of the congregation are asked to raise their right hands and to proclaim loudly three times that JESUS IS LORD.

The service ends at 11.08 a.m., with some commotion as people who have been waiting to enter the church for the Luganda service jostle past those who are trying to leave. The Luganda service eventually starts at 11.20 with a hymn from the Luganda hymn books which, unlike the English hymn books, are individually owned. The clergy who conduct the service are the same as those who had conducted the English service. The general proceedings, tone and readings are identical and the sermons very similar. The same announcements are made.

The main differences, apart from the fact that everything was in Luganda, were that there were fewer people – fewer children in particular – and the church was only two-thirds full; that neither of the visiting preachers was Baganda; one was Musoga and the other Munyankole, and both, before their sermons, asked to be pardoned if their language was not perfect. And finally, when members of the congregation were invited to come forward to be 'saved', there was a larger response than at the English service. Over thirty people went forward, most of them children, the rest quite young men. One boy of about nine insisted that he wanted to be saved, despite the fact that he was from a Muslim home. He was received by the clergyman to extra loud and prolonged clapping from the congregation.

The service ended at about 1 p.m. In contrast to the people who attended mass at the Catholic Church, the majority of adults at both the Anglican services were men.

c. The walls, roof and doors of the *Born Again Church* are made of papyrus mats and the floor is of beaten mud, kept hard by frequent wetting with water. The electric installations look dangerous, one loose socket being used for the public address system. Seating is on rough moveable benches with a few chairs scattered around the altar. On the front of the altar is a large tablet with the words: 'COME LET US WORSHIP THE LORD'. Otherwise the church is a large unadorned hall.

The service is conducted partly in English and partly in Luganda with regular pauses to allow time for interpretation from one language into the other. At 10.10 a.m. the service opens with recorded Christian music played loudly over the public address system. Some time passes as people take their seats. The children go to the front benches. The adults sit behind and there is no segregation between the sexes. The recorded music is followed by spontaneous singing. The words are known to all. There are no hymn books but most members have their own Bibles and a notebook. As the singing continues, some members bow their heads in silent prayer, a few exchange greetings in quiet voices, and some move between benches to be close to others they know.

At 10.25 a.m. five young people – four women and one man – move up to the altar and call the congregation to order. One leads with a prayer of welcome and thanksgiving. All present are requested to smile at, and greet, those nearest to them. Then, led by the choir at the front, they all stand up and begin singing. The singing is immediately accompanied by the gentle swaying of bodies, which soon develops into more energetic movement: dancing, bending, jumping up, and turning towards others in greeting and in praise. People begin to call loudly on God. Some shout and scream and cry. This continues for about thirty minutes when the choir begins to sing more softly and slowly to bring people back to a quieter mood.

Towards 11.00 a.m. many have sat down again and the Sunday School children are asked to sing on their own before leaving the church to join their Sunday School teachers outside. They are replaced by a solo singer until the minister takes his place at the front. Late-comers are still arriving and are led by the church deacons to the front where the children have vacated their places.

At about 11.15 am. new members and visitors are asked to identify themselves by raising their hands. Forms are handed round for them to complete with their names, where they come from, and other details. Singing and praying continue in alternate spells. Then a member of the congregation is asked to give testimony about what God has done for him in his life. He is followed by the formal introduction of a newly married couple recently returned from their honeymoon, who are asked to give testimony. Then special visitors of high status are asked to say a few words.

About 11.50 a.m. offerings are collected by the deacons. This is done by passing round baskets with envelopes marked 'Evangelism and Faith Offerings'. The preacher (followed by the interpreter) then begins to give his message. After an hour he calls upon those who want to accept Jesus to come forward to be blessed in prayer. A few go forward. The preacher then calls upon those who are possessed by demons or who are sick or unemployed to come forward. There are so many of these that they just stand up where they are and he directs his prayers towards them.

The service ends about 1.20 p.m. as people begin to leave.

(iv) Football

The Parish team plays teams from equivalent parts of Kampala. Called 'Kamwokya United', it is one of only two statements of Kamwokya-wide identity (the other being its RC 2 status). Of more interest here are the ten teams within Kamwokya which play in four annual cup competitions. Organized football began in Kamwokya only in 1990,[3] but there is enormous enthusiasm for it. A recent cup final attracted 800 spectators. The great majority were adult men, but some young boys and a sprinkling of young women also turned out. The match was well organized, with an energetic referee, guests of honour who were treated to sodas and cakes at half time, and much shouting, laughter and jocular jeering all round.

Of the ten internal teams, eight represent RC1 zones. Three are named accordingly, the other five to imply ferocity – 'Red Challenge'. 'Eleven Tigers', etc. – or to mark an interest associated with its home zone. 'Youth Alive F.C.', for example, used to be known as Contafrica F.C. since most of its members live in Contafrica zone. But its leading players are also active in the AIDS prevention campaign 'Youth Alive' (based incidentally on the Catholic Church), and the club's change of name reflects the overlap of the two networks. Of the other two teams, 'Intersport' is based in the valley, at the lower end of Kamwokya II, and draws some of its members from the adjoining parish. These players are neighbours, but they can also be identified by (and perhaps identify with?) common residence on swampy, low-status land. Finally, the 'Eleven Stars' team comes from the border area of two zones and recruits largely among the local metal workers (making tin trunks, etc.) who concentrate there.

Teams develop among men with an interest or activity which networks them together. In most cases it appears to be residence which determines which team a man will play for or will support at a match. But ethnicity and work are often implicated, even if not explicitly, and friendship is not confined locally – at least not for men. One informant used to play for a team (now disbanded) whose name can be translated as 'Rest in the Evening'. It was composed entirely of Luo men who drank local beer together. Others say that if a man from one zone has friends playing in another he might well join that other team.

(v) Drinking

Most bars do not have a formal form of advertising for their clients. It is therefore likely that these different bars are generally known to different clients who frequent them as regular customers. One late afternoon in a local brewer's premises – one room only – there was no one there except the male attendant standing behind a small counter. Drink is sold to consume on the premises or to take away. There were only two chairs, no table. The main drink sold is *tonto*, made from bananas. but *waragi* was

[3] The general interest and identity kick of football is, of course, of much longer standing. Parkin (1969) reports that only interest in soccer 'saved the Luo and Lukya tribal associations in Kampala from being virtually defunct' (p. 50).

also available. This was a recognized 'pub', but there was nothing at all to indicate this from the outside. Any new users may generally find themselves attracted to the bars in the main shopping centre, drawn by factors like loud music or flashing bulbs and flickering neon lights. Bars in Kamwokya can be divided into two categories: traditional bars, characterized mainly by the structures in which they are housed and the type of drink sold, and 'middle-class' bars which have a degree of modernity in the drinks sold and the facilities offered. Drinking places are many and widely distributed.

Bars are supplemented by innumerable shops offering all types of drink in addition to essential commodities; even courtyards serve as drinking places. In all drinking places, on all days of the week, men form the majority of the clientele and most people are over the age of 25. Apparently for youngsters drinking is not a priority among their recreational activities. There is no clear indication of the catchment areas of the bars of Kamwokya, but it is probable that people are attracted from other areas because many were observed to drive or walk to the main roads to Bukoto, Kololo, and Kampala after drinking.

In most cases there are no clear-cut lines separating bars as far as ethnicity is concerned; rather, people from various ethnic backgrounds were joined together by a common interest – the pot or bottle of beer. The exceptions are shops which specialize in the sale of drinks associated with particular tribes, for instance, shops advertising *obusheva* from Kabale, this being a drink made by the Bakiga, and *malwa* (locally brewed millet beer) drinking.[4] Kamwokya II is known beyond its own boundaries as a centre for *malwa* drinking places and the quality of the *malwa* brewed in them is said to be better than any. It is said that the drink has gained in popularity in the recent past and that members of all ethnic groups now enjoy it, with the implication that this was not always the case in the past.

Much (most?) *malwa* drinking is done in semi-formal groups or 'clubs'. These are essentially friendship groups whose members know each other well, and joining a group involves a commitment to continuing membership. Each regular member of a group pays a 'fee' every time he attends – usually around Ush.500 per attendance, though it may be as high as Ush.1,500 and is always paid over and above the payment for *malwa* consumed. All fee money is passed to a designated member of the group who 'banks it'. 'Banking' may literally mean what it says; but, more usually, the fees are handed to the owner of the drinking place for safe-keeping. The accumulated funds of a group are used in various ways: to finance feasts on special occasions, such as a public holiday, when a goat may be slaughtered; for distribution among members in rotation on a weekly basis; to help a member at a time of personal hardship or crisis.

The formality of the groups varies, but it is usual for each to have an

---

[4] The drinkers sit together around a single large pot, sipping from it through long straws. Throughout the drinking session the millet brew is periodically warmed and diluted with hot water by the bar owner (sometimes also the brewer) or her assistant.

elected chairman. Some of the groups are made up of members of a single ethnic group, in which case conversations are usually in their own language. But groups are also quite commonly made up of friends with the same or similar occupations (and perhaps working at the same place), or of friendly neighbours/associates. For example, S is Chairman of his *malwa* group. He is Bateso, as are five other members out of a total of twelve. The others are Westerners. The common bond between them is that they all work as security guards somewhere on Mulago Hill. Some live in Kamwokya II, others not, and their meeting place is in one of the Mulago parishes on the borders of Kamwokya. Their subscription is Ush. 1,000 *per week*. They normally meet every evening on their way home from work, and the *malwa* often constitutes their evening meal. S says his wife tries to force him to eat anyway when he gets home; sometimes he does, sometimes not. As the group is multi-ethnic, they converse in English or Swahili or Luganda in that order, but mostly in English.

Apart from their daily drinking sessions, they have a 'formal' meeting to discuss finance every two weeks. If a member has a domestic problem, he is normally allowed to draw Ush. 5,000 from the group's funds, but this must be paid back. When he returns the money, the group 'drinks it'.

Malwa groups range in size from five to twenty members. Women also participate, it is said, but only on rare occasions does a woman actually drink with the men. It is unusual for women to become members in their own right, and the occasional woman seen drinking with an established group is more likely to be the wife/woman of one of the members.

Respectable women do drink *malwa* and other brews without their menfolk, but on the whole they are more likely to drink in their own homes or with friends and neighbours in small groups.

(vi) An RC Court Case
(illustrating one crucial aspect of the Resistance Council's function and the relationship between RC 1 and RC 2)

The defendant was a young man, David, referred to as Dandi during the proceedings, and the plaintiff was Songolo, a man in his forties or early fifties.

Around 100 people assembled round an open space under a tree. About 70 men and a few children were sitting in a semi-circle with two RC 2 officials sitting on chairs together with Songolo (see Figure 4.1). To their right sat the observer and his interpreter. Behind them there were about 30 women sitting in a quarter circle and in a less prominent position than the men (owing partly to the downward slope of the ground). The segregation between the men and the women was almost total, though one or two women were behind the rows of men, some sitting, some standing.

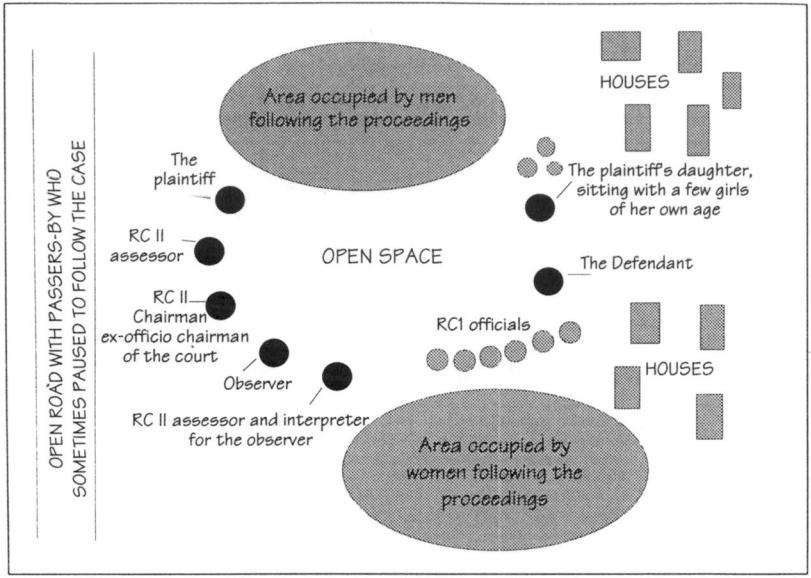

Figure 4.1 *Court case layout*

The proceedings were conducted in Luganda, though there were occasional sentences in English, mainly addressed to RC officials. The RC 2 chairman, Ssenoga, was chairman of the proceedings *ex officio*.

To begin, Ssenoga addressed Songolo (the plaintiff), asking him to state – or to continue stating – his complaint. It was that Dandi (the defendant) was luring his daughter away. They were always together and the daughter had recently been absent from home for ten days without Songolo knowing where she was. By implication they were having sex together. The daughter was still at school (17 years old) and he wanted the court to condemn Dandi and to rule that the couple should not see each other again.

Ssenoga explained about three times that he and the other RC 2 officials present were assessors only: it was for the half dozen RC 1 officials to decide whether there was a case to be answered. Songolo was in an angry mood and kept on interrupting until Ssenoga told him to keep quiet and called for evidence to be given. About 10 to 12 men and one woman spoke up, some more than once.

Some of the contributions took the form of evidence and others were comments on the case. No one could (or would) confirm that Dandi and the daughter were sexual partners. Several people said they had often been seen together. One young man said he had seen them together in a video club (laughter). Another said he had seen them in a certain house. 'What were they doing?' Ssenoga asked. 'Just standing', came the reply (more laughter). Songolo grew angrier and was again told to keep quiet. 'We just want the evidence', said Ssenoga in English and elaborated to the same effect in Luganda.

At one point, Ssenoga addressed Dandi who stood up and moved a few steps towards the centre of the open space. Dandi denied that he was interfering with the daughter, though he did not deny being friendly with her. Everyone present seemed to accept that Dandi and the girl were associates. Ssenoga explained yet again that it was for the RC I officials to decide whether there was a case to be answered. Songolo could see that things were going against him and again interrupted. One RC 2 official stood up and tried to explain once more that it was not an offence for Dandi and the daugher to be friends. Did anyone know anything more? Others spoke to the same effect, including the only woman to speak during the whole proceedings. She was also an RC official.

After what seemed like an hour, Ssenoga asked the RC I officials whether they wanted time to confer. But the RC I chairman said there was no need. They nodded to each other and simply said 'No case'. Songolo was furious. It had now become clear that the 'problem' was that Songolo and his daughter were at odds with each other. At no stage did the daughter say anything and she was virtually ignored by Ssenoga and the court as if she had nothing to do with the case. The general atmosphere was serious but undramatic. At one point a few children who joined the crowd were chased away by Ssenoga, who said this had nothing to do with children, and they scuttled away. At another point, Ssenoga rebuked another girl, about the age of Songolo's daughter and apparently a friend of hers, because she was moving about. 'You are *another* one who does not stay at home. You are always walking around. What for? You should stay at home and get on with your studies.'

Ssenoga summed up, stating that the court had found that there was no case and adding that Songolo could appeal against the ruling of the court. But, standing up again, he commented that the matter was serious even if there was no case to answer. The daughter was still at school and the country needed educated women for the future – to be nurses, and to serve the people. The daughter should not have left her parents' home for 10 days. Where had she been? etc. etc.

He then adopted the role of conciliator and counsellor and asked the daughter to come and sit beside him and her father. 'We want the father and the daughter to be reconciled', and turning towards Dandi, he said something like 'You keep out of this!' The daughter came forward but, as she approached Ssenoga, Songolo stood up and stormed out. There were a few giggles amid the confusion which had built up.

The daughter turned round to resume her original place, but Ssenoga told her to stay where she was, close to him. She sat down, and Ssenoga launched on a fairly long social/political exercise, saying that cases like this should never take place, that the RC authorities were working for peace and stability in the community, etc. etc. He advised the daughter to continue her studies and not to drop out, and he said that Dandi should realize that distracting her from her studies was wrong. He then brought the meeting to a close.

A clutch of RC officials then conferred in private about what to do next. Eventually arrangements were made for Songolo's daughter to stay with a female RC member for a few days. Songolo was to have a couple of days 'to cool down' before they talked to him again. At about this point Dandi came in; he seemed rather amused, but Ssenoga rounded on him. 'You are an RC official and you allow this to happen!' 'We should set an example to the people − it is our job to educate them not to give rise to court cases like this.' 'You must now leave that girl alone − give her up altogether'. Dandi protested meekly that he liked the girl. 'That does not matter', said Ssenoga. 'There are many other women and you must leave this one alone.'

(vii) Neighbouring

Like the parish as a whole, many of its zones are both ethnically mixed and economically diverse. This item focuses on the lives of women in one small neighbourhood[5] in order to show the interplay of ethnic and other diversities and the basis of support in times of general hardship or illness (see further Chapter 10).

Along its outer boundaries there are affluent families who live in permanent houses with good security and ready access to piped water. The heads of these households are civil servants or other workers who receive housing as part of their salary. There may also be office workers, landowners or other sub-elites living there. But the majority of residents live in the densely settled, unplanned 'slum' in the centre of the zone. Here there are no municipal facilities, only a very rudimentary sanitation service and open sewers that cross-cut the area like so many rivers.

People say 'everyone is equal in the slum', implying both that '*we*' share this poor environment, and that membership in the moral community which '*we*' represent is not limited by wealth or ethnic origin. This is not to say that the neighbourhood, *qua* moral community, is open to any old 'outsider', only that 'belonging' is achieved by behaviour, by acting with respect for local ideals.

Primary among these is *empisa* − an ideal combining neighbourliness and respectability. It is a measure applied to men as well as women. But because a woman's livelihood is likely to be narrowly confined to the immediate neighbourhood, she is caught in a double bind − good neighbourly relations are especially crucial for her and a good reputation is impossibly hard to sustain at close quarters. One woman says: *The most important thing for living in town is to co-operate with near neighbours. One must greet*

---

[5] The zone in question is Kifumbira I. This item is directly based on the fieldnotes of Jessica Ogden.

them in the mornings. and everyone must keep an eye on each other and help out if someone is in need. Provided you have been a good neighbour, if people do not see you all day, they will come and check on you. And if they then find that you are sick they will make you tea, clean your house and take care of you… We live so close together that if one suffers, the others will hear her moaning. They will come to your aid because they know you are a good neighbour and they will want to help you…

Greeting demonstrates good neighbourliness and affirms belonging to the moral community. By *not* greeting a woman shows that she rejects that community. Another woman complained that walking the short distance from home to shop and back could take an hour because she had to stop and greet everyone along the way. Behind this 'complaint', of course, is a boast about belonging.

Those who do not greet must be bad neighbours. They are suspect or troublesome, and they have no access to the resources that others depend on. When asked why a woman whose child is plainly malnourished gets no local support, her next-door neighbour says no one will help a person who makes quarrels and disturbs the peace. 'She is always accusing us of stealing her things. She is the one who steals. We just leave her alone'.

The tensions created by someone without *empisa* can stir up accusations of witchcraft. Curiously, in this setting it is the accuser not the accused who is ostracized as a bad neighbour. Only someone who is envious and isolated would deliberately cause a quarrel like this. Mama Beth says: '*A woman who never greets may see you stop for a moment outside her door. Then if her child happens to fall sick the next day, she can even accuse you of harming it by witchcraft*'…

The boundary statement is plain. There are two kinds of women: '*us*', the decent, morally upright people who greet and co-operate with their neighbours, and 'others' who look for quarrels and are jealous of everyone. 'They' stay in their houses and refuse even to greet those who live around. 'We', by contrast, avoid quarrels, greet properly and welcome visitors into our homes.

Five

Household Wellbeing
Ethnographic & Women's
Survey Responses

Here the focus changes from Kamwokya as a whole to households within it. The chapter draws substantially on responses to surveys carried out in the second phase of research in the area (see Chapter 1).

Initially, it was responses to an Ethnographic Survey question about health in the household which alerted us to the essential relevance to this study of the concept of wellbeing which appears as the subtitle of this book. The question was posed (in the English version of the ES questionnaire) in the form 'What is/are the major health problem(s) in your household?' with an invitation to the respondent, by the interviewer's agency, to 'write in' their answer − i.e. there were no pre-coded answer categories imposed. Table 5.1 shows that by far the most common responses given were 'illness' and 'lack of money', both as 'main' and 'second' problems respectively. The apparent illogic of these responses is explained by the fact that in Luganda it is not possible to distinguish between 'health' and 'wellbeing': the word bulamu *signifies either and/or both conditions. In effect, the problems listed in Tables 5.1a,b should be interpreted as threats or impediments to wellbeing in the household.*

The inference drawn from a later question 'The way you see it, what are the major illnesses/diseases in Kamwokya?' is quite different and very much more specific. The medical orientation of the answers (Tables 5.10a, b) may have been encouraged by pre-coding and closing the response options, but, more importantly, the Luganda word for illness and/or disease (endwadde) *is unambiguous − not the opposite of health/wellbeing because it is a concept of a different order.*

These distinctions have implications for the discussion and promotion of 'health', and our experience demonstrates that even semantic error − where respondents are given the chance to correct it − may provoke insights into local meanings which the research had not anticipated.

This chapter considers 'health' in the holistic sense of 'wellbeing', as it is

Household Wellbeing

Table 5.1a Main 'health' problems in the household

Problem	No.	%
Housing	65	8.95
Nutrition	61	8.40
Health care	3	0.41
Illness (specified)	185	25.48
Illness (unspecified)	34	4.68
Child care	2	0.28
Social environment	2	0.28
Physical environment	36	4.96
Crowding	2	0.28
Lack of money	237	32.64
Cost of living	8	1.10
Bachelorhood	3	0.41
Unemployment	3	0.41
Don't know	8	1.10
None	76	10.47
TOTAL	726	100.00

Table 5.1b Households that report a second problem

Problem	No.	%
Housing	3	1.58
Nutrition	8	4.21
Health care	1	0.53
Illness (specified)	15	7.89
Illness (unspecified)	9	4.74
Physical environment	27	14.21
Lack of money	102	53.68
Cost of living	13	6.84
Bachelorhood	2	1.05
Unemployment	8	4.21
Domestic relations	2	1.05
TOTAL	190	100.00

glossed in Luganda and related languages. Under the wellbeing rubric, it is appropriate to include evidence from the various surveys about women's skills and occupations, conditions of housing, hygiene, water and sanitation; and access to income, advice and support along with the health specifics of sickness, immunization, childbirth and the like. Each of these essentials to the household's wellbeing is itemized in the following paragraphs. The final section presents data from the various surveys which suggest affective or social involvement in the area. The sense of being 'at home' is an element of wellbeing, and the fact that belonging is for so many focused

91

on Kamwokya (rather than ethnicity or region of origin) is more evidence of its particular style as an urban system (see Chapter 2).

(i) Income Potential

The mean age of the 203 participants in the Women's Survey is 29. Table 5.2 shows that 75% of the women interviewed are married or co-habiting, compared with 15 per cent who are divorced/separated, and a mere 3 per cent who report being single/never married. Women identify their partners as husbands if they live together on a regular, even if not full-time, basis, and the man makes a financial contribution to the household and the family – in other words, he 'looks after her', 'takes care of her', 'they have a real family'. Women who co-habit with men who do not make such contributions tend to refer to them as *muganzi wangi* ('boyfriend'), as does a woman with a fairly serious partner who does not 'take care of her'. Women in this situation are less 'proper' and less 'well' than those with a husband (see Ogden, Chapter 10). The absence or loss of a serious male partner can be an important threat to economic wellbeing as well as to status and reputation. The discussion of the social penalties of STD infection (Chapter 9) and the individual women's stories (Chapter 10) illustrate this very sharply.

Table 5.2 *Marital status of women respondents participating in the women's survey*

Marital status	No.	%
Divorced/separated	31	15.3
Married/cohabiting	152	74.9
Never married	6	3.0
Widowed	14	6.8
TOTAL	203	100.00

In reality, of course, women's options for income are much wider, and much more independent of men than the local ideals imply. However small the amounts, the money is not insignificant. On this basis the range of *main occupations* is impressive (Table 5.3) – the more so when it is remembered that many are 'occupational pluralists' (Wadel, 1969) and only one occupation is reported here. Note also that for the majority, the main occupation is based within Kamwokya. The opportunity for generating income from a number of sources is enhanced by the concentration of economic activity in or near the home.

Still less visible, as potential sources of income, are skills which might be, or have already been, made marketable under appropriate circumstances. When asked about practical skills, everyone reported having at

Table 5.3 *Women's main occupations and where this work is based*

Occupation	Kamwokya		Elsewhere in Kampala		Elsewhere in Uganda		Total	
	No.	%	No.	%	No.	%	No.	%
Cultivator	1	0.6	0	0.0	1	33.3	2	1.0
Crafts	3	1.7	0	0.0	0		3	1.5
Porter	0	0.0	3	15.0	0		3	1.5
Market vendor	10	5.6	5	25.0	0		15	7.5
Shop keeper	10	5.6	2	10.0	0		12	6.0
Bar	5	2.8	0	0.0	0		5	2.5
Other trade	26	16.3	3	15.0	0		32	15.9
Teacher	3	1.7	0	0.0	1	33.3	4	2.0
Religious leader	1	0.6	0	0.0	0		1	0.5
Cook	2	1.1	0	0.0	0		2	1.0
Child care	1	0.6	0	0.0	0		1	0.5
Domestic	5	2.8	0	0.0	0		5	2.5
Office	0	0.0	4	20.0	0		4	2.0
Cleaner	0	0.0	1	5.0	0		1	0.5
Health practitioner	2	1.1	0	0.0	0		2	1.0
Home work	70	39.3	0	0.0	0		70	34.8
Brewery	18	10.1	2	10.0	1	33.3	21	10.4
Tailor	14	7.9	0	0.0	0		14	7.0
Hair dresser	3	1.7	0	0.0	0		3	1.5
Poultry farming	1	0.6	0	0.0	0		1	0.5
TOTAL	178	88.6	20	10.0	3	1.5	201	100

least one. Most women know how to knit (62 per cent) and make baskets (64 per cent). Sewing, hair-styling and brewing are the second most commonly reported skills, each claimed by around a quarter of the respondents. These were followed by baking (15 per cent), pottery (10 per cent), and being able to be a birth attendant (8 per cent). Almost 8 per cent (16 women) know a specific health practice. They define the nature of their practice as either herbalist or traditional birth attendant (TBA). Finally, of the Women's Survey respondents, two women know how to repair shoes, one woman knows about construction work, and another knows carpentry.

Activity in the area shows the extra inventiveness of some women. For example: *In Green Valley 'artificial charcoal' is drying out. Banana skins are first dried, then burnt and the ash mixed with dust or clay in water. Round lumps are then dried in the sun. They say it is not as good as charcoal but that poor people burn it on top of charcoal.*

Finally, there is in most households scope for selling products or possessions to meet the crisis expenditure needed to treat acute illness, or otherwise to secure or maintain wellbeing (Wallman and Baker, 1996).

It is difficult to quantify levels of income in this setting. In any case we know that money is only one of the essentials of wellbeing. The importance of networks, relationships, etc. is revealed in the discussion of support during illness (below) (see also Chapter 4). More formal social connections are demonstrated by membership of clubs, associations and groups. The Women's Survey sample are relatively little involved at this level. Only 16 women (8 per cent) report membership of a club, association or other group, and only one-third of these hold office in one or more of the groups to which they belong. Perhaps these organizations are peripheral to their central concern with the family's wellbeing.

Table 5.4 *Clubs and associations to which women belong stratified by whether or not they hold an office in them*

Name of club	No	Yes	Total
Akabondo ka Javira (Gyavirra)	3	0	3
Akabondo ka St. Kaggwa	1	0	1
Akabondo ka St. Mugaga	1	0	1
Catholic Women	0	1	1
Christian Church Choir	1	0	1
KWIDA	2	1	3
Mothers Union	1	0	1
Mulago Catholic Society	1	0	1
Society Twezimb	0	1	1
Tukolere Wamu Women's Club	0	1	1
VIWAU	1	0	1
Waddukirwa Group for Women	0	1	1
TOTAL	11	5	16

(ii) Conditions of housing, hygiene and sanitation

This section relates the study population to the 'facts' of the built environment as detailed in Chapter 2. On the evidence of the Ethnographic Survey (N = 726) the vast majority (86 per cent) of people in Kamwokya live in rented accommodation. Eighty-three people in the sample (11 per cent) own the house in which they live, under half of them with title and just over half without title. The remaining residents (3 per cent) 'live' in someone else's house – most often in Contafrica. Those renting accommodation are more common in Church Area, Kisenyi 2 and Central Zone; those owning their houses are most common in Market Area, Green Valley and Kifumbira 2. House rents vary according to the location and the condition of the building.

Some examples
For a 'good' house in the upper part of Kamwokya II, the rent would be about Ush. 200,000 per month, but only, they say, if there is security, i.e.

along the roads where security personnel move, and *if* the house has electricity and access to a stand pipe (few houses have internal water supplied), and *if* it is a 'good looking' house and self-contained. A 'similar' house in the middle of Kamwokya would cost about Ush. 120,000 per month and at the bottom of the valley about Ush. 80,000 per month. A simple room in a 'reasonably good house' in a good location would be about Ush. 30,000 per month; in the middle of Kamwokya Ush. 15,000 to 29,000, and down in the valley about Ush. 10,000 per month. A single room in a mud and wattle house in poor to average condition would be Ush. 20,000 to 25,000 in a good location in the upper part of Kamwokya II, Ush. 12,500 to 20,000 in middle Kamwokya and Ush. 5,000 to 10,000 down in the valley.[1]

Residents say that people live in the very poor parts of the parish only when they cannot get housing in less congested areas; and that the congestion is 'caused by' landowners eager to collect as much rent as possible. Given the variety of housing for rent, it is common for people to start in a poor dwelling and gradually to upgrade – or to hope to upgrade – their accommodation by moving elsewhere within Kamwokya. They rarely set out to leave the settlement altogether. Kamwokya, after all, is 'where the heart is' for most of its residents (Fig. 5.4 below).

With rental accommodation in demand, the enterprising householder is encouraged to reorganize or even to extend his dwelling to take in tenants. Mr T is a good, but not exceptional, example. *He has hired a man to make bricks for a room he is planning to build on to his house and is supervising his work. The bricks have been made from clay/soil dug on his own ground. They have been erected into a rough 'pyramid' about 10 to 12 ft high. Branches of wood are burning inside the 'pyramid' and there is smoke now emerging from the cracks. He says the bricks need about two weeks to dry out before being ready for use.*

Apart from the roof, door and windows, the room will be built entirely from clay/soil dug on his own plot. The man working for him is, he says, not an ordinary labourer, but a 'specialist' brick worker.

At the back of the same house two women and three or four children are clustered around a doorstep. They are tenants who pay a high rent, 'not kinsmen or anyone I knew before' he says, 'just people who were looking for accommodation'. They live in a section of his house with a separate entrance. One room only, it seems.

On the right-hand side of the house as you face it, there is a charcoal seller operating from a rough, poorly built shelter separate from the house. She does not pay rent, she just gives Mr T a bag of charcoal from time to time.

Housing

Table 5.5 shows that most dwellings are made of mud and wattle with an iron sheet roof. The second most common type of house is constructed with blocks or bricks and an iron sheet roof. The great majority of all

[1] The exchange rate for Uganda Shillings was 1,800 = £1 sterling at the start of the project in November 1992. The Ush. rose (as sterling fell against the dollar) in 1993 to 1500: £1 and has held steady around that level to date.

respondents report leaks or cracks in the house roof or the walls. Houses made of mud/wattle and houses with thatched roofs have significantly more leaks and cracks than other houses.

Table 5.5 *Distribution of houses according to the material they are made of*

Material of the house	No.	%
Block/brick-ironsheet roof	317	43.7
Block/brick-thatched roof	4	0.6
Block/brick-tiled roof	5	0.7
Mud, wattle-ironsheet roof	379	52.3
Mud, wattle-thatched roof	7	1.0
Other	13	1.8
TOTAL	725	100.00

The main sources of household lighting used in Kamwokya are electricity (42 per cent) and local lamps (39 per cent). Local lamps are made of tin cans burning paraffin, although some people use diesel. These lamps are known to carry a high risk of fire. They are used·significantly more in houses made of mud/wattle than in brick houses. However, when looking at differences by zone, electricity is the most common source in Market Area, Green Valley and Contafrica, and the local lamp is more commonly found in Church Area, Kisenyi 2 and Central Zone. Another source of lighting common in mud/wattle houses is the kerosene lamp or lantern (used by 18 per cent of households). The remaining households mainly use candles.

Most houses (73 per cent) consist of one room only, and 86 per cent of all households, including those with more than one room, use only one room for sleeping (see Table 5.6). As is shown in Table 5.7 for each zone separately, this has implications for crowding and is a proxy measure of poverty (CHDC, 1994) as well as wellbeing in the sense of health. 518 households (i.e. 71 per cent) have a separate bathroom.[2] The likelihood of having a separate bathroom does not vary with type of accommodation or zone.

By contrast, each type of latrine facility (Table 5.8) is characteristic of certain types of houses and of certain zones. Latrines for exclusive household use are more commonly found with brick houses than mud houses. Most people living in mud/wattle houses share a latrine with other households or report having no proper latrine facility. But it should be noted that four-fifth of households in Kamwokya as a whole share a latrine with other households and that, since comparative sample sizes are very small, it would be incautious to draw any zone-specific conclusions.

As the type of latrine facility has consequences for the health of the people, so do a number of other common items. The Ethnographic Survey

[2] 'Bathroom' refers to a screened ablution area, not to latrine facilities.

Table 5.6 *Number of rooms in house by number used for sleeping*

Rooms in house	1 No.	%	2 No.	%	3 No.	%	4 No.	%	5 No.	%	Total No.	%
					Rooms used for sleeping							
1	531	84.8	0	0.0	0	0.0	0	0.0	0	0.0	531	73.1
2	88	14.1	37	52.9	0	0.0	0	0.0	0	0.0	125	17.2
3	5	0.8	17	24.3	2	10.0	0	0.0	0	0.0	24	3.3
4	2	0.3	11	15.7	5	25.0	1	11.1	0	0.0	19	2.6
5	0	0.0	4	5.7	8	40.0	3	33.3	0	0.0	15	2.1
6	0	0.0	1	1.4	2	10.0	3	33.3	1	100	7	1.0
7	0	0.0	0	0.0	2	10.0	2	22.2	0	0.0	4	0.6
8	0	0.0	0	0.0	1	5.0	0	0.0	0	0.0	1	0.1
TOTAL	626	86.2	70	9.6	20	2.8	9	1.2	1	0.1	726	100

Table 5.7 *Mean household size, mean number of rooms per house, mean number of sleeping rooms per house and mean number of people per sleeping room (per zone)*

Zone	Mean H'hold size	Mean Rooms	Mean Sleeping rooms	Mean no. of people per sleeping room
Contafrica	5.1	2.0	1.4	3.9
Mawanda	4.1	1.5	1.2	3.4
Kifumbira 2	4.2	1.9	1.4	3.2
Central	4.1	1.4	1.2	3.7
Market	3.9	1.3	1.2	3.5
Green Valley	4.2	1.4	1.2	3.8
Kisenyi 2	3.9	1.4	1.1	3.1
Kisenyi 1	3.5	1.4	1.1	2.9
Church	3.2	1.2	1.1	2.9
TOTAL	4.0	1.5	1.6	3.3

Table 5.8 *Latrine facility*

Latrine facility	No.	%
Shared by community	3	0.4
For household use only	95	13.1
Shared with other houses	570	78.6
No proper facility	56	7.7
Other	I	0.1
TOTAL	725	100.0

Table 5.9 Number of households which had specified items in the house

Item	No.	%
Piece of Soap	658	90.6
Jerrycan	697	96.1
Dish Drying Rack	117	16.1
Mosquito Net	168	23.2
Food Cupboard	475	65.5
Container for Boiled water	610	84.1
Candle	676	93.2
Toothbrush	703	97.0

measured a few by asking if, at the time of interview, specific items were present in the house. The items are listed in Table 5.9 which shows the corresponding number of households that had them in the house.

Concerning the use of water, while Chapter 2 includes a description of the water infrastructure of Kamwokya, and Chapter 4 contains observations of the public activity around a particular spring, water and its collection are here put in the context of household wellbeing. The ethnographic survey showed the average number of jerry cans of water that a household collects per day to be just over three. This is an average of three-quarters of a jerry can – i.e. about 15 litres – per day per person. Half of the households draw some or all of their water from a private tap, 24 per cent some or all from a public tap, and 38 per cent some or all from an unprotected well or spring. In addition, 11 per cent of households buy some number of jerry cans of water from a water seller every day.

Most households not only use more than one type of water source, but have more than one way of obtaining water. Three-quarters get it from a place where they pay per jerrycan and 34 per cent collect it (also) from a free source. Almost 18 per cent have their water (or part of it) delivered, usually by a water seller but sometimes by relatives who live in other households, by neighbours or friends.

Most people who reported collecting water do so for their own household. There is a consistent age pattern in these different categories of collectors: household members may be adults or children, but 'other kin who bring water' are mostly children. Water collectors described as 'neighbours', 'friends' and 'water sellers' are largely in the adolescent age groups.

(iii) Illness and Disease

When asked what they considered to be the most common illnesses/diseases in Kamwokya (as opposed to in their own home) 83 per cent of respondents identified malaria and 71 per cent identified AIDS. This was followed by dysentery and diarrhoea (each mentioned by 31 per cent, pneumonia and flu (30 per cent), malnutrition (18 per cent), TB (15 per

Table 5.10a *Major illnesses/diseases in Kamwokya as reported by respondents (N = 726)*

Major health problems in Kamwokya	No. of respondents	%
Malaria	599	82.6
TB	107	14.8
AIDS	516	71.2
STD	18	2.5
Dysentry & Diarrhoea	227	31.3
Cold	224	30.9
Malnutrition	126	17.4
Chest complaints	92	12.7
Other	89	12.3

Table 5.10b *Other major illnesses/diseases in Kamwokya as reported by respondents (N = 120)*

Other major health problems in Kamwokya	No.	%
Not specified	34	28.3
Accidents	1	0.8
Alcoholism	1	0.8
Anaemia	1	0.8
Asthma & diabetes	1	0.8
Asthma	2	1.7
Boils	1	0.8
Children noise	1	0.8
Cholera	1	0.8
Cholera & measles	1	0.8
Drunkards	1	0.8
False Teeth (Ch. 8)	1	0.8
Herpes zoster	2	1.7
High blood pressure	5	4.2
Headache	11	9.1
Hygiene	2	1.7
Kinsimbye (Ch. 5)	1	0.8
Lameness	1	0.8
Leg pain	1	0.8
Measles	28	23.3
Meningitis	5	4.1
Miscarriages	1	0.8
Poverty	1	0.8
Pregnancies	1	0.8
Stomach complaint	1	0.8
Stomach pain	2	1.7
Abdominal pain	1	0.8
Syphilis	1	0.8
Typhoid/measles	1	0.8
Ulcers	3	2.5
Vomiting	6	5.0
Witchcraft	1	0.8
TOTAL	120	100

cent), chest complaints (13 per cent) and STD (3 per cent). 120 respondents also identified 'other' illnesses (Tables 5.10a, b). With responses combined, three-quarters of the respondent in Kamwokya report AIDS and STDs as major health problems, but it is only a tiny minority of them who mention the general category STD as a 'major' or an 'additional' problem . Rather unexpectedly, identifying AIDS as a major health problem was associated with duration of residence in Kamwokya: people who had been there longer perceived AIDS as a major problem more often than did recent arrivals. AIDS was also more likely to be cited by households which had lost a family member in the past two years than by households which had experienced no deaths during this period. The identification of AIDS as a major health problem was statistically independent of age, sex, educational level, ethnic affiliation, illness in the household during the previous two weeks, place identified as 'home', place of birth, mobility, and religion. Reporting STD as a major health problem is similarly independent of all the above variables except age: people who report STD as a major health problem are either young adults (20–29 years old) or over 50 years of age. Finally, there was no association between reporting AIDS and reporting STDs as a major health problem. It may be that there is a tendency to conflate other STD with HIV infection and AIDS, although other explanations are suggested in Chapter 8.

The significance of *other diseases*, however, does vary across Kamwokya. Malaria is significantly more often perceived as a major health problem in Church Area, Mawanda Road, Green Valley, Kisenyi 1 and Kisenyi 2. Dysentery and diarrhoea are most often identified in Mawanda Road, Green Valley, Kisenyi 1 and Kisenyi 2. Most of the 18 per cent who identify malnutrition as a major health problem live in Mawanda Road and Kisenyi 1. Pneumonia and flu are mostly reported by people in Green Valley and in Kisenyi 1. Finally, chest complaints are reported relatively more often in Market Area, Green Valley and Central Zone.

Chronic illness in the household is more often reported in Central and Church zones. Church Zone also has relatively more households with members who have a physical or mental disability. The same is true for Kisenyi 2 and Kifumbira 2. Illness that required treatment costing money in the two weeks before the survey was more often reported in Kisenyi 1, Contafrica and Kifumbira 2.

Concerning *mortality*, 160 of the 726 respondents in the sample had experienced death within their household during the previous two years. 69 per cent of these households had had one death, 20 per cent two deaths, 7 per cent three, and the remainder had lost between 4 and 6 people in the household. Together, they numbered 229 deaths. Fifty-five per cent of the people who had died were male and 43 per cent female. The sex of the remaining 2 per cent was unknown because the reported death was prenatal (i.e. caused by spontaneous abortion).

Table 5.11 gives the full list of reported causes of death stratified by sex and age of the deceased. It should be stressed that 'cause of death'

Table 5.11 *Mean age at death by reported cause of death (N = 229)*[a]

Reported cause of death	Female No.	Female Mean age	Male No.	Male Mean age
Measles	10	1.5	9	2.1
Malaria	21	13.2	34	18.8
Toothbuds	1	2.0	2	0.04
Headache	6	22.5	3	50.7
Chest pain	1	25.0	2	57.5
AIDS	23	25.9	29	27.1
TB	2	14.5	7	33.8
Cancer	2	47.5	4	40.8
Heart failure	3	43.0	1	34.0
Blood pressure	3	42.7	1	67.0
Sickle Cell	0	–	2	22.5
Drowned	0	–	1	21.0
Motor accident	0	–	6	24.0
Witchcraft	3	40.3	2	34.0
Asthma	0	–	1	1.0
Old age	1	103.0	2	64.5
Meningitis	4	16.5	6	22.0
Pneumonia	1	0.03	2	16.5
Poison	0	–	1	66.0
Snake bite	0	–	1	25.0
After operation	1	35.0	1	28.0
Drug poisoning	0	–	2	18.5
Abnormal head	0	–	1	0.01
Dehydration	1	0.01	1	3.0
Typhoid	2	14.0	1	85.0
Affected liver	0	–	1	7.0
Diabetes	1	80.0	1	29.0
After childbirth	4	20.8	0	–
Long illness	2	42.5	0	–
Natural cause	2	0.01	0	–
After immunization	1	0.09	0	–
Don't know	1	35.0	5	11.0

a) Data on 4 abortions missing

refers to what the respondent said, not to a medical diagnosis. On this evidence, the major *perceived* causes of death in both sexes are AIDS (23 per cent), malaria (23 per cent), measles (8 per cent) and meningitis (4 per cent). The fact that men travel out of Kamwokya more often than women may have a bearing on the disproportionate number of them that have died by road accidents and drowning. Otherwise, apart from indications that men are more likely to die of malaria and women of 'headache', there are no unexpected differences between causes of death reported for men and women.

The age distribution shows that measles and dehydration are major killers of infants and children, while AIDS is the major cause of death in young adults. Malaria and meningitis hit both children and young adults.

Deaths in the previous two years were significantly more common in households where there are now children without their own parents (Fig 5.3). The major causes of death reported in these households are AIDS and malaria. Defined as the number of reported deaths divided by the number of people in the survey population of each area, mortality was higher in some zones of the parish than others. Again it should be emphasized that sample sizes for each sub-parish (RC 1) in the ethnographic survey are extremely small and may not be a reliable indicator of patterns in those areas or in the parish as whole.

The next section covers health and illness in more detail. (A still finer focus on paediatric crises and STD is given in Chapters 8 and 9.) It is compiled from responses to the Women's Survey. Because the 203 women interviewed for it had also been respondents in the Ethnographic Survey, each is by selection head of her own household, or the senior wife of a head of household. These are therefore women of authority in their homes.

Women's illnesses

All respondents were asked questions about their most recent episode of illness. Well over a quarter of them (56) claimed never to have been sick, underlining norms which require women to 'keep going as long as they can walk' (Bantebya-Kyomuhendo, 1994: Chapter 10). Amongst those who had 'ever' been sick, the largest number (67) had had their most recent illness episode during the week of the interview, 22 had been ill in the previous week, 14 others three to four weeks before the interview, and 44 had been ill more than a month prior to the interview.

The most common symptoms were fever, headache, cough, abdominal pain and 'flu' (reported in the category 'other'). Amongst the 147 who reported having been sick, 19 did not seek treatment for their last illness. For 13 of them, the main reason for not seeking treatment was lack of money. Three women did not consider treatment necessary, one said she would get better anyway, and one said she was not allowed to go for treatment. Whether or not treatment was sought/given was apparently independent of socio-economic status (no behavioural difference was found in different educational, occupational, marital and age groups) and of the timing of the last illness.

By contrast, the type of person providing treatment did vary with the educational level of the respondent. Those who were more educated were more likely to report going to the doctor or the hospital, while those with less formal education tended to go to a nurse, or to shops and pharmacies. In all these respects the survey data match the case study and discussion findings in later chapters.

The decision to seek treatment was for most respondents their own. This was true for 81 of 147. For 10 women it was a decision taken jointly with the husband, and one took it together with a neighbour; 34 women say that their husband took the decision. For one woman, the decision to seek treatment was taken by her father, and one other reported that it was made by a relative other than her parents, husband, or children. Whose decision it was to seek treatment was independent of the kind of symptom present.

The most common treatments received were tablets (94 per cent) and/or injections (36 per cent). Nobody said they used herbs, surgery, or massage. Eleven women had used liquid medicine, one used powder, one prayed, and one had a tooth extraction. Injections were administered more often as treatment for fever than for other symptoms. They were reported given in hospitals and clinics. Tablets and other treatments were not specific to any symptoms. Tablets were taken both at home and in hospitals/clinics.

Concerning the place where treatment was received, four-fifths of the women who reported any past illness said that they had gone to a hospital or a clinic for their most recent episode. Another 17 per cent had treatment at home, three women went to a private practice and one received treatment at the church. Satisfaction with the treatment for the last illness was high (86 per cent). However, not everybody was cured: 88 people recovered completely, 34 improved but were not cured, 3 did not notice any change and one did not know what the result of the treatment was.

Children's illness is examined at length in Chapter 8; comparisons of action taken by women for their own illnesses and for those of their children are made also in Chapter 10. According to WS responses, in the two weeks prior to the survey, a total of 183 children of the 203 respondents were said to have been sick, 107 of them (58 per cent) boys, and 79 (42 per cent) girls. Ages were similar for both groups. The average age of the child reported sick was 2 years and 3 months.

The most common children's symptoms were fever (67 per cent), cough (62 per cent), diarrhoea (16 per cent) and vomiting (10 per cent). One child had 'false teeth' (see Jitta, Chapter 8), another had worms, one felt dizzy, three children had a headache, four children had general weakness and five had abdominal pain. Eight children had skin-rash, and flu was also commonly reported (21 children).

Twenty children had not been given treatment, the most common reason given being lack of money (true for 70 per cent). In four cases, the mother did not consider treatment necessary; one child was considered too young for any kind of treatment, and in one instance, the woman was not allowed to seek treatment. In two-thirds of those cases where treatment was sought for the child, it was the respondent herself who decided to provide it. In most of the rest (32 per cent), the child's father had made the decision. Decisions for treatment of the remaining three children were taken by other household members, in one case by the respondent's mother.

As in the case of the respondent's own illness, most reported that their children were treated by a modern doctor (57 per cent), or a nurse (24 per cent). Fifteen per cent were treated by the pharmacist, one was treated by the TBA, two received treatment from a friend of the respondent. and four children were treated by the respondent herself. Treatment was most often said to be provided at the hospital or a clinic (true for 83 per cent). The next most common place was the child's home (15 per cent). The rest were treated at a private practice. Tablets, injections and liquid medicine were the most common treatments (respectively given to 72, 50 and 46 per cent of the sick children). Injections and tablets were given especially for fever, and liquid medicine for cough.

At the time of the Women's Survey, more than half of the children who had been sick in the previous two weeks had recovered from their illness, and about a third had improved but were not yet better. In 7 per cent there was said to be no change, and three children had got worse.

(iv) Immunization of Children

In relation to questions about the immunization status of their children, the 203 respondents reported a total of 201 children. This must be a gross underrepresentation of children under five years of age since the same respondents reported a total of 302 children under five years of age in another context (i.e. in the ethnographic survey). Again, it may be that a survey associated with government health services (i.e. the Child Health Development Centre at Mulago Hospital) left respondents embarrassed to admit to their children not being immunized. Whatever the explanation, when asked to do so by the interviewer, respondents were able to show an immunization card for only 189 children. But of these, 52 children (27 per cent) had not yet completed their course of immunization, and for more than half of them, the main reason given for incomplete immunization was that the child had not yet attained the appropriate age. The second most common reason (given in 15 per cent of the cases) was illness of the child. Nine per cent of the women said they had simply postponed immunization. In addition, two women were confused about its contra-indications; one said she was too busy; another believed that the right vaccine was not available; and one reported 'family problems' as the main obstacle to completing the child's immunization.

(v) Fertility and Childbirth

Respondents were asked what they considered the ideal number of children, first for urban and then for rural areas. The average ideal number reported for urban settings is four children (a figure given by 66 per cent of the women); for rural areas, the ideal is six children (given by 45 per cent). In both urban and rural areas, the ideal family was further specified as consisting of an equal number of boys and girls. The tendency to report an ideal family size of four children in urban settings was common across different socio-demographic groups, but the ideal given for rural settings was associated with the respondent's educational level: the higher the educational level, the smaller the family size.

Regarding pregnancy, 200 of the 203 respondents had ever been pregnant.[3] Their mean age at first pregnancy was 17 years, with better educated women having slightly higher ages at first pregnancy. The average age at last pregnancy was 26 years and this was not associated with educational level. The average number of pregnancies was 4.5 and of live births 4.1. Table 5.12 gives age-specific fertility rates (i.e., the number of live births per woman). While the number of children born is related to age, it is not associated with educational level. Considering that education is positively associated with age at first pregnancy but not with age at last pregnancy, it appears that better educated women space their children closer together. The number of children that women have is similar for all marital and occupational groups. Mortality amongst children is reflected by the average number of children still alive, which is 3.5 – that is, against an average of 4 live births per respondent.

Table 5.12 *Age-specific fertility rates*

Age group	Sample size (total = 200)	Mean No. of live births
14–19	10	1.2
20–29	117	3.1
30–39	49	5.4
40–49	18	7.8
50+	6	6.5

Twenty-eight per cent (56) of the women in the sample had experienced miscarriage. Of these, two-thirds had had one miscarriage, a quarter had had two miscarriages, and four women had had three miscarriages. The number of miscarriages was not related to the total number of pregnancies. Eight women had had still-births: amongst them, two had had two still-births, one woman four still-births, and the remainder one.

The great majority of women (93 per cent) reported having obtained ante-natal care during their last pregnancy; 82 per cent said they received ante-natal care at a clinic or a hospital, while the remainder had such care at home. At the delivery, close to two thirds of the women were assisted by a nurse-midwife, 14 per cent by a modern doctor, and slightly fewer (13 per cent) by a TBA. Four women had been assisted by a friend, two by their mothers-in-law, and five by other relatives. One woman was also assisted by her own mother. Seven per cent were alone when they gave birth.

While 82 per cent had had their last baby in either a clinic or a hospital, 18 per cent of women had given birth in their own or a relative's home. Not surprisingly (given the place of delivery), the majority of the women

[3] Respondents for the Women's Survey were selected on the grounds that each had at least one child under five years at home. The three who said they had 'never been pregnant' are assumed to be caring for children born of someone else.

were assisted during birth by a modern doctor or nurse. However, 13 per cent reported having been assisted by a traditional birth attendant. Given that TBAs are legally banned from hospitals in Uganda, it is striking that so many of the women who said they were assisted by a TBA also reported having had their child in hospital.

Concerning help during the first month after the latest delivery, 39 women (20 per cent) said that they did not receive any help from anyone. The rest were more or less specific about the helper. Most often specified was the husband (by 28 women), the sister-in law (by 19 women), or a friend (by 16 women). Eight women were helped by their mothers-in-law. But the greatest number (66) said they got help from another relative (unspecified). In addition, five women were helped by a TBA, one by a doctor, and five by a nurse.

(vi) Support and Advice During Illness

About two-thirds of the total (133 women) have relatives whom they can go to for help or support in times of illness. These relatives most often live in Kamwokya (34 per cent) or elsewhere in Kampala (33 per cent). Only 11 respondents go to relatives who live in their own or their husband's home area outside Kampala. The remaining 33 (25 per cent) can resort to relatives who live elsewhere in Uganda.

More specific details about family support during illness were asked in reference to the last time the respondent was ill. On that occasion, the majority of those who reported that they could go to a relative went to their mother (40 per cent) or sister (25 per cent). But 37 respondents who sought help from a relative during their last illness went to more than one. Seven women received no help from the relatives they had approached. Where help was provided, respondents were asked to indicate the type or types of help they were given. In decreasing order most women (73 per cent) asked for and were given economic help (cash or kind), 22 per cent were given practical assistance and 19 received emotional support. As regards the combination of types of help, 7 women reported getting both economic and emotional help, 9 women received both practical and economic help, and 4 women obtained all three types of assistance.

In the matter of giving rather than receiving help, 31 of the 133 respondents who said they could go to relatives in times of illness did not provide help to those relatives when they in turn fell sick. On the other hand, 139 respondents did report assisting some of their relatives in times of illness: 102 of them reciprocated in more or less equal exchange, while the other 37 who reported helping their relatives did not approach them in turn for help. Amongst respondents who help their relatives, 81 per cent provide economic help, 30 per cent provide practical assistance and 11 per cent give emotional support.

Seventy-six women (37 per cent) can approach people other than relatives in times of illness: two-thirds of them identify Kamwokya as the place where these people live, and a quarter go to people who live elsewhere in Kampala. One respondent (who comes from outside Kampala) has such a person in her home area, and the people who give support to the remaining six respondents (8 per cent) live elsewhere in Uganda.

Table 5.13 gives the frequency of respondents seeking advice or help for illness from a number of health services and support groups. It shows that the modern health sector is the most commonly reported source for advice or other help in times of illness, and the indigenous health system is reportedly used less often. This 'modern' preference may, again, represent an idealized view of what *should* happen – or what respondents think the Survey sponsors want to hear (see further Chapters 6, 8 and 9). In any case, all types of support or treatment source as well as religious organizations are frequented by some treatment seekers 'occasionally', and

Table 5.13 *Percentage of respondents using specified health services/places/people during illness for treatment (N = 203)*

Place/person	Never	Occasionally	Regularly
Hospital	3.4	55.2	41.4
Clinic	5.9	75.7	18.3
Diviner	95.0	5.0	0.0
Herbalist	74.3	25.2	0.5
Saved spiritual healer	62.9	32.7	4.5
Community health worker	72.8	25.7	1.5
TBA	79.2	18.8	2.0
Market/shop	39.6	33.2	27.2
Pharmacy/drug store	7.4	80.2	11.9
Religious leader	67.3	29.2	3.5
'Kabondo'	82.6	11.9	5.5

by many more according to the treatment providers quoted in Chapter 6.

The reported preference for modern health services is also apparent from answers to questions about where respondents would advise people to go for help or what to do to treat specific diseases or illness. The modern health sector (hospital, doctor, clinic, blood test, quinine) is most commonly recommended for children with high fever, persistent high fever, cough, persistent cough or convulsions, and for adults, both male and female, with a sexually transmitted disease (STD) (but see Chapters 7 and 9). The hospital is also most often recommended for treatment of bone fractures, although nearly as many recommended the traditional bone-setter. For the problem of infertility in women, while most respondents say they do not know a place or person to recommend for treatment, 24 per cent say that one should go to a clinic doctor. Thirteen per cent recommend infertility treatment at the hospital, and a significant number would advise the sufferer to accept the situation, to pray, or to visit a traditional healer.

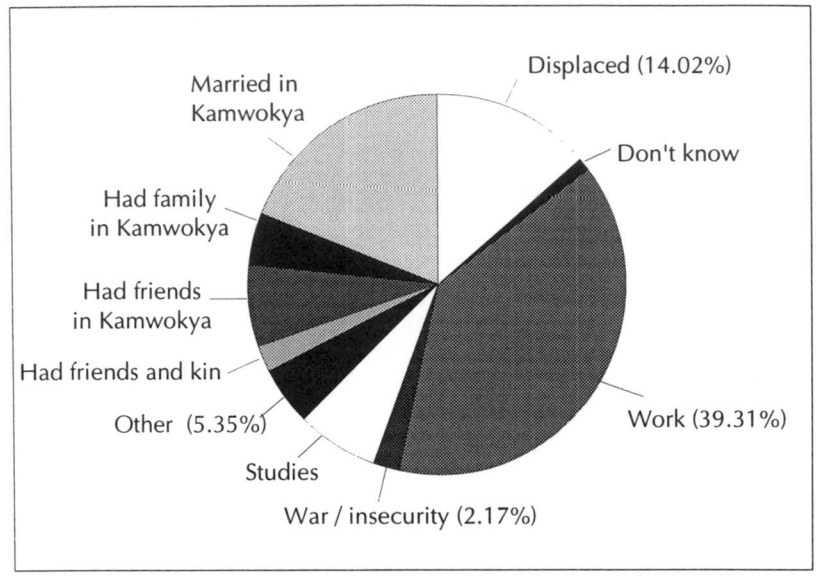

Figure 5.1 *Reasons for coming to Kamwokya*

Nevertheless, while traditional and alternative treatment options do not top the list as the most commonly reported places to go to, they are all recommended by significant numbers of respondents. Worth noting is the range of advice given for women who have an STD, and for women whose partners have an STD. Women with STDs are mostly advised to seek treatment in the modern health sector. If that fails, a small proportion would recommend them to take traditional herbs, but more than a quarter (55 women) say they would not know what to advise next. However, a woman whose partner has an STD is advised by many to go for modern treatment but also or alternatively to insist on separate beds. Ten respondents (5 per cent) would advise divorce (see further Chapter 9).

(vii) Feeling Good about Kamwokya

Survey evidence for feeling good about Kamwokya – or about the household's situation in Kamwokya – can only be inferential, but even to identify items which may affect attitudes to the place is to say something about wellbeing in it. We would do better if we knew more of the past circumstances and future aspirations of respondents: Does living in Kamwokya represent an improvement or a disappointment? Is it a sign of success or of failure? The majority are quite recent migrants: What (not where) did they come from? (cf. Wallman, 1977: 13, 14).

It helps that we know *why* they came. Figures 5.1 and 5.2 show ES

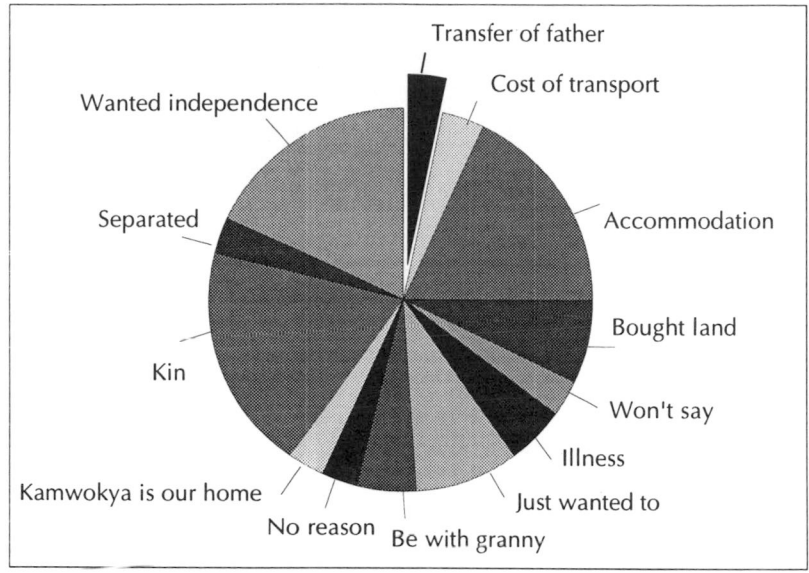

Figure 5.2 *Other reasons for coming to Kamwokya*

responses to that question and suggest that most had hopeful if not positive motivations: only '*war / insecurity*' and '*displaced*' sound wholly negative, but even in these cases the respondent may intend to imply relief that he/she is now in Kamwokya and away from the turmoil of another place or a previous time.

Similarly, it is our assumption that a household's position on the typology shown in Figure 5.3 is relevant to its sense of wellbeing in Kamwokya — and the same caveat about interpretation applies. Only those in the lower right-hand quartile ('Both parents in household') are optimally 'well'; households without children (37 per cent) or without parents (9 per cent) almost certainly feel less good about their situation and (probably) about their general wellbeing in Kamwokya. Again, we do not know if things have got better for them or worse, for whom '*no children*' means barrenness or abandonment and for how many it is an entrepreneurial strategy. Is '*no parents*' the result of AIDS or the normal lifecycle?

The final figure (5.4) is less complicated. It needs only to be juxtaposed to the one showing Home Area in Chapter 2 (Figure 2.3) for its point to be made. Residents being trained as interviewers encouraged us to ask the question '*Which is the place where your heart is?*' on the grounds that this proxy for 'Home' exists in Luganda as it does in English and that answers would say something about people's attitudes to where they live. Apparently more than half of those born elsewhere — all in-migrants of shorter or longer standing — feel at home in Kamwokya. The sense of belonging implied is another dimension of wellbeing.

109

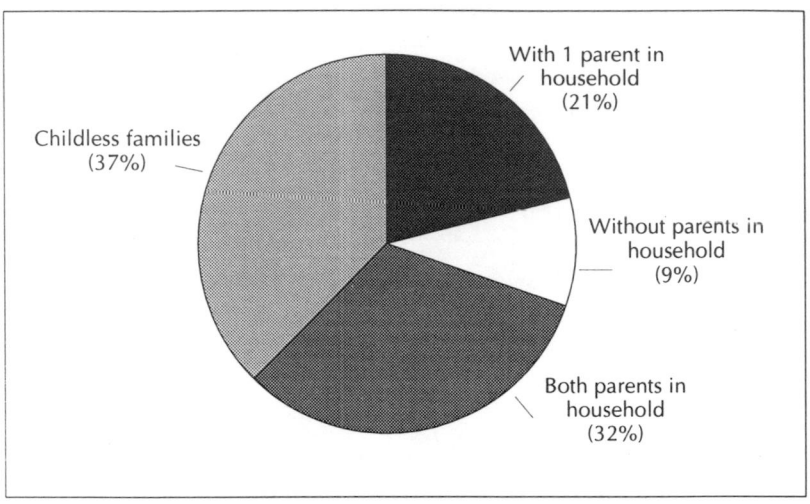

Figure 5.3 *Household types: status of children in relation to parents*

Inevitably questions of feeling are subject to interpretation and not suited to empirical survey. The strategy in this section has been to impute more than empirical meaning to questions of fact. In the context of other layers of data about Kamwokya becoming progressively more qualitative as the book proceeds, the inferences drawn here are substantiated.

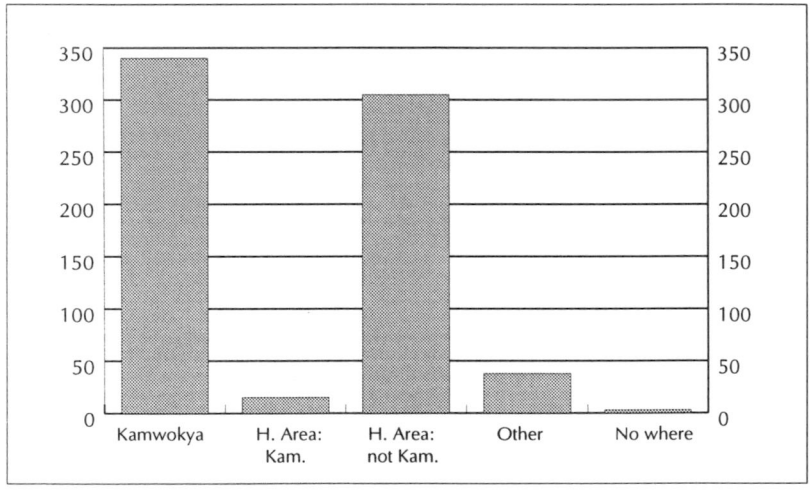

Figure 5.4 *'Where the heart is'.*
Data from Ethnographic Survey 1993

Six

▽▽▽▽▽▽▽▽▽▽▽▽▽▽▽▽▽

Treatment Options

The four sections making up this chapter together represent the scope of treatments recognized by residents of Kamwokya. It will be clear that only a very small proportion of them fall within the scope of conventional, officially sanctioned biomedical practice. The importance of what we are calling the 'informal economy' of disease management is therefore made plain. We have emphasized the need to take these usually unenumerated options into account when seeking to improve, even just to understand, health-care delivery in a setting of this kind.

The first section sets out the approaches most commonly applied to accounts of treatment selection — arguments based respectively on theories of modernization, economic development and homophily. References to a wider literature than we have been able to review here are, of course, provided.

The second section reports the methods, procedures and results of the Treatment Sources Survey carried out in Kamwokya in the second (surveys) phase of the overall project.

The third section under the title 'observations of the Visible Health Units' gives observers' accounts of people coming and going in advertised clinics, drug shops and the like. By means of listening to open transactions and talking to those involved in getting or giving treatment, the observers (all of them non-medical, by contrast to the researchers in Chapters 8 and 9), found it possible also to note the specifics of which medicines were obtained for what symptoms, and with what economic implications.

Finally, the fourth section presents interviews with ten traditional healers — some 'pure' herbalists, others combining the use of herbs with psychological or spiritual treatments of one sort or another. In contrast to those in the third section, the traditional healers might be described as 'invisible' since their places of work are not normally signposted, some are consulted only indirectly, and all of them get new patients/clients by word of mouth.

Degrees of secrecy in their practice vary, but it is important that reputation in every case is achieved by past performance, and that all of them are legitimated by being embedded in and recognized by the community in which they work. These healers are

Treatment Options

a very important source of primary health care in Kamwokya; some expressed a particular eagerness to have their methods or remedies 'tested' – and hopefully ratified by – the bio-medical institutions. In Uganda, given the scarcity of 'formal' treatment resources and personnel, there is increasing official willingness to involve them in primary health care.

Theoretical Perspectives

The approaches from medical anthropology concerned with treatment selection can be condensed into three main categories: modernization theories, economy-based theories and homophily theory.

Early etic approaches to understanding the relationship between Western biomedicine and African indigenous healing systems were put forward by colonial anthropologists. These models focused on the cognitive *differences* between Europeans and Africans as being central to differences in aetiologies of illness (see e.g. Levi-Bruhl in Horton, 1973). In contrast to this view were those approaches noting the resemblances between African and Western (cosmopolitan) disease aetiologies (e.g. Gluckman, 1982). They argue that the form of 'rational thinking' depends on cultural context, or on the social environment. An adjunct to this paradigm stressed the possible complementarity of Western scientific and indigenous theories: African healers can answer the *why?* of illness causation, Western science the *how?* (e.g. Marwick, 1982). This approach is taken a step further by those who argue that the 'extra-biological' explanation provided by indigenous therapy is integral to the healing of the whole patient (Eisenberg, 1977).

(i) Modernization
These explanations all argue that therapeutic choice is based on the aetiological convictions of the patient. Recent theorists have noted that these concepts of disease may be to some degree a function of formal education, people with higher levels of formal (Western-type) education tending to believe in natural causes of illness and those with lower education in supernatural causes (Nanchengwa, 1984). Therapeutic choice, however, remains pluralistic. Irrespective of beliefs about causation, people tend to utilize 'modern' health services but would also consult traditional healers when the former fail to bring them relief (cf. Kalumba, 1982; Nyamwaya, 1992).

(ii) Economic approach
Approaches based on concepts of rationality consider views of illness and health to be the products of a social and economic environment. Health-care utilization and decisions are constrained, according to this model, by economic options. The 'rationality' involved here is not aetiological (as above) but economic, essentially disregarding cultural and conceptual explanations of disease. This paradigm stresses the importance of financial and resource constraints in the choice of health-care options.

A middle view recognizes that the patient's environment embraces cultural as well as economic factors. Changes of either sort may precipitate shifts in choice of health care, but aetiologies remain essentially intact. The actual choice of therapy is necessarily governed by economic and geographic possibility, but is part of the social process of everyday life. It is, in short, the interaction between the social environment and disease aetiology that shapes the process of treatment choice (Janzen, 1978).

(iii) Homophily

The third perspective adds homophily ('the degree to which pairs of individuals are similar in certain attributes, such as beliefs, values, education, social status and like') to the list of factors affecting treatment choice (Rogers and Shoemaker, 1971: 210; Jonker 1988: 21). This emic approach considers the rationality of patient behaviour to be based on a combination of aetiological conviction and social values. In this view the importance of social/cultural values can outweigh monetary costs, and the choice of health practitioner depends upon the degree of homophily between the patient or treatment seeker and the treatment options available (cf. Sargent, 1982).

There is still no satisfactory framework to integrate shifting disease aetiologies and convictions, economic factors, social structure and the personal environment of the patient in a single explanation. But it is clear from a range of evidence that indigenous African therapeutic systems continue to co-exist with Western biomedical practice throughout the continent, despite the fact that Western medicine enjoys considerably more legitimacy, public support, funding and status. These systems, themselves not undifferentiated, are complementary, and seem to correspond to the illness categories held by people in both urban and rural areas.

The two systems are used simultaneously or sequentially by most Ugandans, and 'traditional medicine' exists alongside the modern system as it is said to do in all African countries. Observers do make the point that patient flow and reverse flow between the parallel systems constitute a much neglected and highly complex process about which more information and sound theory are needed . One essential basis, both for the categorization of disease and for the treatment sought as a result, is the distinction made between 'African' diseases, those that are culturally based, and 'European' diseases, that are pathogenetically derived. Although an individual may pursue a spectrum of options, the treatment sought (resources permitting) will correspond, at least initially, with the way the sickness has been classified.

These details of interpretation aside, it is important to underscore two general points: i) African cities are, by any measure, 'viable and vigorous' arenas of traditional medicine; and (ii) traditional medical practitioners are among the largest categories of self-employed persons in the informal urban economy.

People seeking treatment anywhere like to choose among a range of options and/but can only take up options which are there. Amongst these options in Kampala is a plethora of different categories of 'healer' – some legitimate, others charlatan. Before proceeding to report the findings of the Treatment Sources Survey (TSS) carried out in Kamwokya II, it may be noted that the WHO definition of *legitimacy* matches the popular Kampala version very closely. Both have confidence in a traditional healer who is recognized as such by local people and can be trusted to the extent that he or she is embedded in networks of local relations.[1]

Treatment Sources Survey, Kamwokya II (1993)[2]

The Treatment Sources Survey (TSS) was designed to achieve a general understanding of the number, range and operations of all treatment sources in Kamwokya. It also served to identify persons and places appropriate to the case and the situation study phases which followed (see the following sections below. See also Chapters 7–9).

Our original list of treatment sources was derived from the early mapping and Broad Brush Survey (BBS) exercises. At that stage it included only those that were plainly advertised or otherwise visible to passers-by (see next section). The list was gradually extended, first by residents working as interviewers on the Ethnographic Survey (ES), each of whom produced a list of all the treatment sources they knew in and around the parish, and then by follow-up in the field – most fruitfully during the course of the TSS itself. Two local residents, one woman and one man, were selected out of the ES group and hired to conduct the interviews. They used a short, largely open-ended questionnaire, in English or Luganda, depending on the preference of each respondent, and every interview was afterwards 'debriefed' by one of the researchers.

The local treatment sources are of two types: the formal biomedical (clinics and drug shops) and the informal/traditional (herbalists and diviners). But too rigid a formal/informal distinction is misleading because the traditional system is, in many cases, highly formalized, and the 'formal' relies heavily on informal networks. Mulago doctors, for example, regularly refer patients to their own private clinics for further treatment. The drug shops are especially ambiguous: they are used primarily for home treatment, they tend to sell antibiotics for which they are not always licensed, and the manner in which the drugs are obtained regularly involves some kind of informal networking between Mulago Hospital and the community.

Nonetheless, all the formal biomedical treatment sources in Kamwokya could be classed in one of the two main categories: the clinics and the

---

[1] This point is central in any operational definition. Mbiti (1969: 166) identifies a traditional healer as: 'a person recognised by the community in which they live as being competent to provide health. They (may) use vegetable, animal or mineral substances, and other methods based on social, cultural and religious background (prevalent in the community) to treat physical, mental and social ills.' See also Nyamwaya (1992).

[2] The input of Catherine Barasa, Makerere Department of Sociology, was invaluable throughout the Treatment Sources Survey.

drug shops. All of the clinics in Kamwokya are privately owned and provide services for cash. Often the owners and primary providers of the clinics are doctors, medical assistants, clinical officers or nurses who also work at Mulago Hospital. The clinics provide an important income-generating function for those government employees who cannot get by on what they are paid for their work in the formal sector (Obbo, 1991). The drug shops are also privately owned and are stocked with both prescription and non-prescription drugs. They fall under different licensing classifications, but some, as indicated above, sell drugs for which they are not licenced. Those in our sample were largely run by certified nurses and midwives. Often, however, an assistant is hired to work at the counter. These assistants may be untrained (even uneducated) young people who nevertheless dispense drugs to customers. Some drug shops also provide consultations – which is to say that they offer advice about treatment – but for this service no fee seems to be charged.

The fieldworkers identified 31 clinics and drug shops in Kamwokya and interviewed all but four (two clinics and two drug shops). Most interviews were conducted in English.

The distinction between 'herbalists' and 'diviners' is also problematic. Both tend to use herbal medicines as a part of the treatment. The 'herbalists', however, define themselves as strictly pharmacological, using only *materia medica* in the treatment process, whereas 'diviners' rely additionally on spiritual/supernatural resources when seeking to diagnose the *why?* or the *how?* of an ailment, and not simply the *what?* – i.e. where they consider the ultimate cause of an illness to be some spoiling of the relationships between the patient and his/her ancestor spirits, or between the patient and others who may be wishing him/her harm (Nyamwaya, 1993; see further section four).

The fieldworkers identified 12 diviners and 12 herbalists in Kamwokya. They interviewed all but three of the diviners and all but 5 of the herbalists.

We were surprised by the difficulties encountered with the people identified as 'herbalists'. Intuition had led us to expect more trouble in encouraging the 'diviners' to participate. Also surprising were the responses of the herbalists to the symptom list presented to them (see Table 6.4). They did not, overall, claim to treat the symptoms presented in the list; at least half of them responded 'never treat' to every symptom listed (including the commonest crisis symptoms in children: fever, cough and diarrhoea, which the other categories treated either regularly or occasionally without exception).

It may be that the problem is one of language. Only half of the herbalists in the sample had any formal education. All the 'diviners' on the other hand, had been educated at least through to Primary 3 (half of the sample went through to Primary 6). A second possibility is that the herbalists identify *causes* rather than symptoms, *per se*, and so may not recognize 'symptoms' as being what they treat. A third possibility is that most mothers will treat these common complaints at home, seeking treatment outside only if the symptoms worsen (become 'serious enough') (see Chs 7–10).

Many women already know herbal treatments for these complaints and use the herbs or obtain the medicines from drug shops independently. If the symptoms persist they may take the child to a clinic, hospital or diviner, depending on their perception of the cause of the illness and its seriousness. Lastly, it may be that the herbalists did not respond as expected because of some fear that the project was suspicious or disapproving of their work. There is still a general feeling that outsiders think of herbal medicine as 'backward' and 'un-Christian', and this may have contributed to under-reporting, even among those who agreed to be interviewed. It is anyway clear that, in addition to the 'visible' herbalists identified for the TSS, there are more secretive others who have no practice as such, but who do grow and sell or give away herbs.

One such person recorded in one researcher's fieldwork is an old woman living alone in Kifumbira 1:

She is childless and after her husband's death his other children drove her out of his house. She now sells charcoal and grows medicinal herbs around her house. She insisted that she is not a doctor but that if people come to her and ask if they can pick some of her herbs she will let them do so. She does not charge them (because, she says, she is a Christian). When I expressed an interest she went out and collected four specimens, each with a different curative effect:

a) one used by women who have given birth to twins.

b) a strong-smelling herb used by people who are being 'chased' by ancestral spirits. If you stuff the herb into your nostrils it will force the spirits that are bothering you to tell you clearly what it is they want you to do, or what they want done by the clan.

c) a succulent used by Banyankole women to wash their genitals with when they smell. I asked if the smell or the treatment was associated with STDs and they said no.

d) another succulent used by pregnant women who ache and are uncomfortable. They squeeze the juice from the leaves and rub it on their bodies.

The old woman said people were afraid to come to her place to buy charcoal and that her business was not doing well. I wonder if the community thinks there is more to her growing of herbs than meets the eye, or than she is willing to discuss...

Unlike the diviners who seem to inherit the gift of healing, the herbalists have mostly learned it from their grandparents or other elders. Some are even now teaching the skills to their grandchildren.

In the event, data from 14 clinics, 13 drug shops, 9 diviners and 6 herbalists were analysed. The main points are shown in Tables 6.1–6.4 and are discussed, with other findings, in the following sections; Personal Characteristics; Therapeutic Situation; Forms of Payment; and Symptoms Treated. Under each heading observations on providers in 'traditional' and 'modern' sectors are sub-divided.

Personal characteristics of the treatment providers

(I) HERBALISTS AND DIVINERS

A number of interesting differences between these two categories of 'traditional' health provider emerged from the data.

The herbalists were on average older than the diviners. All were over the age of 35, the ages ranging up to 75 with an average age of 50. The diviners' ages ranged from 28 to 70 with an average age of 39. Almost all the herbalists were women (only one man in the sample), whereas the diviners were almost evenly divided, with a slightly greater number of men (six men and five women). Two-thirds of the herbalists were single. The 'diviners', on the other hand, were more likely to be married; only one-third of these practitioners were single. All the diviners, but only two-thirds of the herbalists, reported that they had children.

There were some notable differences in ethnic affiliation. The majority of the diviners were Baganda, with one Musoga and one Munyoro. Only two of the herbalists were Baganda; three were Banyankole and one a

Table 6.1 *Characteristics of health providers of Kamwokya*

	Clinic (n=14)		Drug shop (n=13)		Diviners (n=9)		Herbalists (n=6)	
	No.	%	No.	%	No.	%	No.	%
Sex: M	1	7	2	15	5	56	1	14
F	13	93	11	85	4	44	5	86
Age – range	22–45		17–64		28–70		35–75	
Mean Age	32.2±7.1		33.5±13.2		38.5		49.6	
Residence – Kamwokya	10	71	11	85	9	100	6	100
Outside Kamwokya	4	33	2	15				
Health Care as Main Occupation	13	93	11	85	9	100	2	29
Years of Practice					8 –?63 av.19		10–40 av. 25	
Specialization			5	38	8	89	4	57

Table 6.2 *Clientele attending different treatment sources*

	Clinic		Drug shop		Diviners		Herbalists	
	No.	%	No.	%	No.	%	No.	%
Residence Kamwokya	3	21	7	54	9	100	7	100
Outside Kamwokya	11	79	6	46				
Patient range (per week)	10–210		8–200		4–30		0–10	
'Seasonal' patients	13	93	7	54	9	100	4	57

Joluo from Kenya. Religious affiliation also differed slightly. The majority of the diviners were Muslim and one-third Christian (two Protestant and one Catholic). There was only one Muslim herbalist, the others being Christian (two Protestant, two 'Saved', and one Catholic).

All the diviners had some formal education; five had attended school up to Primary Six, and one had Senior One education. By contrast, two of the herbalists had no formal education, one was schooled in catechism, one had Primary 5 and two Primary 6 level. All the respondents in both categories were resident in Kamwokya. The herbalists had been living there longer on average, but this may be due to the fact that as a group they were older.

Both the herbalists and the diviners had been practising medicine for years – the herbalists for an average of 25 years (range: 10–40) and the diviners an average of 19 years (range: 8–63). Only one-third of the herbalists interviewed said that health care was their main occupation. One woman who treats 'false teeth' (see Chapter 8) actually had to be interviewed at her market stall where she works every day from dawn until late into the evening. By contrast, all but one of the diviners said that health care was their main occupation.

(II) CLINICS AND DRUG SHOPS

The personal characteristics of these 'modern' categories are more difficult to assess. Often the respondent was simply the only person free at the time the interviewer called, and not, therefore, the primary provider at the facility. As noted above, the person attending the drug shop counter was often an unskilled assistant. The owner of the shop was not always available (many of them are nurses or doctors with practices at Mulago or other hospitals). Similar conditions pertain at the clinics; the doctors themselves were not available in most cases. All personal data obtained therefore refer to *the respondent* who may or may not have been the primary provider in a given facility.

Most respondents were women (one male respondent among the clinics, two at the drug shops). The ages of the clinic respondents ranged from 22 to 45. The drug shop respondents ranged from 17 to 64 years of age.

The ethnic affiliation varied a great deal. Among the clinic workers, however, there was a preponderance of Basoga people – almost half the sample. The other dominant group was the Baganda. Among the drug shop respondents there was greater variation, the only clusters being among the Baganda and the Banyankole. Religious affiliation was similarly varied.

Five of the clinic respondents had certificates in midwifery and two were certified nurses. The remaining respondents had either Senior 3 or 4 education, and one had been to university. Among the drug shop attendants, 8 had formal health-care training and one is currently a medical student at Mulago/Makerere University. Of the remaining four respondents, one had Primary 6 education, two had Senior 4, and one Senior 3.

All but two of the drug shop respondents and all but four of the clinic

118

respondents live in Kamwokya. 13 of the 14 clinic respondents and 11 of the 13 drug shop attendants stated that health care was their main occupation.

Therapeutic situation

(I) HERBALISTS AND DIVINERS

The herbalists reported seeing very few patients per week. Although one reported seeing ten, the others either did not know (1), saw two patients (2), or 'sometimes none' (1). By contrast, the diviners' answers ranged from 4–5 to 30 (two were uncertain). Most herbalists and all diviners said numbers vary with the time of year.

The majority of the healers in both categories treat primarily from their homes, or in a combination of places. One respondent from each category could treat patients 'anywhere'. None of the herbalists and only one of the diviners had a place for patients to stay overnight.

All the herbalists reported that they allow people other than the patient to sit in during consultation and treatment. The diviners generally do not.

(II) CLINICS AND DRUG SHOPS

All but two of the clinic respondents had regular assistants. The drug shops were more evenly divided in this regard; 7 had assistants and 6 did not. The majority of both the clinics and the drug shops had only one assistant.

None of the clinics reported allowing people other than the patient to sit in during consultation. Four of the drug shops allowed this. The question of allowing others to sit in during treatment is again difficult, especially where drug shops are concerned, since the 'treatment' involved is usually simple dispensing. Interestingly, however, four of the drug shop

Table 6.3 *Facilities reported*

Facilities	Clinic (n=14)		Drug shop (n=13)		Diviners (n=9)		Herbalists (n=6)	
	No.	%	No.	%	No.	%	No.	%
Treatment at healer's home	–	–	–	–	6	(67)	5	(71)
Instruments[a]	–	–	–	–	5	(56)	2	(29)
Assistants	12	(86)	7	(54)	–	–	–	–
No assistants[b]	2	(14)	6	(45)	9	(100)	6	(100)
Credit	13	(93)	10	(76)	9	(100)	4	(57)
Cash payments advance	3	(21)	9	(69)	3	(33)		
After treatment	6	(43)	1	(8)				
Set fees	1	(8)	–	–	–	–	–	–
Barter	–	–	–	–	9	(100)	1	(14.2)

Notes: a) Instruments used by the healers included: razor blades, 'spirits', and a holy book (the Koran).
b) Traditional healers had no assistants. They could have been unnecessary as the client load was low. The effect is that skills which might be acquired are not being passed on.

respondents said that they did not allow others to be present. Only three of the clinics permitted this. One of the clinic respondents added the proviso that if there was a language barrier between the provider and the patient, a close relative would be present in order to translate.

Payment

(I) HERBALISTS AND DIVINERS

All but one of the herbalists insist on payment in cash; the exception provides her services free. The diviners also prefer cash payments, but *all* sometimes accept non-money payment. Likewise two-thirds of the herbalists and all the diviners sometimes extend credit. All herbalists/ diviners were unwilling to discuss how much they charge. A consultation fee or its equivalent (*ekikubansiko*) was mandatory and ranged from Ush.200 to 500. Payment procedures for services differed amongst the healers, from payment in advance, payment in kind, payment in instalments to non-payment. Reasons for non-payment included default by patients and the providers' moral attitude of not asking for payment.

They pay in instalments, some pay all, some do not give any money. I do not charge them for treatment because I was shown these herbs by my grandfather and some spirits.

The herbalists had higher starting fees, but generally charged less at the upper end. Generally the diviners had wider ranges of payment, and one reported that fees were negotiable. Both herbalists and diviners sometimes add on extra fees here and there which can increase the overall cost to the patient. These extras (for example a white hen or goat, or some food) were probably not included in any estimates given.

(II) CLINICS AND DRUG SHOPS

These providers are unanimous in accepting only cash payment. Most respondents, however, conceded that credit will be given in emergency cases and/or when the patient is known to them. One clinic respondent said that in the event of a client being unable to pay cash, he would accept non-cash payment to be held as collateral until the patient was able to pay him whatever balance there might have been.

Symptoms treated

Finally, Table 6.4 shows the numbers in each category who reported regularly or occasionally treating the symptoms listed. It is important that the various providers are unlikely to share a single symptomatology: differences in the way signs and symptoms are classified cast doubt on the value of too literal a comparison between clinics and drug shops on the one hand, and herbalists and diviners on the other. We have already noted the apparent reluctance of those identifying as 'herbalists' to admit to treating common and quite ordinary symptoms – cough, diarrhoea, fever, headache – in which many are known to be expert. And the clinician specifically concerned with STD treatment in Kamwokya (Chapter 9)

Table 6.4 *Numbers treating listed symptoms regularly and/or occasionally*

Symptoms	Treatment sources			
	clinics n = 12	drug shops n = 12	diviners n = 9	herbalists n = 6
In children <5				
cough	12	12	9	3
fever	12	12	8	2
convulsions	9	4	9	3
measles	9	4	6	3
diarrhoea	11	12	6	1
depressed fontanelle	6	1	0	2
false teeth	1	0	3	2
AIDS	3	0	1	0
skin rash	9	11	6	2
In adults				
fever	11	12	6	2
getting thin	6	4	4	0
diarrhoea	11	12	7	2
bad sleep	7	4	5	0
cough	11	12	8	3
love problems	4	1	9	0
headache	11	12	8	3
AIDS	3	0	1	0
stomach ulcers	11	11	2	0
pulesa (pressure)	9	7	3	0
diabetes	1	2	0	0
broken bones	1	0	3	3
skin rashes	10	11	6	2
syphilis	10	8	7	2
gonorrhoea	10	5	4	0
swelling of glands	7	4	3	1
genital ulcers	8	3	5	2
other STD: candida,trich, UTI	3	–	–	–
emambega (genital itching)			6	–
other general:worms	1	–	–	–
kinsimbye (pneumonia)		–	–	1
In men only				
impotence	2	1	8	2
men-only STD	3	0	3	2
other: *ekiwungwe* (breathlessness)	1	–	–	
In women only				
pregnancy	5	0	8	3
delivery	2	0	4	1
heat in womb (*ekigalanga*)	3	1	8	3
infertility	1	0	5	0
uterine shape/size	0	0	3	0
anaemia	9	10	7	3
enseke (tubal pregnancy)	7	4	6	2
women-only STD	3	0	3	2
other: weak uterus	–	1	–	–
amakiro (pre-eclampsia)		–	1	–

observes that diagnosis of a particular disease is not invariably based on the same combination of signs, not even by the same category of treatment provider.

General differences between 'modern' and 'traditional' providers show where all, or nearly all, of one category, and none, or nearly none, of another say they ever treat a particular complaint; *stomach ulcers* are a case in point (Table 6.4). More provocative, however – and perhaps medically more important – is the likelihood that the same symptoms are treated quite differently by the various types of practitioner because each ascribes a differently by cause or kind of cause to the disease they represent. Given the possible range of disease aetiology applied by the four TSS categories, the assumption should not be made that, for example, *getting thin* is one symptom, one ailment across the board.

The following sections throw some light on the problem by focusing on various of the treatment sources in action, and later chapters provide a context for the processes by which women, faced with symptoms of one sort of another, come to choose among the treatment options offered.

Observations of the 'Visible' Health Units

The health units identified during the initial mapping exercise by the BBS represent those among the total eventually studied which are obvious to an outsider – either by being clearly signposted, or by showing products through an open door. Of the 29 indicated, 17 were classified on first sight as clinics, 8 as drug stores (selling drugs and medicines but not making these up on the premises), 2 as pharmacies (making up prescriptions as well as selling either prepared or patent medicines), and 2 as traditional healers' premises.

But both the total and the classification were later discovered to be inaccurate. Firstly, later field-work revealed the many health units which had not been identified because there was no external evidence that they provided any type of health service. Secondly, the observers later concluded that the only self-styled pharmacy in Kamwokya II was in effect a drug store according to the official definition, i.e. it did not make up prescriptions. Thirdly, the observers reported that they had not identified any resident herb-sellers, but had seen itinerant herb-sellers from other areas visiting Kamwokya II (selling herbs mixed with clay, known locally as *emmbwa*, especially for pregnant women). The notes refer only to sources of treatment visible to the outsider – first the clinics, then some of the drug shops. Less visible, not to say secret sources of treatment are described in the sections on Traditional Healers (the following section) and Home Treatment (in Chapter 7).

Clinics
According to the advertisements and signposts seen, the clinics varied

appreciably in the services they offered. Out of the total of 17, 13 were advertised as general clinics, 10 as offering laboratory services, 3 as dental clinics, 2 as paediatric clinics, 2 as maternity clinics, and one as having X-ray facilities. All appeared to be larger than the drug stores and had at least two rooms, one always serving as a waiting room. On closer observation, however, some of the 'clinics' appeared to have few patients requesting clinical services or attention and the observers concluded that some were little more than drug stores.

The following more detailed observations made outside four clinics (two in Kamwokya II and two in Kamwokya I) give an indication of differences between clinics within the two wards.

(a) *'Kamwokya General Clinic'* is situated in the Market Area of Kamwokya and faces on to Kira Road. It forms part of a row of shops and advertises itself as 'a general clinic and dental surgery'.

This clinic was observed from outside from the time it opened at 10.00 a.m. on a week-day until it closed after dark in the evening. During the whole of this period there were only two or three visitors who appeared to be 'patients' as distinct from 'customers'. For example, a young girl who seemed unwell was escorted to the clinic by an adult woman. They spent some time in the clinic and the observers assumed that the girl had received some form of medical attention. Throughout the rest of the day, people calling at the clinic normally left after a few minutes carrying a variety of bottles, tubes or containers. Many were served on the verandah without even entering the building, and there was no evidence of anyone attending for dental surgery.

The observers estimated that the clinic had approximately 75 customers during the whole day: 39 (52 per cent) were women, 21 (28 per cent) were men and 15 (20 per cent) children. One of the observers reported her conclusions as follows:

Kamwokya General Clinic seems more of a drug store than a clinic because almost all clients stood outside and were served with drugs on request, which implies that they came for some specific drug or with very minor complaints which could be catered for without any examination.

(b) *'Silent Clinic'* is situated in Kamwokya II on the outskirts of the market zone and in a slightly less commercial area than Kamwokya General Clinic. It consists of two rooms — a laboratory/consulting room-and a waiting room which form part of a three-room building. The third room is a shop which we have called 'a unique shop' because of its character as a social gathering place with free television and video services. Other buildings in the immediate vicinity of Silent Clinic are mainly residential houses. The clinic offers laboratory and general services and has one male and one female attendant. Their white coats gave the impression that they were medically trained.

At 2.10 p.m. we saw two patients waiting inside after having had blood samples taken. About 30 minutes later the male attendant came out of the laboratory room to hand papers to the female attendant who then gave both patients drugs to take away. At 3.30 p.m. two boys came and bought drugs and left immediately... Approaching 4.00 p.m. a man who looked weak and ill arrived and was taken straight to the inner room. He stayed some time and we think he was given an injection... About 4.30 p.m. a boy aged around 17 years came to the clinic accompanied by an elderly man. The boy was dressed in a towel. He walked with difficulty and was clearly in a lot of pain. He was immediately met by the male attendant and taken inside. He stayed some time and we think he had a wound dressed. Perhaps he had (previously) been circumcized. There were no more visits by people who appeared to be patients, but a number came to buy drugs. Throughout the afternoon there were few patients, but it may be that there were more during the morning. The clinic was still open when we left at 7.00 p.m.

(c) *The Family Doctor's Clinic* and the *Kololo Polyclinic.* Both of these are situated in a block of 12 purpose-built commercial premises in the Kisementi area of Kamwokya 1 – i.e. on the upper side of Kira Road, and outside the area of this study. There is a general merchandise store between them and a pharmacy next door to the Family Doctor's Clinic. The Polyclinic advertises X-ray, laboratory and physiotherapy services. From the outside there is no indication of services offered at the Family Doctor's Clinic. Our observers thought there might be a connection between the two clinics, but had no firm evidence of this. There is good road access to the block of premises and ample parking space.

Two observers were asked to record comings and goings at the two clinics and the pharmacy for a whole morning, but the pharmacy was closed throughout their time of observation and for several days after it.

The Family Doctor's Clinic was opened at 8.25 a.m. by a woman who arrived by car and the Polyclinic at 9.20 a.m. by another woman who also arrived by car. The first visit to the former was by a woman with a baby at 8.30 a.m. and to the latter by 'an older school boy' at 10.00 a.m. From then on, there were regular visitors to both clinics. By 1.00 p.m. there had been 14 visits to the Family Doctor's Clinic and 21 to the Polyclinic. There were only a few cases of people who went in and came out quickly. Many visitors stayed inside for an hour or more. The overall average length of visit was 40 to 45 minutes.

There were appreciable differences between the two clinics in the composition of their visitors. Nine of 21 visits to the Polyclinic were paid by individuals on their own, and only 4 of the 21 involved children. In contrast to this, only one of 14 visits paid to the Family Doctor's Clinic was by a single person, and 12 involved a child or children accompanied by one or more adults. These figures suggest that the two clinics have different functions.

The observers had no way of knowing where the visitors came from, but they noted that 18 of the 35 visits to the two clinics were by people who arrived by car – often good quality vehicles (BMWs, Pajeros, etc.) and/or 'official' cars or pick-ups bearing the identities of Government

Departments or non-governmental organizations. They also noted that all the visitors were 'well-dressed' and 'looking smart' from which they concluded that the clientele was 'mainly medium or high class'.

These few observations underline the stark contrast between the clientele of health units in Kamwokya I and Kamwokya II. The clinics in Kamwokya I are within easy walking distance of Kamwokya II, but in the light of this admittedly limited evidence it seems that few, if any, of the visitors came from Kamwokya II.

Drug shops

In contrast to the clinics, many of the drug stores show no name and no advertisements; they can be identified by drugs and medicines visible through windows and open doors. Some appeared to be operated by 'medical personnel' (wearing white), others not. And, even when 'medical personnel' were apparently in charge, the stores were commonly left for long periods with junior shop assistants to serve customers. Most of the drug stores do not offer 'clinical services', but some were seen to give clinical attention or advice. (See further Chapter 7.)

JUKIRA NSUBUGA NA BAANA DRUG SHOP

This is situated at the roadside and in a noisy environment; outside it, there is a market where a variety of foodstuffs are sold, e.g. tomatoes, fish, cassava chips, sweet potatoes, etc. Licences are seen hanging inside. There is a variety of drugs, but the largest quantity are locally made ones. The shop is well painted and generally clean. It has two rooms, the front one is a drug shop and behind there is a bedroom. It has a papyrus ceiling. When the observer reached there, the owner began cleaning some containers and the shelves in order to remove dust.

I reached there at 11.50 a.m. and at 12.45 p.m. a woman came with Ush. 100 and asked for tumboack (stomach ache pills) (1 pair). She looked sickly and poor. Also the man who came at 12.50 p.m. with a prescription on a piece of paper showing expen (penicillin for injection). He was given it ... Another man came to ask whether they inject and the attendant told him that they do not. Looked better-off according to the way he was dressed. He went away, but later came back to ask for medicine for backache and was given panadol and aspirin, but was advised to go to see the doctor. He was charged Ush. 550. He went to eat food outside the clinic (i.e. in the market) ... (1.25 p.m.) A third man came for bandaging, but was told that they don't do it. The man asked for drugs, but was advised to go to the clinic to see a doctor. He bounced back later and asked for chlorophenical or ampicilin, but it was not there. He insisted on being bandaged, but the attendant told him to buy a plaster, since it heals wounds, but the man refused and went away. He did not even have any prescriptions from the doctor... At 2.00p.m. a man came looking for Camaquin and he was told to pay Ush.350 for a dose, and he bought some for 700/-. He was advised to buy panadol or aspirin to take with the drug, and he bought some for 200/-, each tablet costing 20/-.

Treatment Options

This is located near the road and many taxis pass, and cause a lot of dust. The drug shop is attended by a nurse of around 30 years of age, and the owner is a woman who works in town. The shop has a variety of drugs which are locally made, and some are imported. It is not a well-stocked drug shop and is in an old building, with a papyrus ceiling. Outside it is noisy because there is a video centre directly opposite, with many people. There is also a drain with dirty water which smells badly.

The nurse said that the owner buys drugs from any cheap pharmacy in Kampala, since she is after making a profit. She reported that they are licensed, but not to sell antibiotics. Nevertheless, according to the observation made, these are sold on request.

When asked whether she treated STD, she said that she did, but added that this was a rare case. She said that people rarely admit this, but she can tell because some of them come looking for a specific drug and a few others come with prescriptions. Others are frank with her and come complaining and she gives them treatment.

A man brought Ush. 200 and asked for tablets for flu. A woman came with prescriptions, and the nurse asked her who wanted the medicines and the woman said that they were for an old person. The nurse asked whether the patient suffered from blood pressure, and she said this was so. The woman said yes the old person understood because when they brought him drugs, he refused to take them thinking they would make him mad, and that he was supposed to take drugs for two months. The nurse advised her that if they could not raise the money at once, she should keep on buying until the dose was completed. For example, one type of drug cost 6,000/- but the woman brought only 500/-. She was given folic acid for anaemic people and aldomet for blood pressure... A woman came with a child and brought 2,000/-. It seems she had received treatment on credit before, and now the baby was OK. She looked like a working woman. Another came looking for tablets for nausea. The nurse explained that there are certain drugs they do not sell because of the expiry date since not many people ask for them... A man came looking for ceptrin, but the nurse did not give it to him. She said that he was a drunkard and disturbed people and he even wanted free treatment. Another woman came asking for advice regarding the drugs she had got from the hospital, i.e. frygyl, tetracyclin for stomach pain. Her child was also sick, with diarrhoea and malaria. The nurse gave her chloroquin. She looked a low-class person... Another man brought 100/- and the nurse gave him ventolin. She said that he was a daily customer. He looked a working-class person... A lame girl came with a prescription for 32 tablets. Each tablet cost 50/- so when she asked how much and the nurse said 1,650/- the girl went away without the medicine. A woman came looking for advice about a hoarse voice, and she was given strepsils for 300/-. She said that her 6-month-old daughter was also sick (cough). As it was a dry one, the nurse gave her cough linctus for the cough... Another woman came looking for modium capsules, but they were not in the shop. A woman sent a young boy who said things which the nurse could not understand. The nurse sent him back and the woman came and said that she wanted septrin and took 200/- worth. She wanted more on credit, but the nurse refused because she was not sure of getting the money. A young girl also came with 500/-. She had been sent by her mother who had malaria. She wanted septrin and the nurse gave it to her.

P AND N DRUGSHOP

The person selling is around 28 years of age and she is the owner of the drug shop. She also works in Mulago Hospital. Her drug shop is separated by shelves from a curtained-off room, but she does not sleep there. She is a licensed person and she gets her drugs from town. Her drug shop is well arranged and neat, and she sells locally made drugs and imported ones. She receives all classes of people, i.e. working people and other low-class people.

Two men came at 6.25 p.m. looking for deep heat, which costs Ush. 3,500. They said that it was expensive, so the nurse suggested the alternative of salimia which is relatively cheap and serves the same purpose, but they went away without buying... A woman came with a child and brought 100/-; she had previously bought panadol on credit and had come to pay... A young girl also came looking for panadol for 100/-, each tablet costing 25/-. The nurse asked her who wanted it, and she said that it was for an old person. She was asked the sickness but she didn't know... A man came with a young girl looking for chlorophenical and when asked for what sickness, he said that it was typhoid. He had bought some drugs but they were not enough. He was buying them for an adult aged 17. When the nurse asked for a prescription, he said that he had left it at home... Another man came complaining of nasal discharge, but said that he just felt it, it did not come out. He also had a slight headache, but he did not know why, so he was asking for advice. He also complained of jaw pain, but had no tooth problems. The nurse said that maybe he was going to develop mumps, so she advised him to take pain killers like panadol or aspirin, but the man said that he wasn't sure that these would heal him. He said that his problem had been chronic since Primary 6 and he used to take chloroquin, but he no longer wanted to because it made him itch. He asked the nurse whether she could give him a substitute, so she said that she would give him phenobarb. The man said that the itching lasted four days, so he was advised to take camaquin and the nurse gave it to him. She advised him to take it with aspirin and the man said that he had some at home. He had brought photographs for the nurse so he did not pay any money. It was just an exchange.

PATIENCE DRUG SHOP

This is located in Contafrica Zone but it is not registered. It is in a slum area, near the dirt road. The owner is a nurse who had been working in Kadi and Sons drug shop in the same zone. She was later mistreated and suspected of stealing money. She had to leave her position and decided to set up on her own. The shop is in a filthy place and the general environment is bad. The observer noticed a terrible smell from the surroundings because nearby there was a dustbin where people pile up rubbish; the shop is also near a path so it is exposed to dust, especially when a vehicle passes. It consists of two rooms, the back one being the owner's bedroom and the front one the drug shop.

The clinic is not well-stocked and it is not arranged neatly. She normally gets her drugs on credit from a certain pharmacy in Kampala city because when she explained her problem to them, they agreed. After selling she takes them their money.

A boy came looking for ampicillin but it was not there, and when the nurse asked him, he said that he was buying it for somebody else... At 4.05 p.m. a girl who was also accompanied by five children came for magnesium. When she was asked who wanted it, she said that it was for an old person and she had only 50/- and each tablet cost 20/-. The nurse said that she knew the person who wanted it because she had been coming to her for treatment. The patient had been advised to take magnesium whenever she felt uncomfortable... A second man came for Aspro at 6.06 p.m. but he did not say what he was suffering from.

On the whole the drug shop has few customers. The owner said that she is aiming at survival. What she earns is for her children's food.

SEMAKULA AND BROS. DRUG SHOP

This has two rooms, the drug shop being in front. Still in the drug shop, a small section is separated off by a curtain. On one side of it there is a bed and on the other a sewing machine which the attendant uses for making clothes, since she is also a tailor. Behind is a bedroom because a bed was seen, also chairs, plus a sideboard. The attendant cooks there on a coil. The shop is in a slum area near the dirt road and is therefore exposed to dust. There are many children around. The general appearance is not good. It has a papyrus ceiling and there are bats in the roof, so dust falls on the drugs. The owner of the shop is a doctor who used to work in ward 16 of Mulago Hospital, but apparently he has gone on a course so it is his daughter aged about 24 who is running it. She told me that she does not normally get customers in the daytime, but they may come after 5.00 p.m. Anyway, sickness increases at night.

The drug shop has both locally made and imported drugs, but it is not well stocked, even though it is licensed.

At 11.05 a.m. a young boy came looking for aspirin and she gave it to him... At 12 noon a girl came asking for Hedex. She was told that a pair cost 150/- and the attendant asked her who wanted it. She said that it was for her mother... At 1.30 p.m. a man came looking for medicine for the chest but it was not there. He was offered cough linctus, but he did not take any. At 2.10 p.m. a poor old woman came complaining of malaria and general weakness. She was advised by the attendant to take glucose and to drink a lot, and she was given chlorophenical and panadol. She did not have any prescription but just asked for the drugs... A young boy came with a written note addressed to the attendant, but the person's name was already in the debtor's book and the boy was sent away... At 3.25 p.m. another young girl came asking for ceptrin and took some. At the same time an old woman came asking for ceptrin and panadol and she got some.

FRANK AND MAY DRUG SHOP

This is a well-organized drug shop selling locally made and imported drugs. It is licensed, but not for antibiotics. The attendant (a nurse aged about 30) says they have not paid for this year. The environment is generally good. The shop is located a few metres from the main road, and the next houses are bars selling soft drinks and beer. The nurse said she normally gets customers in the evenings. Her drug shop has a proper ceiling. The owner is a dispenser and mixes her own drugs as well as buying from pharmacies in town. She has a proper pharmacy in another part of Kamwokya. The nurse said that she normally receives patients complaining of coughs, malaria, headaches and abdominal pains.

A man came complaining of abdominal pain but the nurse advised him to go to another clinic in the Market Area... A woman came looking for medivers but she did not have enough money... A woman came complaining of headache and she was given tablets and the nurse advised her to go for a blood check-up. There was a possibility that she had malaria... A man asked for a drug for treating itching feet, but the nurse had none and advised him to go to the other pharmacy belonging to the same owner... A woman also came asking for panadol for 100/- and she was given some. She did not say what she was suffering from... A young girl also came complaining of abdominal pains and the nurse said that she would send her to see the doctor. The girl said she had already been to Mulago Hospital and they had given her two injections. The nurse said that her problem was that she did not finish the dose. She had even come with 100/- for ampicillin antibiotic but there was none left. The nurse said the girl had gonorrhea and she told the observer that she had frequent abortions and therefore had problems. She looked about 17 and poor.

Interviews with 10 Traditional Healers

It is said to be the stigma attached to traditional healers in sections of Ugandan society that makes them reluctant to advertise themselves with signposts or placards outside the residences where they operate. Local knowledge confirms that even respectable members of society, educated people, church leaders and ordinary Christians visit them, but traditional healers and their methods are a source of conflict within the community and for the individual.

However, it is official Ugandan government policy to harness the resources of the traditional sector in recognition of its being closest to the people. More than two thirds (70 per cent) of births in the country are assisted by traditional birth-attendants (TBA) and it is beginning to be accepted that some herbal treatments may be useful in the treatment of chronic diarrhoea and herpes Zoster in AIDS patients. There is some indication that these treatments 'are as effective as Acyclovir, which is very expensive (over US$80 a course) and generally not available nor accessible to patients in Uganda'. And Acyclovir is the treatment of choice in the biomedical system. There is also an indication that much of the treatment of mental health issues in Uganda, as in other parts of East Africa, is provided by spiritual healers (Nyamwaya, 1992).

In March 1994, in-depth interviews were conducted with ten of the healers identified and interviewed in the Treatment Sources Survey. Each interview took place at the healer's premises and lasted between one and two hours. All practitioners were asked basic questions regarding training, illnesses treated, types of treatment, fees and personal questions as to age, religion, etc. In recognition of working time lost, the interviewees were given presents of soap, sugar, disposable gloves or token monetary contributions of Ush. 1,000 some time after the interview.

They were all co-operative and talkative. A number of them belong to, and are registered with, an association of healers. Some said that they refer patients to Mulago Hospital as required, and two wanted to have their herbs tested for efficacy in the treatment of AIDS-related conditions so that they could be brought into wider use. The TBA had once thought of joining the association but her brother, also a healer, had declined to become involved so she deferred to his judgement. She was the healer who also felt a need for somewhere closer than Mulago to which she could refer patients with immediate serious problems, such as mothers giving birth with excessive bleeding.

There are several differences to be noted with respect to gender. Firstly, all five of the herbalists were female, while three of the five diviners were male. While all five of the herbalists were taught their trade by other females, (grandmothers, or in the case of one, a great aunt), the male healers inherited their traditions from their grandfathers, as did the remaining two female healers.

While all three of the males described very similar training and preparation rituals including being taken into the bush and left on their own, neither of the two women healers had had this experience. Both mentioned marital problems provoked by their progressions, and the fact that, since in Uganda children are children of the father's village, they would not be allowed to pass on their skills to any children they bore. One of the women expressed a belief that the spirits did not want her to marry and had prevented her from having children within her marriage. The other said that her husband and in-laws insisted that she make a choice between her work and her marriage. She chose the work and lost her husband.

Amongst the herbalists, there were three Protestants, one Catholic, and one Muslim. All five of the herbalists were careful to describe themselves as only herbalists. They insisted that they only prescribe herbs and do not possess supernatural gifts or use spirits in any way in their work. Those who were most concerned that they should not be seen as diviners were also those who noted that their churches had no problem with their work.

Four of the spiritual healers are practising Muslims, although one of them said that he had been to several other churches initially. The fifth belongs to the Church of Uganda but says she has a problem with gossips there. It is because of this that she only treats patients from outside Kamwokya. Generally speaking, the Muslims had no difficulty in combining their chosen religion with a healing profession which involves the use of supernatural powers, spirits of their ancestors, and other spirits; one of the Muslim healers uses the Koran in his divinations, if requested.

All the spiritual healers/diviners listed health care as their main profession, but only two of the six herbalists interviewed in the TSS were full-time. A major difference between them is that the traditional healers all felt that they were being used by the spirits in their work. Most of them had at some time experienced illnesses which they said came to let them know that they had been chosen and that they must allow the spirits to work through them. All the traditional healers said that they would not refuse to treat patients because of lack of money. One noted that he gathers the herbs from the field free of charge and that his ancestors would be annoyed if he refused to treat people, with or without money. He said that where there are big problems, there is often no money. He mentioned that when someone was brought to him in a coma, he had to go ahead and treat the patient and trust him to pay after his recovery. He said that his ancestors are sympathetic.

Only one of the herbalists said she would not treat without a fee, although others said they must have a small initial payment in every case; the patient is then asked to return with a larger fee following successful treatment. Another said she would accept non-money payments of sugar, meat or soap and that she sometimes allows credit. She said that she could not refuse to treat because of lack of money, especially when, as she put it, it is for the children of the Nation and the mothers cry...

Profiles

Kavina Naduma: herbalist

Mrs Naduma is a Muganda who was born in Kamwokya. She learned her skills from her grandmother. She says that her only formal education was the Catechism of the Catholic Church. She has been a practising herbalist for 35 years. This is her main occupation. Her clients come from Kamwokya as well as outside Kamwokya, although these days she has very few clients 4–6 regular clients a week. She generally treats only pregnant women, although she sometimes treats men and women for gonorrhoea (*Nziko*). She does not treat physical pain.

Women come to her when they are pregnant and feel that they are going to miscarry. She specializes in treatment of heat in the womb (*Ekigalanga*) which she treats with a herb that reduces the heat over a period of three days. She does not carry out any physical examination of her patients. She often begins treatment in the the third month of pregnancy. A herb is given to prevent protracted labour when the time comes. Women are given the herb, which has been mixed with clay and shaped to preserve it. This is later ground by the women and mixed with water to provide a herbal drink which is taken three times a day.

Mrs Naduma gathers her herbs from a nearby field with the assistance of her grandson. When she treats gonorrhoea, she gives the patients two bottles of a herbal drink which she has prepared. Women occasionally come to her for treatment of menstrual pains and infections. She says that she does what she can and refers them to hospital if they are not helped.

She does not treat people without charging a fee. There is one set fee (Ush. 2,000) which is paid after treatment. Patients usually return later to let her know the outcome of the treatment. They usually bring her a gift of sugar at that time. She showed us one of the herbs that she uses which looks very similar to mint. She would have shown us other herbs but she said that they were too far away.

Miriel Kamanembo: herbalist

Miriel is 41 years of age and was born in the Bushenyi District of Western Uganda. She has been a resident of Kamwokya for the past twenty years and she has no children. She has no formal education but her paternal grandmother was a herbalist. She says that she began learning about using herbs from being with her grandmother; however, her abilities are a 'gift of God'. She is a Protestant. In fact, she started at the age of ten and spent a lot of time with older women who had these gifts. It was an exchange of information in which she could also tell these women things which they did not know about herbs and treatment. She suffered from stomach aches which forced her to learn about many herbs. She is now a registered herbalist.

Miriel treats a number of conditions.

1. People who have problems with joints, particularly the lower limbs, come to her to eat cow's foot and shin which are prepared by her. Some of these people are referred to her by medical personnel. Others come because of her reputation. This remedy is also good for hangovers and people in need of this also come to eat this dish. She does not actually prescribe this, but people consume the dish until they feel better.
2. Headaches affecting one side of the head (migraines?), sometimes accompanied by pains which affect the arm. These patients usually come after failing to receive effective treatment at the hospital or clinics. Patients have often suffered with these headaches for up to three months before coming to Miriel. The headaches are treated with herbs which have been ground and wrapped in a banana leaf which is then heated on the fire. The patient then lies on his back and drops from the banana leaf are applied to the nostrils. This causes sneezing in the patient and the headache clears. If not, then other herbs are collected and put into a basin. The patient then puts his head over the basin covered by a towel to cause sweating as he inhales the mixture.
3. Backaches – 2 types. She does not treat what she refers to as water in the back resulting from hospital treatment. She treats other kinds of backaches, which might result from spending a long time in bed after malaria or physical strains, by rubbing herbs on the back at least three times.
4. *Ekineyo* – treatment for children who are not growing. She squeezes a herb and gives it as a drink and to apply in the nose and as a wash. Another group of herbs are given to the mother to put in food to increase the appetite. If this is not successful, she tries different herbs. She also treats worms in children.
5. Symptoms of AIDS – Miriel states that she is HIV positive herself and that some of her patients come from the AIDS clinic. When patients with lung problems come and tell her the truth about their illness, she treats the

problem and then advises them to go to Mulago to be treated for TB. If the patient does not tell her the truth, then she simply treats the diarrhoea and gives no other advice. She also treats the rash with a mixture of vaseline and herbs which is rubbed on the body. Swellings which are common with HIV are treated with herbs to draw out the swelling, then lanced with a sharp instrument which is heated in the fire as she says that if the swelling disappears within the body it causes more harm. There is also a herbal drink which is boiled for three hours and used for the pain which accompanies AIDS. She applies powdered rock salt for thrush.

6. *Kiwo* (STD) – Normally women come to her with this complaint. She uses herbs in a basin which the patients then sit in for at least 30 minutes. She gives them more herbs to take home. These are inserted in the vagina and left overnight and removed the following morning. The herbs extract the infection. She then advises the use of a form of Nystatin which can be obtained from the drug shops. Men occasionally come. She says that the men are not shy to show her their wounds. 'At the time of delivery, you do not remember that you are naked.' She does examine the patients and pays attention to breaks in the skin. Sometimes she notices water discharge in the wounds. She says that the discharge in women can lead to prolonged periods and swelling.

Miriel is not a full-time herbalist and she says that most of her patients are not regular. They come from outside Kamwokya as well as from within. Sometimes a week goes by without any patients. Her fees vary depending on the treatment. They range from Ush. 500 to 2,000. Sometimes she will accept non-money payments of sugar, meat or soap, and she'sometimes allows credit. However, Miriel says that she can not refuse to treat because of lack of money, especially, she says, when it is for the children of the Nation and the mothers cry.

Joyce Teddy Kokulowoza: herbalist

Teddy is a 45-year old woman who was born in Tanzania. She has four children and has lived in Kamwokya for twenty years. She is Protestant, a member of the Church of Uganda. She has no formal education, but she learned how to treat women for infertility and has been a practising herbalist for 8 years.

She only treats women, the majority of whom have never been pregnant. She also treats women who have never delivered and those who have given birth but who have become infertile.

For women who have never conceived, Teddy gives them a herb to drink. She says that if they retain that drink then she knows that she can treat them successfully. However, if they do not retain it (results take place within about five minutes), then according to her and her aunt's experience there is no hope of successful treatment and she advises the patient accordingly. She does not treat them further.

A different herb is administered to women who have given birth successfully at least once. It is taken each night until the woman has conceived. If the infertility is due to the husband, she does not treat him. Generally, by the time a woman comes to her, she has exhausted all other possibilities and knows that the problem lies with her.

Teddy has regular patients and they come from both inside and outside Kamwokya. She has no set fees. Patients pay an initial fee at the consultation and then more after the cure She does, sometimes, extend credit but she does not take patients who cannot pay for her services.

Kosomo: spiritual healer

Kosomo is a hereditary traditional healer who examines patients through powers given to him by his ancestral spirits. He says that through prayer he receives information in several ways: i) at times the ancestors tell him; ii) or he may have a vision which shows him what to use to cure patients; or iii) he uses his prior experience (for example, with impotence he does not have to be told by the ancestors how to treat this nor does he need to examine the patient). He does not need to touch his patients to examine them. He says that supernatural powers are needed for this.

Kosomo says that when he was in Primary 4, he found that his sight was affected and he could not see the blackboard. He went to the Catholic Church to have prayers said for him. He was not assisted by these prayers. He also went to Protestant churches. He is now a Muslim. Later he dreamt that he must go to his grandfather. The grandfather then told him that he must carry on his healing tradition. Kosomo says that he was afraid. He thought that he would never have a wife and that he would not have friends. He also said that his business was not succeeding.

He then told how he had to go into isolation. He went out somewhere (he does not know where) with only a spear. He was told that he was gone for nine days with nothing to eat or drink. Family members kept watch for him and played special musical instruments. Upon his return, several miracles took place during a special ceremony in praise of the ancestors. Kosomo says that the ancestors will come when called, but it is necessary to have a shrine 'to give what is due to be given' and if the spirits are satisfied, then he is in full control. He also mentioned that if a woman goes to the shrine 'when she has her period, she will never finish the period'.

Kosomo says that he has five ancestral spirits that he can call upon in his work. They each have specialities, so he knows which spirit will be dealing with the various situations. Most of his patients come from outside Kamwokya. His speciality is headaches and other chronic problems which are not successfully treated by others. He treats only adults, not children. He also treats mental problems.

Kosomo prescribes many kinds of herbs. He gives both powdered and fresh herbs for drinking and washing the body. He expressed a desire to know how to preserve these herbs so that he could be more efficient in curing coughs and weaknesses.

Kosomo says that he treats those who come to him whether they have money or not, because the herbs that he gathers from the field are free of charge and because his ancestors would be annoyed if he refused to do so. He has no set fees but will give the treatment and then the patient can bring gifts later. He says that where there are big problems there is usually no money. As an example, he cited someone brought to him in a coma; he had to go ahead and treat the patient and allow the patient to return to pay after his recovery. The patient can pay according to his means when he is ready. He says that his ancestors are sympathetic.

Kosomo does not regard his powers as satanical. He says that he tried a number of churches for prayer but his prayers did not work until he allowed his ancestors to come to him to do their work. He says that they do have the power to destroy but that they do not use the powers in this way.

Abdul Zake Kazada: spiritual healer

Abdul Zake is a 42-year-old male traditional healer who is married with children. He has been a resident of Kamwokya for two years. He is a Musoga with Primary 6 education. He is a hereditary healer with 22 years experience. This is his main occupation. He has regular patients as well as passing trade and generally sees around 45 patients a week, although this varies with the time of year. He also has one regular assistant who treats patients when he is away from home.

Abdul Zake treats a number of conditions: diarrhoea, pregnancy, mental cases, epilepsy (*nsimbu*), skin rashes, *ekigaranga* (causes deformities in the foetus), chronic fevers, swellings in women, kidney diseases, and symptoms of AIDS-related diseases. He does examinations of two types. During the first type, he consults the Muslim Holy Book or Koran. This is used for less serious problems. The second type of examination consists of a consultation with the *Mayembe* or spirits. This consultation is used for more serious situations. Patients specify which kind of examination they desire. There are also times when patients come knowing what the problem is and he simply dispenses the herb needed to treat it.

When we were interviewing Abdul Zake, a patient was present. This man had been brought to him some six months previously, tied with ropes because of his mental illness. The patient said that he had been mentally ill for six years and had tried everything he knew to get better before coming to Abdul Zake, but all the earlier treatments had failed to help. He stayed with Abdul Zake during the six months of his treatment and he is now almost cured. Indeed, he was no longer restrained and sounded quite lucid even though he did appear to need further treatment. He is being treated with a potion made from four herbs.

Herbs used by Abdul Zake are sometimes gathered from great distances. He maintains quite a stock for dispensing to his patients. He also expressed an interest in having better preservation of his herbs as well as better distribution of them. He sends some herbs to doctors in Tanzania who are treating patients suffering from AIDS. He says that he does not have herbs to treat AIDS but he can treat various symptoms such as diarrhoea, skin rashes, thrush, herpes, and can prescribe a herb to increase the appetite. He does not tell patients that they have AIDS because he says that only adds to their stress. He does counsel them on how to reduce risks in sex. He knows from his own experience that there are many AIDS cases in Uganda and he believes that they are caused by immorality. He says that many people are doing whatever pleases them, and that there is a long way to go to solve the AIDS problem.

Abdul Zake says that even as a child he knew that he was a healer. He has inherited the gift from his grandfather and there are others in the family who are healers, including females. He says that he was never afraid of it even though, like Kosomo, he had problems with his eyes as a schoolboy and could not see the blackboard. He says that *Mayembe* (spirits) would attack him. There was also an initiation for him when he was sixteen. He was taken to the Lake and left on his own for 7 days; he does not remember much of it but he did have dreams while he was on his own. Rituals were performed. His grandfather left all the things that he had for healing to Abdui Zake when he died.

He says that he obtains his healing powers from the spirits and that he prays to them. He first prays to the Creator for blessings. Then there are the ancestral spirits which were once all living members of his family. These are the spirits which work through him when called upon for an examination. They will also make a sign to him when they wish to come. He says that his mosque does not put restrictions on his work. But he does not do abortions because it is a sin to do this.

His initial fee is Ush. 500. After that the rest is negotiable. He does help even those who come without money; they are expected to pay later. He says that he is not in the business for the money; he wants his reputation to grow. He also offered to provide us with herbs that could be tested scientifically for their efficacy.

Asuman Matoyu Musawo (Jajja): spiritual healer

Jajja is a 34-year-old male hereditary healer who has lived in Kamwokya for the past five years. This is his main occupation which he has been practising for nine years. A good number of his patients come from outside Kamwokya. He has both regular patients and passing trade and, although it varies with the time of year, he treats at least nine patients a week. He can accommodate patients overnight in an emergency. He treats individuals alone and he uses *Mayembe* (spirits) for the examination. He gives patients the choice of leaving the door open (unlike many diviners) and he says that most frequently he does treat with the door open. He does not always examine the patient. Sometimes he just looks at the patient and knows what to do. The patient is allowed to choose the method. He also provides herbal mixtures that are requested by the patient without examination.

His specialities are yellow fever (*enkaka*), impotence, rash (big patches that discharge water), heat in the womb, pleurisy (*Akabengo*), genital ulcers, swollen legs and swollen breasts (abscesses), pregnancy, convulsions and headaches. He specializes in shifting swellings to a different part of the body that is more suitable for treatment. He usually burns the localized swelling so that the pus can come out.

Jajja says that he treats with one type of herb,which he collects himself from as far away as Tanzania. He gives the herb in powdered form, which must be dissolved in water. It is the same for all. He belongs to the Uganda Herbalists and Culture Association. And he says that they work together. Kosomo is his friend and they consult with one another.

Jajja believes that AIDS is caused by immorality but he also says that not all of the cases that are reported as AIDS are in fact AIDS. Some people simply get sick and neglect to seek health personnel and it simply appears to be AIDS.

He says that he does not discriminate in treating people; he treats everyone. He says that sometimes people fail to pay but he does not mind because everything comes from God and he does not see why he should make a lot of money from what he has been given free. He says that whatever grows on the land belongs to God and is a free gift. If he were to refuse people, the ancestors might get angry and punish him for some time.

Jajja says that he must go to the mosque or church because there is only one God. The spirits that he works with are ancestors, not God. There are two

136

types of spirits according to Jajja, Lubale and Mayembe. He describes the Mayembe as angels which can be sent out to get the information they are ordered to get, and the Lubale as providers of treatment. He inherited everything from his grandfather who died when Jajja was only six years old. He already knew that he was a healer and he had no initiation, but he has the power to initiate others. He can train one of his own children, but it is the ancestors coming into the child that will let him know which one is to be.

His fees range from Ush. 500 to 30,000.

Mukuuma: spiritual healer

Mukuuma is a 42-year-old female traditional healer and Traditional Birth Attendant with a Primary 6 level education. She has twelve children but separated from her husband when he and his family objected on religious grounds to her work as a traditional healer. There was a misunderstanding concerning her supernatural powers and she had to choose between her husband and her work. She discovered that she had inherited her grandfather's healing tradition when she suffered a long illness when she was 28. The illness lasted a year and she was feverish and had lots of dreams. She consulted medical doctors but they failed to help her. Later, she was told that she had spirits inside who wanted to use her for healing others and that she was not ill at all. Her parents were 'saved' Muslims and objected to her working with spirits. There are others in her family who are traditional healers; however, she is the only one who delivers babies as well. She has been practising since 1979 and this is her full-time occupation. Her main work is with women in helping them to deliver. She says that in 1966 she was delivering her third child alone. She remembered how to follow the procedure. Using this experience, she delivered almost all of her subsequent births on her own and became interested in helping other women to deliver. Mukuuma has a sister who works at Mulago Hospital, so she went to see how babies are delivered in the hospital.

Mukuuma says that she does not normally need to consult the spirits for labour pains. Most of her patients are treated at her home but if the birth looks as if it is too complicated then she goes to hospital with the patient and leaves her in the hands of the doctors. Patients are delivered lying down face up as they do in hospital. She makes them change their position if the head of the baby is not engaged. Another complication that she encounters is when the cord is wrapped round the baby's neck or the mother fails to give support by pushing. She gives herbs to the mothers to help them to relax.

Mukuuma uses gloves to avoid infection. The mothers also bring polyethylene sheets and other equipment for the births. She advises them to keep their things because she might have to examine them again and she will not do it with her bare hands. She keeps spare birthing sheets on hand for those who do not have them. She has done things this way since 1984. She records each birth. At times, she delivers three babies a week. Others come to her for treatment before going to hospital. But if the hospital fails them, then they return to her for further assistance. She has regular customers. There are those whom she has delivered five times. She also gives follow-up treatment. The mothers bring their small babies back for treatment. She sometimes comes across babies with AIDS but she does not tell the mother, because, she says, she does not want to worry them. She advises women with AIDS to go to the hospital. She treats toddlers as well and she treats men, usually for STD. Sometimes partners come together for treatment. She treats syphilis with herbs. She prepares two types of medicine; herbs for drinking and for rubbing on the body. She says that she will not reveal these herbs to anyone other than those who will take over when she is dead. And these will be chosen from amongst her brother's children. She cannot choose from her children because they are not children who belong to her family.

Mukuuma also deals with swellings and other complications of the body that are the result of spiritual problems. She says that, if you lose your appetite, it is a result of these kinds of problems. She likes to treat problems in a physical way with herbs first, but if the worst comes to the worst, she will contact the *jajja* (spirit). For example, if someone comes to her with a headache she will touch the head to see whether there is a high temperature and then use herbs. If these fail, then she consults the spirits.

Fees are set in accordance with the condition of the patient. She says that she will not refuse to assist a person who has only part of the fees but that she will not continue to treat them. She says that there are others (like her brother) she can consult in especially difficult cases but they are a long way away. She wanted to become a member of the Association but as her brother refused to become a member and she respects him she decided not to. However, she does say that she would like to have access to someone closer who could assist mothers with immediate serious problems such as excessive bleeding.

Olive Murramer: herbalist

Olive is a part-time herbalist with thirteen years experience. She is 34 years old and the mother of six children. She has resided in Kamwokya for sixteen years and has a Primary 7 level education. Her maternal grandmother taught her how to practise as a herbalist when she was about sixteen years of age; however, she did not practise then because as a teenager she felt it was unimportant. When she was pregnant she came back to it. She belongs to the Church of Uganda and she says that they have no quarrel with her work.

She treats convulsions in children, heat in the womb and *Enoga* – a rash in babies that can threaten the life of the child. She says this is a result of the mother having untreated syphilis. This is a pretty common situation and in subsequent pregnancies, she treats the mother and there is a successful birth. She has treated a man for STD. She has also assisted at a couple of births. She found it exciting but does not wish to become known as a *besawo* (healer) and she does not want to have too many patients. She would be interested in training as a Traditional Birth Attendant. She only treats residents of Kamwokya. These patients are regulars and have all been referred by someone who knows her.

She treats women who have miscarried (due to heat in the womb) with a herb to wash out the remains of the pregnancy. They are treated once a week for three weeks with three types of herbs. She also treats women with AIDS who are pregnant. She does not tell them that they have AIDS. She does examine women by touching them and if a pregnant woman is threatening to miscarry, she advises her to attend the hospital.

Olive is paid well for her work. Her initial fee is small. When the patient is recovered, she will bring more. The amount depends on the original condition of the patient. It may be as much as Ush. 5,000. And if the service is appreciated, the patients sometimes give more. She says she will treat women who do not have the money.

Olive does not belong to the Association but does consult her friend and fellow herbalist, Mama Khadijah on difficult cases. She obtains her herbs from her grandmother.

Gertrude Ndagire (Mama Khadijah): herbalist

Mama Khadijah is a 30-year-old mother of five children and was taught to be a herbalist by her paternal grandmother when she was twenty. She is a Muganda from Luwero and has lived in Kamwokya for twenty years. She attended school up to Secondary 3 level. She has been a practising herbalist for five years and it is her main occupation.

Her specialties are the treatment of burns,convulsions in children and haemorrhoids (*Ememe eyemabega*). She also treats itchy rashes affecting the feet, hands, and buttocks. She says this usually affects those who are in the bush. It is treated with a powdered bark and applied with vaseline. She and Olive both treat convulsions but have no idea what causes it. Sometimes when they are called in the child will have been ill for as long as five days. She says that the mothers usually attempt to treat the children before they are brought to her. If there is no fever, the illness will be treated by them because these kinds of convulsions are not accompanied by fever. If fever is present, they suspect malaria and advise the mother to take the patient to hospital right away. They both say that it is dangerous to wash a child with convulsions; death might occur if they do so. So they give a very bitter herb to the child to drink.

Mama Khadijah only treats a few cases a month and all of her patients come from the Church area of Kamwokya. Like Olive, she does not treat people at random. All the patients are referred to her. She also fears being called a *besawo* as she does not know how to examine in this way. She says that she is inexperienced. She does consult her grandmother and Olive on difficult cases.

Mama Khadijah treats both sexes and treats from her home She receives fees of Ush. 2,000–3,000. She does not extend credit and does not accept non-money payment.

Bavidi: spiritual healer

Bavidi says she is 29 and was born with the power to heal. From early on she experienced difficulties: she became lame, unable to see and suffered from mental problems. She could not attend school. It was thought initially that she had been bewitched but her paternal grandfather who was also a traditional healer heard a voice calling. He told her things that she could not understand when she was around seven years old She often spoke spontaneously about things that had happened long before. Her aunt knew the history of these things and advised the elders to take care of this girl. She developed a huge swelling on her neck, something like a boil. Her father advised others to let her die saying 'if one grass comes off the thatched hut, the roof doesn't leak'. For three years she walked with a limp and up to about the age of ten, there were different problems for her month after month. Her father fled the family and went to Kenya but he returned when the powers chased after him and turned his skin white for being disobedient. Her subsequent initiation involved preparing a shrine and eating from twelve dishes of food prepared by a traditional healer.

She started working as a healer from the age of ten. Within three days, she could move but she was still blind. She does not remember all that happened but she was later told about these things. She remained in her father's house. Even though she was blind she could go into the bush, pick herbs and return to her family to teach them about these herbs. Something, she says, allowed her to move on her own, pick these herbs, and return to the family with this knowledge. Later she dreamed of a woman standing in front of her who directed her to pick a certain herb and use it to wash her face. She then almost fell asleep again when her head was grabbed by a strong force. She shook her head and immediately she could see again.

She says that conditions were imposed on her by this female spirit who came to her with a man as she slept. She was told not to dig in the garden and not to fish from that time on. Her father rejected the story and insisted that she go digging. The spirit man came back again, told her that she was forbidden to dig and she was banged about by spirits. She was then taken to Mulago Hospital. Since that time her arm was affected and she cannot dig or do that kind of work. She also has a hole in the back of her head which she says prevents her from carrying water. Water flows from the hole in her head if she attempts to carry water.

She had a child when she was thirteen, at about the time she was banged about by the spirits. She is now married but there are no children of the marriage. She says that the spirits have prevented it. At first she did not fear her gifts, but she began to be afraid when she married because the spirits did not want her to marry and she had lots of problems in the marriage. She says that she is pretty much confined to her home. If she is needed in the village, she is picked up and brought back to her home as she does not travel on her own and does not stay away from home. The father of her child can come to visit her but she can not go out to find him.

She treats heat in the womb and any problems that threaten to interrupt a pregnancy. She also treats infertility but she is not paid until the child is three months old. She says that she cannot refuse to treat an infertile woman unless she examines the woman and finds that she cannot help her to conceive.

When she conducts examinations, something comes into her head to let her know whether she can help. She treats any problem that comes her way. She treats a wasting disease in children by making a soup from the insides of a goat and herbs. The child takes the soup for a period of one week. This situation generally comes from spiritual problems, a bewitching or sometimes the child is born infected with AIDS. If it comes from AIDS (and she knows the difference just by observing), then she simply treats the symptoms and advises the mother to consult the hospital. She treats the diarrhoea, loss of appetite, and a constriction of muscles inside the abdomen. She believes that AIDS comes from immorality. She does not tell patients that they have AIDS. She believes that it can be an example of being bewitched but does not know whether to call it a medical or a spiritual problem. She regards medical treatment as useful.

She uses a separate room for examining patients. It is not a real shrine but more of a laboratory. She no longer closes the door when examining patients. She says that she was a diviner with oracles, but then she wanted to become saved and join a church (mushroom or Protestant). Later she returned to her senses.

She invites her spirits to come into her head and then she begins to tell your life story. She experiences different spirits working with her in the manner of a prompter in a play. She is told something like 'This is Ivan and this is how we can serve him'. Her powers are always male, so she hears male voices. They give her a sign when they are going to come.

She goes to the Church of Uganda now. She enjoys Church but says that there are gossips there. But she says that God is her priority and she asks God to intervene with her patients. She says she does not belong to the *Mayembe*, she is *Lubale*.

She says that her spiritual powers are not needed to treat pain. It is simply a matter of giving herbs to drink or to rub on. She treats emotional pain by preparing a drink for psychological effect and a wash and makes the patient lie down. She does not take cases of people who are mad, but refers them on.

She only attends to patients who come from outside Kamwokya and far away in order to avoid rumours. People are referred to her. She belongs to the Association and has a certificate. Her fee is generally Ush. 2,000. She used to defer payment until the patient had recovered but she discovered that they do not always come back.

She would like to have her herbs tested for their efficacy. She is concerned that so many people claim that they can cure AIDS. She does not want to do this and spoil her reputation. However, if the herbs are proved to be effective, it will create a name for her that will never be forgotten.

Seven

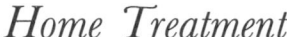

Home Treatment

JESSICA OGDEN & GRACE BANTEBYA KYOMUHENDO

Home treatment is a common first response to the onset of an illness episode the world over. In industrialized countries a plethora of over-the-counter medications are available to treat the symptoms of colds, flu, arthritis, hayfever and other common, non-life-threatening illnesses. As a matter of course, we self-prescribe: we go to our local chemist and buy remedies we recognize and know will relieve our symptoms. We might treat our illnesses at home in other ways as well: with warm baths or cool cloths, bowls of chicken soup, dry toast, days off school or work. We undertake these measures, saving ourselves the considerable expense and inconvenience of going to the G.P. or clinic, while affirming our own agency in maintaining wellness in ourselves and the members of our household. We eventually go to the doctor should home treatment fail to bring relief 'soon enough'. It is with some degree of confidence that we undertake this step. The expectation is that the cost of going to the doctor (in terms of time, if not money) will be offset by satisfactory results: we will get well.

In Kamwokya, home treatment occurs in a context where the expectations of wellbeing and cure are very different, and where the formal health-care system has broken down as a result of two decades of civil war and economic mismanagement. In Uganda, home treatment and the over-the-counter purchase of prescription drugs (including antibiotics) have significant public health implications. This chapter discusses the significance of the household as a locus of health care; the nature of the home treatment process (including the importance of drug shops); the relationship between home treatment and autonomy; and the role that 'invisibility' plays, especially in the (home) treatment of sexual infections.

The Household as the Locus of Health

This section gives a brief review of the literature concerned with the role of women as health-care providers in their homes and the importance of 'home' as locus of wellbeing.

Maintaining good health entails more than the management of disease and illness. Most household chores, in fact, contribute to household health management. Cooking, washing the family's clothes, keeping the home environment clean and safe, managing the household expenses, and keeping networks and relationships functioning and healthy: all these activities contribute to the maintenance of good health and wellbeing in the household (Graham.,1984; Raikes, 1989; Browner, 1989). In Kampala (as elsewhere) these chores are performed primarily by women. Treating the sick can be best understood as an extension of this health-producing work that women undertake in their households on a daily basis.

Berman *et al.* (1994: 206) have called this process the Household Production of Health (HHPH), and define it as:

> A dynamic behavioural process through which households combine their (internal) knowledge, resources, and behavioural norms and patterns with available (external) technologies, services, information, and skills to restore, maintain, and promote the health of their members.

They note that such an understanding is useful also as a challenge to the 'single disease approach' (common in biomedical analysis) where ill health is analysed in terms of a particular nameable disease rather than of the absence of or threat to wellbeing.

In her discussion of household health in Latin America, Browner (1989) emphasizes the centrality of women's roles and activities. She notes that in her field area (as in ours), sickness is a fact of daily life, and 'women possess significant specialised knowledge concerning health care... It is usually women who prescribe remedies, decide at what point in an illness to seek outside attention, and what type of practitioner to consult' (p. 145). She writes that

> When we recognise the extent to which illnesses are treated at home, we gain an even better understanding of the significance of women's role in household health (*ibid*).

It could be said that in Kamwokya the inverse of that statement is more to the point: that in recognizing the importance of women's work as health-inducing we are struck by the extent to which illnesses are treated at home. Having a healthy family reflects on a woman's fitness as a wife and mother, and enhances her status as a 'proper woman' (*omukyala omutufu*) and a good neighbour. Although in general extremely poor women are excused and pitied if their families are sickly, if a particular woman is not popular in the neighbourhood and her family – particularly her children – are unwell, she will be sharply criticized by the other women.

Another key element of the household as a locus of health care is the fact that, in general, what is treated in the home is treated in secret. This is especially important for the treatment of stigmatized illnesses such as sexually transmitted diseases and those illnesses brought about by witchcraft or some transgression of traditional morality. This important aspect of home treatment is treated in greater detail below.

Treating illness episodes in the home, therefore, tends to be an extension of women's activities, and it is generally women who undertake the responsibility for it. It must be noted, however, that in households that have a resident man, this man is included in the decision-making processes that surround home treatment, especially if money is going to be spent. The importance of home treatment in Uganda, of course, extends beyond the fact that it is an important area of feminine decision-making. The current pattern and extent of home treatment in Kampala reflect a more sinister state of affairs. As Berman *et al.* (1994) indicate, in addition to knowledge, beliefs and cultural norms, expectations of efficacy underlie health-seeking patterns. In Kampala people have extremely realistic expectations of their struggling health service, and tend to use it only as a last resort. Thus home treatment is not only a logical first response to illness in this setting. It is often the most effective. Susan Whyte (1991), also discussing contemporary Uganda, writes:

> In the face of continuing high morbidity, people are taking health care in their own hands and are pleased to find the tools they think they need available in shops and markets (Whyte, 1991: 192).

Because of what has essentially been the collapse of the formal system, Whyte observes that a system of lay medicine has arisen. People in this setting want health, but they do not want *health care* as it is delivered in the formal system. They want medicines but they do not seem to want *medicine* (in the institutional sense). She continues:

> The ultimate in privatisation is not the obvious mushrooming of private clinics but the tendency of people to avoid the clinical relationship altogether by acquiring medicines and treating themselves (*ibid*,:141).

This rise in 'pharmaceutical self-help', Whyte argues, reflects a 'family care' pattern, present in many African cultures, where 'the family, not the specialist, had the primary responsibility to decide on a diagnosis and treatment' (*ibid*). It has taken on new significance on the contemporary stage, however, with the existence of easily available antibiotics and other potentially dangerous prescription drugs.

Pharmaceutical availability, and the population's use of this resource, is introduced here to highlight an essential aspect of health care in the home; although home treatment occurs the world over, it has an extra new dimension in Uganda. Here the lay public take the health of their household members into their own hands, not just as a first line of treatment, but as the main form of treatment for all kinds of illness, of all degrees of severity.

The Home Treatment Process

From our various data sources it emerged that the specific pattern of treatment-seeking varied largely according to: type of symptoms presented; who was suffering; socio-economic level (and status aspirations) of the household; and whether or not the patient had a chronic condition. This section begins with discussion of an important link in the chain of treatment-seeking factors, the drug shop, and will briefly deal with the two main types of illness investigated in this study – paediatric and sexual infections – and how they are treated in the home.

Medical anthropologists and sociologists have long regarded Africa as a special case for understanding treatment-seeking and therapeutic choice. There is a sizeable literature analysing the ways in which African peoples of various countries and situations pick their way through the complex of options now available to them. Much energy has been put into understanding when, why and in what order a patient decides to go to a traditional healer or the local government clinic. Staugard (1985a) quotes a Motswana informant saying that he feels he has one foot in the traditional system and one in the modern system, and is unsure which foot to trust. It seems from our work, however, and the work of a number of other writers in recent years, that choice of treatment is not a linear process nor a 'black and white' alternative of modern or traditional systems. Rather, people are pragmatic and opportunistic in their therapeutic choices. There seems to be a continuum or a movement amongst the available systems, and in Uganda the informal economy has done a lot to fill in any gaps in between. Most people do not use one or the other 'system'; most use both more or less simultaneously. And more and more in the urban Ugandan context, the distinctions between them are becoming less precise. As Last (1992: 402) notes,

> what may seem to the outsider as a Babel of different medical ideas is, to an insider, an adequately homogenous means of coping with illness in all its forms.

He argues that patients do not necessarily see the different systems as 'alternatives', and some of the doctors do not act as part of a 'system'.

> Instead there is a whole medical culture within which the various systems or non-systems have affected each other over time, to the extent that a segment of the medical culture can flourish in seeming anarchy (*ibid.*: 403)

Berman *et al.* (1994) proffer a Health-Seeking Behaviour Framework which outlines the illness episode as entailing a complex 'treatment path'. They divide this 'path' into a common-sense sequence: onset, recognition, diagnosis, treatment, and outcome. At each stage decisions are made and action taken. The third and fourth stages, definition/diagnosis and action/treatment, are the focus here. In general, at the onset of symptoms a home diagnosis is made, and a degree of seriousness is ascertained. In some households in our study immediate professional help was sometimes sought at this initial stage (especially among those with higher socio-economic standing, or with status aspirations). In the majority of cases, however, the symptoms are first treated at home in two ways: with non-medical remedies and treatments, and/or with medicines purchased, without prescription or advice, from drug shops, pharmacies or clinics. These drug shops have a key position as a link between the formal biomedical system and self-treatment. Because of their importance, both to home treatment and to the health system in Kamwokya in general, the drug shops are discussed in some detail below, and also in Chapter 6.

Drug shops, clinic dispensaries and pharmacies

The history of Uganda's health service crisis is documented by Dodge and Wiebe (1985), and Susan Whyte (1991) offers an illuminating discussion of the resultant growth in private biomedical care. Most important here are the mushrooming of drug shops and pharmacies in Uganda's towns and cities, and the competition for drugs between the government services (which receive drugs as aid from external donors) and these drug shops, whose owners often have links with the formal system and may acquire some of their supplies illegally. Whyte discusses this in the context of the 'privatization' of health care in Uganda. It can especially justifiably be put into the context of the country's informal economy of health, and much of our data support Whyte's findings.

The drug shops in Kamwokya were examined in two ways. The Treatment Sources Survey questionnaire was administered to 24 of the area's 31 drug shops and clinics (12 drug shops, 12 clinics). Of the 12 drug shops, 7 were selected for further observation and more in-depth study. A Makerere graduate was hired to observe in the drug shops and record her observations in detail (Chapter 6). During the observation period the observer also had the opportunity to talk informally with the drug shop attendants. The following discussion is based largely on these two studies.

In the licensing process for opening a drug shop or pharmacy, no special licence is required to sell class 'C' drugs (aspirin, Malaraquin, vitamins, cough sweets, etc.), but only a licensed pharmacist should sell class 'A' and 'B' drugs (prescription medications including antibiotics and injectables) (Whyte, 1991:135). In reality, these laws are not enforced, and almost all of the drug shops observed in our study, regardless of whether they had the necessary licence, sold prescription drugs to customers requesting them, even without the necessary prescription. Clinic dispensaries and establishments calling themselves pharmacies also sold prescription drugs to customers without prescriptions.

A second issue that should be raised in relation to the drug shops is the way in which they are owned and generally operated. Most drug shops, and all private clinics, are owned by a physician, at least in name. Often these private enterprises are the main source of income for health-care professionals working in the public sector. In the examples we observed, however, the physician him/herself was working at Mulago or another hospital, and was rarely, if ever, in attendance. The shops were run by a variety of people ranging from untrained young people to medical assistants, nurses and midwives. The clinics and drug shops are simply important means of supplementing the income of health-care professionals who do not earn a living wage in their main job (cf . Obbo, 1991).

Whyte (1991), for example, found a direct correlation between the drugs missing in the public sector dispensaries and those available in private clinics and drug shops. This finding was echoed in our research. Respondents regularly claimed that doctors at Mulago Hospital prescribe drugs not available at the hospital dispensary. This forces the patients to use the private sector to buy medications that should be available to them free of charge. Some of our respondents suspected that the clinics and drug shops recommended were those owned by the prescribing physician. We have only verbal testimony to support these claims.

A third key issue in understanding the nature and role of the drug shop in the home treatment system is the way drugs and medicines are paid for. All drug shops require payment in cash, although almost all the attendants interviewed, and all of those observed, did give credit to some customers. Two of the drug shops in the study had a credit book, and the researcher observed a number of customers come in to repay their debts. One of the local clinics enjoys huge popularity in the area due to the fact that the attending physician finds it difficult to refuse credit to anyone in need. Still, cash flow is a problem for many Kamwokya residents seeking medicines. If credit is refused, or if the customer does not want to incur a debt, then she is likely to purchase only the amount of the required drug that she can afford. For example, a woman comes into a drug shop requesting septrin for a patient with a cough. She places Ush.500 on the counter and the attendant gives her 500/− worth of septrin (this may be a few tablets or one day's worth), despite the dangers involved in incomplete doses of antibiotics. The attendant might advise the customer about the requisite dose, and urge her to come back for more tablets the following day. Alternatively, a mother might know that the last time her child had a cough he got well after two days, or 1,000/- worth of septrin, even though the doctor prescribed five days of the drug. She will then go with confidence to the local drug shop and buy two days worth of antibiotics, knowing that it will be sufficient to make her child well. This is common whether the ailment being treated from home is a cough or gonorrhoea. The medical implications, though not well understood, are nonetheless cause for concern.

In effect, the Kamwokya residents use the drug shops and dispensaries in at least three different ways:

(i) The customer knows the drug she wants and either knows the amount needed or buys according to the cash she has available rather than according to appropriate dosage. Whyte (1991) notes in her study that

147

half of all transactions conducted in drug shops, and a quarter of those in clinics, were undertaken by customers who were self-prescribing.

(ii) The customer is ill or has a patient at home but does not know the most appropriate medicine to buy and asks for advice from the attendant (who may or may not have any formal medical training).

(iii) The customer has a wound or injury and is seeking treatment.

Only the first of these three is considered to be related to home treatment. The customer seeking advice or treatment from the drug shops, however, as in (ii) and (iii), has already considered his/her condition to be beyond the immediate control of household members.

In the Treatment Sources Survey the providers were asked to respond to a list of symptoms stating whether each symptom was treated regularly, occasionally or never. The symptoms most commonly treated in the drug shops were coughs and fever, diarrhoea, headaches, stomach ulcers and skin rashes. All types of STD are treated by some of the drug shops. None of the drug shops claimed they ever treated 'false teeth' (see Chapter 8), AIDS, broken bones, pregnancy/delivery, or infertility in women, though one drug shop did say it ever-treated 'love problems' and male impotence. The observation exercise revealed, however, that customers did not always disclose the nature of the symptoms being treated, but simply asked for the drug they wanted. Where the attendant was a trained health professional, the customer might be questioned as to who the drug was for and what symptoms were being treated. Often, however, the drugs were simply sold to the customer with no questions asked.

Chapter 6 and this chapter take up the role of home treatment as one option in the management of paediatric illness and of STD. The following section deals with its particular 'private' quality and the preference for it when faced with shameful or morally compromised infection.

Illness as a Moral Category:
Invisibility, Stigma and Secrecy

There are a number of ways in which illness can be seen as morally defined. We have noted, for example, the moral imperative to have healthy children. The way in which the presence of illness in a home is seen by the rest of a community can reflect on the moral status of the parents and *vice versa* (cf. Graham, 1985). It does not appear, however, that this leads mothers to treat paediatric illnesses, *per se*, in secret. Home treatment for most paediatric symptoms is primarily about efficiency. Mothers feel they can handle most problems at home without undue expenditures of time and money. The home treatment of STDs is a different matter: it is about shame and secrecy because the disease stems from moral transgressions. Most paediatric crisis symptoms are not considered to stem from a breach in the moral code, but a number of common childhood symptoms are linked to cultural causes, and these too can be stigmatizing. Although certain 'traditional' or Kiganda diseases may in some cases be shameful, however, they are shameful in a different way from STD, and are therefore treated differently. STDs should be treated in secret. *Kiganda* illnesses in most cases require a traditional healer and cannot by their very nature be treated at home. The principal moral dimension of illness is causation. This section discusses the ways in which causation is linked to stigma and how it in turn seems to affect the nature of, and reasons for, home treatment.

Our data substantiate claims in the literature that some childhood diseases are seen to be caused by a breach in the moral code about which the ancestors are unhappy. These illnesses can be stigmatizing for the parents of the sick child, and they require special treatment from a traditional healer. According to Hogle *et al.* (1991) Ugandan traditional healers (*basawo*) recognize four categories of illness. One is trivial illness (such as colds), for which there is no special treatment; the second category comprises European diseases which include pneumonia, malaria and syphilis, for which biomedical practitioners should be consulted. The third is broadly considered to be 'traditional Kiganda' diseases (*enwadde ez 'ekiganda*). These include more trivial complaints (such as swelling of the feet caused by standing too long on cold ground) as well as a full range of conditions caused by bewitchment, the displeasure of the ancestors for inappropriate behaviours and breaches of tribal taboos, for which traditional healers of various kinds are consulted. 'False teeth', for example, is a disease, commonly recognized in Kamwokya, which causes diarrhoea in infants, but which can be treated only by specialist traditional doctors. Mothers cannot treat 'false teeth' at home, but must take their infants to a traditional healer to have the teeth removed. Convulsions, on the other hand, are believed to stem from 'traditional' causes, but are often treated at home with bitter herbs and steam baths. Mothers in this case do not avoid modern health facilities because of stigma, but because they do not believe their convulsing child will respond to modern treatments (see Jitta, Chapter 8).

Sexually transmitted diseases are, by and large, recognized as being 'European' diseases. They do not require the intervention of a traditional healer; indeed, some respondents felt that traditional healers might even make the situation worse. STDs are caused by a moral transgression, but a transgression of a different sort. People know that STDs (other than AIDS) will respond to modern medical treatment (see Chapter 9). The current state of the public health service has enabled Ugandans to maintain the 'secrecy' of their sexual infections by making it possible for them to obtain antibiotics without prescriptions. Because it is a private matter individuals can even try to ignore it and hope that it will go away. They can hope that denial of diagnosis and treatment will mean that their worst fears will not be realized and they will not be told that they have AIDS. All of these 'strategies' are possible with sexual infections up to a point – until they become serious enough to interfere with normal life. The implications of this complex of stigma, shame, secrecy and self-prescription/self-medication for STD are cause for concern.

Health and Agency: Home Treatment and Autonomy

The role of agency in home treatment is not well understood. The general impression one gets from talking to mothers about home treatment is that they have a certain amount of pride in their medical knowledge and effectiveness as health-care providers in their homes. We have noted that part of being a good mother (and by extension a good woman and a good neighbour) is maintaining one's family's health. Maintaining one's own health is also essential in so far as it is possible, for few women in this area can afford to be sick. There is a saying locally that 'proper women do not fall ill'. The ways in which women themselves respond to illness (other than STD) depend somewhat on the nature and severity of the symptoms, a woman's socio-economic status, and whether or not she has a chronic disease. One of the case-study women, for example, is a mother of eight and is relatively well-off financially. This woman says that she goes immediately to hospital when she feels ill and does not waste time self-treating for anything more serious than a headache. Other case-study women, however, did not prioritize their own health in this way, and regarded time spent on themselves as time wasted. These women tended to self-treat or go without treatment until the symptoms became so severe that they required hospitalization (see Chapter 10). It has to be said, again underscoring the general point made by Whyte (1991), that people's overall competence, or their belief in their own competence, must go hand in hand with the ever decreasing levels of competence (and confidence) in the formal health-care system. Whyte found, as indeed we did, that there is very little sense that people are incapable of managing their own health problems.

There is little help elsewhere in the literature. Graham (1989:186–7) outlines two theoretical models that have tried to provide a framework for understanding health behaviour and behavioural change. These are the Belief Model, and the Locus of Control Model. The Health Belief Model, derived from patient compliance studies, places a person's perceptions (seriousness, risk) of the ailment from which she is suffering at the centre of the analysis. The Locus of Control Model has as its key variables the individual's general perceptions about herself: whether or not she believes that she can control the outcomes of her actions.

> where individuals believe they can achieve what they want (internal locus of control), the prognosis for changes in attitude and behaviour is promising. However where people believe that their lives are controlled by forces beyond their control (external locus of control), the incentive to seek information and make changes is limited (*ibid*).

In this view, however important perceptions and attitudes may be, health choices and health behaviour 'are shaped by material as well as mental structures' (*ibid:* 187) and are primarily pragmatic. Over time, and in economically constrained settings, health choices become health compromises which, in turn, become family routines.

But while the evidence from Kamwokya confirms that much of self- and home treatment has to do with the overall need for pragmatism and routine in daily life, there are other processes also at work. It is our sense that a fuller understanding of the place of agency in home treatment may open important avenues to changing potentially dangerous behaviour patterns (eg. Blaxter, 1983; Berman *et al.*, 1994; Graham 1989; Steptoe, 1989).

Conclusion: Implications of Home Treatment

In conclusion we offer a few summary points about the implications of home treatment as it has developed in Uganda.

- Home treatment is an extension of the 'normal' health-producing behaviours of household members, especially women.
- Because it is the first response to an illness episode, success or failure at this juncture can affect the course and eventual outcome of the illness.
- Because home treatment is private and relatively invisible it is a socially convenient, if not always clinically effective, way of treating sexual infections.
- With the decline of the formal system home treatment has become undeniably central in everyday life but is very poorly understood. Most home treatment involves the informal health sector which is largely unenumerated and in some respects illicit.
- Home treatment is also a response to the economic environment. Although people have the means to treat themselves with controlled medicines such as antibiotics they do not necessarily have the knowledge to administer these drugs. A combination of ignorance and poverty (on the part of the patient as well as the service provider at drug shops) leads to the situation we currently have in Kampala where people are receiving inadequate doses and often inappropriate medicines. This may only lead to further problems both in terms of antibiotic resistance and of more serious strains of disease moving into the community.

The stigma surrounding STDs, in combination with the general crisis in health care and the presence of antibiotics readily available without prescription, is a potentially deadly state of affairs. Inadequate partner notification, incompletely or inappropriately treated sexual infections and a moral climate that makes discussion of sexual risk difficult, combine to provide a ready climate for the transmission of HIV.

Eight

Children's Illnesses

Mothers' Definition & Management of 'Serious Enough' Symptoms

JESSICA JITTA

Almost half of the developing world's urban dwellers are children whose vulnerability has increased with the rapid urban growth, cities in economic and environmental crisis, and recurring conflicts. The problem continues to grow: it is estimated that by the year 2000, there will be more poor urban households (72 million) than those in rural areas (56 million). With urban centres growing at an annual rate of 5 per cent in Africa, more than half of the absolute poor will be concentrated in cities; and the available data indicate that urban children fare worse than rural children in many respects. The infant mortality rate among these children is often higher than the national average, in some cases higher than that of their rural counterparts. Poor urban households have less access to safe water and spend up to 40 per cent of their earnings on water, while malnutrition and anaemia are rampant in slum areas (UNICEF, 1993).

The situation is compounded by the frequency of acute illness afflicting young children, especially those under the age of five. Studies conducted in African cities have documented diarrhoea, coughs and fever as the most common symptoms (Watts et al., 1990).

In a study conducted in Mulago village[1] a typical Ugandan urban slum area, 35 per cent of all children under the age of five were reported sick during a period of two weeks. The most common symptoms included fever/malaria (in 40 per cent), coughs, respiratory symptoms (30 per cent) and diarrhoea and vomiting (16 per cent) (Zirabamuzaale and Jitta, 1989). These happen to be the symptoms of the most serious conditions responsible for the main causes of childhood morbidity and mortality. In Uganda, among infants the main causes of death include respiratory infections (18 per cent); diarrhoea (15 per cent) and malaria (12 per cent). During the second and fourth year, malaria is responsible for 18 per cent of deaths, while respiratory infections contribute 10 per cent. The morbidity patterns, based on the reasons for admission to hospital, are similar (UNICEF, 1989).

Because mothers are primarily responsible for looking after sick children, the outcome of these acute illness episodes is influenced by their management of the condition(s) in

---

[1] The parish around the hospital is always referred to as a village.

the home and decisions about when symptoms are 'serious enough' to warrant treatment outside the home. Late presentation of sick children to health units is a major factor contributing to high mortality from acute illness.

Chapters 6 and 7 examined the treatment options available to mothers; this chapter allows some assessment of how appropriate these options are seen to be. Since both traditional and modern types of health care are available in most African countries, an understanding of what leads to the choice of one over the other is essential for health-care provision (Akhtar, 1987: 34).

Introduction

This chapter discusses mothers' perceptions of acute illness in their children and their assessment of the symptoms which are serious enough to warrant treatment outside the home. Understanding mothers' health-seeking behaviour in this respect allows us to predict their actions when faced with illness crises, and may be helpful in identifying factors which impede their early and effective management.

Health workers need to know what mothers and their families believe causes the symptoms, and how they deal with them. Knowing why and when mothers and their families seek, or do not seek, help for sick children can be helpful in designing more effectively targeted education messages and more appropriate improvements in health service.

The general objective here is to describe urban mothers' perceptions of common acute symptoms in children under the age of five and to relate the perceived seriousness of these illnesses to their subsequent management. The specific objectives are:

a) To describe mothers' perceptions of and beliefs about the causation of acute symptoms of illness in children aged under five.

b) To determine the factors they consider when rating the severity of such illness and at what stage they regard symptoms as 'serious enough' to warrant treatment outside the home.

c) To determine to what extent mothers' assessment of symptoms and choice of treatment options aid or impede taking biomedically appropriate decisions in young children's illness episodes.

Focus group discussions, using a short topic guide, were conducted among mothers from different socio-economic backgrounds and community leaders of the area. The following topics were discussed:

- mothers' perceptions and beliefs about the types and causation of common acute symptoms in children under five;
- factors mothers take into consideration when rating symptoms 'serious enough' to warrant treatment outside the home;
- treatment options that are available outside the home, and factors influencing their choice among them;
- mothers' perceptions and interpretations of a satisfactory treatment outcome.

Participants were recruited in five groups, each comprising 6–10 discussants, and each homogenous in background. They included: a) professional women: b) market/small business women: c) housewives: d) female youths; and e) mixed male and female community leaders. Most participants were parents, including some of the 'youth' participants ('youth' covered the age group 15–20). Detailed written transcripts were taken of each discussion by one of the moderators, while the second moderator concentrated on promoting active discussion of the topics. The planned tape recording of discussions did not take place due to objections raised by several participants. Analysis was carried out based on the methods used by Krueger (1988). Participants were from a mixture of tribes, although the majority were Baganda, the numerically dominant tribe in the Kamwokya area.

Participants seemed to welcome the opportunity to discuss acute illnesses of young children. They participated eagerly in the discussions, sharing their anxieties regarding the formal health system in general and their concern about the ineffective communication between mothers and health workers in particular. At the end of each discussion, participants posed their own questions about childhood conditions, mostly voicing myths about symptoms of acute illness and the role of modern medicine in curing culturally specific '*kiganda* diseases'. Questions asked reflected the community's desire to acquire more knowledge about these symptoms with a view to reducing the harm they cause.

Findings

Common perceptions and belief about acute symptoms in young children

Participants spoke of five common acute symptoms/illnesses which affect young children: measles, diarrhoea and vomiting, fever, coughs and convulsions. Although fever and coughs were cited as the most frequent symptoms, the three most feared were measles, diarrhoea and vomiting, and convulsions, in that order. Other serious but less common symptoms included refusal to eat, skin rashes and 'false teeth'. 'False teeth' is well conceptualized by the community and believed to be a serious condition. The discussions of 'false teeth' generated a lot of anxiety among the participants because, as they explained, many modern health workers did not want to believe that such a condition existed. The illness is commonly perceived as a cause of several conditions in children between the age of three months and two years. The symptoms of 'false teeth', which usually include diarrhoea, are believed to lead to fever, convulsions and death, if not treated promptly (Anguyo, 1993; Bwengye, 1989). The signs used to diagnose 'false teeth' are the normal erupting of primary canines in the lower jaw of young children. The scientific explanation given is that dehydration, caused by diarrhoea, dries the gums, making canine teeth inside the gums more pronounced and the gums pale (Bwengye, 1989). Frequently, the treatment is extraction of the milk teeth believed to be 'false' by traditional practitioners using pointed knives, sharpened bicycle spokes or even finger nails (Anguyo, 1993). Modern medicine is believed to be useful only in treating the complications of the condition, such as stopping excessive bleeding or infection of the wounds after extraction.

From the discussions, it was clear that mothers do not differentiate clearly between illness and symptom. In Luganda, both are expressed by one word *endwadde*. Here, therefore, the words 'symptom' and 'illness' are used interchangeably. It is common for people in the community to refer to a sickness of the head, chest, stomach, etc., relating illnesses to the felt anatomical distribution of pain rather than its cause.

Measles (*olukusese*) is an illness which is very much feared because of its severity and because it is a frequent cause of death in young children. These mothers were not very sure about what causes measles, but were firmly aware that it is contagious.

Measles just comes. It can spread to the whole village.

Mothers know that measles can occur in infancy, when the child is just beginning to sit up and that it tends to be more severe in younger infants than in older children. Measles is so feared that it is often not referred to by its name but by more grandiose names such as *Omulangira,* translated as 'the Prince.' The reasons given for fearing measles can be summarized in the words of the housewives group.

It hides in the body. It is contagious. It is not easy to treat. It is associated with many other illnesses like colds and fever. When it is about to be cured, it brings terrible fever which can kill the child.

They seemed to feel that there was very little they could do to prevent it: a lot of emphasis was put on treating the condition, with little mention of how to prevent it. This can be attributed to gaps in knowledge about the value of immunization. Mothers do, however, have adequate knowledge about the infectious nature of the condition, and about some of the factors which contribute to its severity.

Diarrhoea and vomiting (*okudukana n'okusesema*), commonly referred to in combination, were described as affecting infants and young children under three years of age. Participants felt they were serious conditions because they rapidly make children weak and can lead to sudden death. Diarrhoea and vomiting were much feared because it was difficult for a mother to ensure that her child retained either food or medicines. In Uganda, diarrhoea is referred to as a single illness, unlike in certain other African countries where it is known and referred to as as many as eight illnesses (Yoder, 1989). This at least simplifies the task of translating health education messages, in that it is not necessary to choose between several terms.

Participants believed that common causes of diarrhoea were poor hygiene (children eating dirty things, poor sanitation and garbage disposal), poorly prepared food (poorly cooked or containing a lot of fat), and worm infestations. Other causes they considered important included bottle feeding or not breast-feeding infants, poor child care, leaving children in the care of very young house-girls while the mothers go out to work, and teething. On this evidence, mothers' perceptions of the causes of diarrhoea and vomiting in young children correspond closely to those of modern medicine. They also recognize the potential dangers of the condition and are aware of some of the ways of preventing it.

However, in many Ugandan traditions, especially among the Baganda, diarrhoea in young children is (also) considered to be due to a number of behavioural errors in marriage and conjugal ceremonies, 'false teeth' (see below) and the onset of pregnancy in the mother (Namboze, 1983). While discussants in this study did not entirely dismiss these traditional causes of diarrhoea, they put more emphasis on scientific causes of the condition. One possible explanation is that traditional beliefs are less strongly adhered to in urban communities because of the influence of education and frequent interactions with modern health services. Another is that they were aware of, and responding to, the biomedical status of the seminar facilitator.

Convulsions (*okwesüka*) in children cause a lot of fear among mothers because a convulsing child is considered a dying child. In addition, spirits and witchcraft are believed to be common underlying causes of convulsions. Convulsions are also feared because they can develop into epilepsy. Participants explained that when convulsions occur in young children, they are sometimes accompanied by very high fever and in many cases it was difficult to distinguish convulsions from malaria and other causes of fever. When convulsions occur with fever, the condition is referred to as *eyabwe*, meaning 'that sickness of theirs' referring to its frequent occurrence in children. Other perceived causes of convulsions included poverty and delay in seeking adequate treatment for fevers; the use of drugs past their expiry date to treat fever; and the combination of high fever and poor nutrition.

Mothers' beliefs about the nature and causes of convulsions are a mixture of the scientific and the traditional. Convulsions is one symptom where traditional causes are believed to be more important, even though the role of malaria and other fevers is recognized. Other studies of health and culture in Ganda society reported similar findings (Namboze, 1983). In some cases even if malaria is known to be an immediate cause of convulsions, the possibility that spirits and witchcraft caused the malaria which leads to convulsions is not ruled out. Fever (*omusujja*) was reported as the symptom most commonly affecting all children, regardless of age. Among its specific causes are malaria, diarrhoea, measles and coughs. Other associated factors included poor child care, poor nutrition, drinking unboiled water, presence of stagnant water and mosquitoes and neglected wounds. Generally, fever was so common in children that mothers worried about it only when it was unusually high.

Coughs (*okukolola* or *ekifuba*) were reported to be a very common acute symptom, especially in children attending nursery school. Some of the important causes were listed as dust, especially in the dry season; children infecting each other; overcrowding in houses; and poor ventilation of houses. They explained that some parents neglect to treat their children when they have coughs and these children become a perpetual source of infection to other children. Many participants pointed out that the infection in coughs was air-borne. On the whole, a cough is like fever in that mothers do not pay much attention to it until it becomes serious.

Home treatment of acute symptoms in children

When a child becomes ill, the mother may seek advice from several sources and by a variety of methods. The first step is usually home medication, based on local beliefs about the illness and the advice of friends; as a rule mothers try some form of home treatment before they seek treatment outside the home. Many symptoms are treated with herbal baths and drinks. Buying drugs from the drug shops is a common first step in the home treatment of most of the acute symptoms (see Chapter 7).

Very often the mother asks a shopkeeper for specific drugs, which she then administers in the home. If she is uncertain, however, she may explain the symptoms and condition of the child to the shop assistant who may or may not have any medical training and who then hands out drugs for the child. In the latter case, home treatment is combined with treatment sought outside the home. Whatever the distinction between them, it is important to note that drug shops are a vital link in the search for treatment for acutely sick children, and should be more specifically targeted for training or upgrading the quality of care they offer.

Diarrhoea is often treated in the home with a combination of home remedies and modern medicine. Oral fluids (herbal, fruit juices and salt solutions) are given for both diarrhoea and vomiting. A variety of cereal mixtures or extracts, such as rice water and wheat flour mixed with cold water, are also said to be given to children suffering from diarrhoea. Some foods, such as ripe bananas and orange juice, are deliberately withheld when a child has diarrhoea. Breastfeeding normally continues despite the diarrhoea, although other types of milk may be withheld if it becomes very severe. Mothers who can afford it will buy modern medicine, usually antibiotics such as Cotrimaxazole or other antimicrobial drugs such as Metronidizole, from drug shops if the diarrhoea does not respond to other treatments. Similar enquiries in other developing countries yielded very similar findings (Levine, 1992).

The attribution of severe diarrhoea to 'false teeth' does not help mothers to appreciate or take appropriate preventive and therapeutic measures for the diarrhoea. The accepted therapeutic procedure of extracting normal young children's teeth, without anaesthesia, leads to many children suffering from pain, bleeding, wound sepsis or damage of the underlying gums and the permanent canines and subsequent failure of the eruption of permanent canines.

Fever will first be treated with herbal baths and drinks. A bitter herb (*omululuza*) is often given if the fever is thought to be due to malaria. Children with high fever may be steamed (covered with a blanket over steaming herbs) or tepid sponged. Aspirin and anti-malarials such as chloroquine or quinine are bought from a drug shop and may be administered to begin with, or given with or after administering herbal medicine.

Measles had a variety of home treatments, which include smearing the body with sheep fat, and giving the child animal fat (sheep) preparations, fish especially *enkejje*, honey, raw eggs, and fruit juices. Herbal drinks and baths made from different roots are prepared, and in cattle-keeping tribes such as the Iteso and Karamajong, cow's urine is used for bathing or smearing the patient. A number of food items such as meat and salt are withheld from children suspected of having measles. Aspirin and Cotrimaxazole bought from drug shops are given. More often than not, measles is treated with both herbal and modern medicines because of people's fear of it.

Convulsions, although one of the most feared conditions, are often treated in the home. The implication is a potential danger of mothers delaying or not seeking appropriate treatment for convulsing children. The reason given for avoiding modern health facilities in this case is that convulsions are thought to be due to traditional causes and therefore not likely to respond to modern methods of treatment. Also some mothers consider injections dangerous when the child has convulsions. Bitter herbs are given to drink; they can also be smoked or put in a steam bath for a convulsing child. Even anti-malarials such as quinine are sometimes given. Other remedies reported include crushed onions put on a child's nostrils or given to the child to drink. On the whole home treatment is unlikely to lead to proper management of the convulsions or their underlying causes.

Cough is the least treated symptom. A variety of local herbs is used, usually by cooking the roots and/or leaves and making them into cough mixtures. Raw eggs and honey are given where the cough becomes difficult to get rid of. Eventually, if it becomes serious enough mothers buy cough mixtures from drug shops.

The findings show that, generally, home treatment for most of these symptoms is a combination of herbal remedies and modern medicine bought from drug shops. Mothers who are pressed for both time and money do not, on the whole, seek help outside the home until these home treatments have proved useless. It is clear that some remedies are beneficial, such as Oral Rehydration Salts and fluids for diarrhoea, but many are either uncertain in effect or harmless (as observed by Namboze, 1983). Some practices are undesirable: withholding nutritious foods from sick children and thus depriving them of the essential nourishment required for recovery is an obvious example, and the administration of unprescribed drugs, especially antibiotics and anti-malarials, may be medically unnecessary or insufficient for full treatment of the conditions.

Factors mothers consider in determining severity of symptoms
Participants identified general as well as specific factors which indicate the severity of symptoms, but agreed that the newborn period was assessed using a slightly different combination of factors. Mothers seek help outside

the home when their sick child fails to respond to home treatment, especially when the condition gets worse, but also when there are no signs of improvement. According to our findings, it is common practice to allow 2 to 3 days of home treatment before looking elsewhere, although the time allowed for different symptoms may vary.

The persistence of symptoms throughout the day or/and night is observed as one of the danger signs.

At times a child with fever may not be taken to hospital because the child may be well during the day, getting serious at night, but if a child is hot throughout the night and morning, mothers take them to hospital.

Refusal to feed was taken as a cardinal sign, especially in very young infants. *If a child refuses to take anything at all, I would take him to a clinic or a hospital.*

The presence of a chronic or any other known debilitating condition is often taken into consideration in determining whether the child should be treated outside the home. There was general consensus among participants that children who had chronic diseases like asthma and sickle cell disease are usually rushed to health units when they fall sick.

While mothers did not notice any differences in the way acute symptoms affected children of different sexes, they believed that age is important in determining the severity of symptoms. Generally, all symptoms are thought to be more severe in young infants than in older children, while some conditions like 'false teeth' are known to affect only infants and very young children. Most participants considered the newborn period as posing special problems and they admitted that danger from these acute symptoms in the newborn is more difficult for them to assess accurately. They noted that well babies often become seriously ill within hours and that deterioration is rapid. This was a problem particularly in babies born prematurely (low birth-weight infants).

Factors taken into consideration for each of the symptoms to be serious enough to warrant seeking treatment outside the home are summarized in Table 8.1. Singly or in combination, these factors were described as major criteria for determining the seriousness of the symptoms.

In the case of measles, mothers were more likely to seek help if their children had persistently high temperatures. Also help would be sought if there was bad diarrhoea and/or vomiting, if the child developed a severe sore mouth, making it difficult for him to feed, and if there was a persistent dry cough, interfering with normal rest and sleep.

Children with diarrhoea and vomiting would be rated as having severe forms if they developed sunken eyes. This was said to be the most recognized and feared sign of severe diarrhoea. The duration of diarrhoea was also important if it lasted more than a week. Other factors used to rate the severity of diarrhoea included the development of severe general weakness, the loss of normal skin elasticity and the passing of very little urine. The latter three factors were described by the professional women's group as useful criteria for assessing severity. Regarding vomiting, weakness and

Table 8.1 *Factors considered in assessing the severity of symptom or illness*

SYMPTOM	Factors considered
Measles:	• persistent high fever • presence of severe diarrhoea and vomiting • severe sore mouth • presence of severe persistent cough
Diarrhoea and vomiting	• eyes become sunken • duration of diarrhoea exceeding one week • child becomes very weak • loss of skin elasticity • child passes very little urine
Convulsions:	• when occurs with very high fever • sudden development in a child who was well
Fever:	• steadily rising temperatures • convulsions develop • presence of deep fast breathing • child becomes confused
Cough:	• difficulty in breathing • child cries when coughing • associated with high fever • associated with vomiting • presence of wheezing • persistent dry cough interfering with sleep
Newborn:	• refusal to feed • develops vomiting • difficulty in breathing • crying excessively • restlessness and not sleeping well

failure to retain food were much more important signs of severity.

Vomiting makes the child very weak. It becomes more serious when the child vomits whatever it is given, in the way of food and drugs. You need to take such a child to hospital.

The danger signs for fever included a persistent and steadily rising fever, the development of convulsions, the child becoming confused and, in younger infants, the presence of deep fast breathing. Because fever is one of the most common acute symptoms most mothers assess the severity of a fever using the above factors before seeking help outside the home.

A cough is very common in young children, and mothers worry if it is associated with difficulty in breathing, the presence of a high fever and if the child cries when coughing, indicating presence of pain or severe discomfort. Other factors which may be considered include the presence of a wheeze, if the cough is associated with vomiting, or if it is persistently dry and irritating and interferes with the normal rest and sleep of the child.

Any of these same factors might be used to assess the symptoms in a newborn baby. Participants felt that during this period, help would be sought outside the home if babies refused to feed, had difficulty in breathing, cried excessively, became restless and had persistent vomiting.

There is a high level of consistency in the way symptoms are assessed by mothers. A number of these factors are signs of severity used in standard medical practice as indicators for mothers to seek treatment from health units particularly those listed in the case of a newborn and for diarrhoea and vomiting (Table 8.1).

But it is important that some of the factors mentioned occur in fairly advanced stages of illness, such as sunken eyes and the child passing very little urine in the case of diarrhoea. This may partly explain why help is sought too late for some symptoms and would lead to late presentation at health units. In some cases, the medically most critical signs recommended for the recognition of severe symptoms, such as chest indrawing for a cough and frequency of stools in diarrhoea, were never mentioned.

It was not clear to what extent mothers can distinguish the legitimate signs of severity of symptoms for seeking help from those which are less important. For example, in the case of a cough, it is not very clear to what extent mothers can distinguishish a cough and cold from pneumonia. None of the signs listed, including difficulty in breathing, are specific for lower respiratory infection (pneumonia), for which WHO recommends seeking treatment from health units (*ARI News*, 1989). Furthermore, mothers using the blanket term 'difficulty in breathing' may not be able to distinguish chest indrawing from fast breathing.

The study also shows that mothers give special priority to seeking help for the newborn and children known to have chronic diseases, and that they recognize the role and importance of nutrition in recovery and will seek help immediately when a child is not feeding.

Health education messages need to be more specific and information more focused on danger signs for each of these symptoms to be made clear to mothers. If the views of the people are known, messages can be developed not only to help mothers recognize the danger signs, but also to help them take appropriate measures. In addition, understanding the reasons why and when mothers seek or do not seek help for their children can be applied to designing health services which are more relevant and effective.

Treatment options and factors influencing choice of treatment

When a child's symptoms become serious enough to warrant seeking treatment outside the home, the family may seek advice from several sources and try a variety of treatments (see also Chapters 7 and 10). Mothers accept the diagnosis and advice that make the most sense to them.

The study showed that both traditional and modern types of health sources were consulted. Mothers sometimes consult and use both services concurrently or they may consult one first and, if it fails, they will then consult the other.

Some people start with medical units; when they fail, the mother may go to a traditional healer.

The choice between modern and traditional services is greatly influenced by the way they and their families perceive and describe the symptoms.

Findings from this study reflected the complex nature of health needs and the extent to which people use both systems.

In the modern sector, the study revealed that there is great variation in personal preferences for the choice of the specific modern health facility for each of the different symptoms. The source of treatment for modern health care included private clinics and government health units and hospitals. Advice from other people on the best place to go to was important, but many participants stressed the fact that mothers would go to where they expected to obtain the maximum attention for their sick children. Because of this, many mothers will choose to go to a unit where they know someone who will assist them to be attended to quickly and to ensure that the best care is given.

Numerous other factors were described. Major among them are availability, affordability, and the quality and acceptability of the care and services given. The distance to a health unit was important. Private clinics are the nearest, some of them being within Kamwokya parish. Where hospital care is desired, mothers consult the government and private hospitals which are nearest to them. Access to cash enabled mothers to consult paying clinics and hospitals in town; these were preferred to government units because the waiting time before the child was attended to was much shorter. Where cash was a constraint, Mulago, the government hospital, was consulted because, as they explained, the costs were likely to be much lower. But the fear of being admitted to hospital kept some mothers from taking their children to hospital in the first place.

Sometimes you may be admitted, but without anyone to attend to your home. You may have five other children left at home.

Concerning the quality of care, paying units were considered to offer better quality services overall. Shortage of drugs at Mulago Hospital was one reason for mothers not taking children there if they could afford to pay private clinics or hospitals. On the other hand, participants explained that if more technical procedures were expected such as intravenous fluids or if the child was very sick and admission was anticipated, mothers would go to the big hospitals where such services could be offered. Very young babies (newborns) were preferably taken to hospital rather than clinics since mothers were more certain to have them attended to there by a doctor.

Discussion of traditional healers showed that mothers consult them primarily when they suspect evil causes. *There is a lot of evil in people nowadays. So when I suspect witchcraft as a cause, I will consult a traditional healer.* Some symptoms or conditions are known to be handled better, or only, by traditional healers, such as a patient who is confused and talks nonsense, children with epilepsy or with serious convulsions, and 'false teeth'. Participants explained that false teeth were among the symptoms ignored or rejected in modern medical units and were therefore necessarily taken to a traditional healer.

The majority of mothers anyway consult traditional healers if their sick child fails to improve with treatment from a modern health clinic or hospital. In some cases, this may lead to mothers 'running away' from hospitals. Participants recognized that failure to respond to treatment given in a modern medical facility may be due to incomplete treatment or poor feeding (poor nutritional status) of the child. In many cases traditional healers are seen as a second choice, and there are a few mothers who do not like to take their children to traditional healers at all. Many mothers preferred to take children with measles or convulsions only to traditional healers. Yet others described themselves rushing to hospital at the first indication of convulsions.

When the eyes of the child change you just rush to hospital. You may even forget to dress yourself.

On the whole mothers consult a combination of modern and traditional medicine sources to ensure a successful outcome for the treatment of their children. Treatments are also combined when one type fails or if the cause/nature of the symptom is thought to be a mixture of both traditional and modern causes. Very dangerous illnesses such as measles are more often than not treated with combinations to guarantee a successful outcome.

With measles if you do not put in a lot of effort the child dies.

In the case of 'false teeth' a combination of treatment sources has become the norm. The child is taken to the traditional tooth extractor and afterwards to the clinic to stop excessive bleeding. Also in the case of coughs, both modern and herbal medicines are given fairly routinely.

What we want is to cure our children. It is not good to depend on one type.

Mothers also change from one kind of treatment source to another. Reasons given for changing from one health unit to another include mistreatment by health staff or when unsatisfactory treatment is obtained. Some hospitals have a better reputation for the treatment of specific symptoms, so that friends advise them to change. In other cases, mothers change hospitals when they become scared at the rate at which other children are dying. And in paying hospitals, quite simply mothers may have to change because of inability to meet the cost of care.

In the case of traditional healers, mothers will change from one to another when they are unhappy with the way the traditional healer has diagnosed and/or treated the sick child. Again, certain traditional healers have specific conditions they are known to handle specially well and mothers may be advised which one to consult. And, as in the modern sector, the money or other costs of some traditional healers is so high that the mother is forced by circumstance to change from one to another.

Perception of treatment outcomes

The study revealed that most mothers considered good recovery to have occurred when the sick child gained appetite, began to play well, put on weight and became happy and laughed. Of these general signs of recovery, gaining a good appetite and being able to play were considered the most important, but amelioration or disappearance of the original symptoms was also taken into account. For example, a cough is considered to be improving when the child stops coughing at night and the cough becomes wet or loose. Reduction in frequency was a specific sign of improvement in diarrhoea, and regaining normal eye position was seen as a sign of recovery.

The eye of the child could have gone in, but you may recognize them getting back to normal.

Recovery or improvement is expected to be at different speeds: fever would be expected to have improved in one to three days, convulsions should improve immediately, diarrhoea and vomiting should reduce in one day, and measles is allowed five days to one week. But participants were aware that in illnesses such as measles it is difficult to predict whether conditions are improving or not.

A child with measles may seem to be recovering, but may get fever suddenly and this may take the child.

Respondents' recommendations for improvements in caring for sick children
The following recommendations and suggestions for improving the health status of children were made by the various groups. A number of these recommendations were directed to mothers and their families and others were directed to health workers and health units.

- More specific health education on good child-rearing skills, and on how to take care of sick children, should be given to communities, targeting parents and those who look after young children.
- Mothers should be encouraged to take their children for immunization, to practise good personal and environmental hygiene and to feed their children well in order to reduce the frequency and severity of any of the symptoms discussed.
- Mothers should seek help from health units promptly before the symptoms become too severe, and the treatment prescribed should be completed. Sick children should not be left in the care of young house-girls; mothers should look after children when they fall sick.
- Health workers should carry out more effective counselling of mothers who bring sick children to them. They should show concern and attend promptly to the sick.
- Health units, especially government units, should be better equipped and staffed to be able to offer quality care to sick children.

The recommendations made by the women and community leaders imply that this urban community, at least, realizes that solutions to the problems of child health rest not only with the formal health services but also with the mothers, the families and the community. The participants were quite silent on how the traditional healers and herbal medicine could meet some of the health challenges posed by sick children. Although the community strongly believe in the positive role which traditional medicine plays in the provision of health care, they do not look for change in the traditional system but rather in the modern health system, to bring about the desired improvements in health provision. This is an aspect which can be positively exploited in order make improvements in health provision.

Conclusions and Recommendations

Urban mothers recognize measles, diarrhoea and vomiting, convulsions, fever and coughs as the most common acute symptoms/illnesses that affect young children below the age of five. Their perceptions and beliefs about the causes of these symptoms/illnesses often influence why, when and where they seek help for the treatment of sick children. Usually the first step is to administer some form of home treatment using traditional remedies and/or drugs, bought directly from the drug shops.

Failure to respond to home treatment, refusal to feed and symptoms occurring in a newborn baby were the most general factors in determining help being sought outside the home. Cultural beliefs are a major cause of delay in seeking the right help for the sick child, a factor which directly contributes to the high morbidity and mortality from these conditions.

Although mothers can identify some legitimate signs of severity for each of these symptoms or illnesses, there were knowledge gaps in their ability to distinguish the really dangerous stages from the less dangerous ones, and this affects the decisions they take to seek help. The commonly recognized danger signs relate to fairly advanced stages which lead to delay in seeking help.

The choice of the source of treatment is greatly influenced by cultural beliefs about the cause of the illness and the accepted treatment of the symptom, together with the availability, affordability and acceptability of the services offered. The most common reason for combining traditional and modern medical treatment is to increase the chances of curing the condition.

The two most important signs of recovery are resuming normal feeding and resuming normal play. Mothers recognize the role and importance of a good diet, proper child care and keeping the environment clean, and to a less extent immunization, in preventing these symptoms and ensuring rapid recovery in the case of sick children.

These summary observations allow two general recommendations and one specific one to be made. The general points are (i) that health messages targeted to mothers and child carers should be more specific and comprehensive in the areas of good child rearing, care of the sick child, the role of immunization and the importance of ensuring good personal and environmental hygiene; and (ii) that there is need to improve the quality of care in government health units and in particular to improve the communication between providers and carers. Specifically, (iii) alternative health providers such as shopkeepers, traditional healers, etc., should be specifically targeted for training as a way of improving services to meet the enormous demands for health care in these emergency situations. (The same recommendation is made in respect of STD treatment at the end of Chapter 9).

Nine

Private Disease
Perception & Management
of STD

FRANK KAHARUZA
& OTHERS

This chapter brings together a number of different perspectives on the perception and management of sexually transmitted diseases (STD), and their relation to HIV (which is itself, in this setting, most often sexually transmitted).

The first section is an introductory summary of the now extensive general literature on links between them — i.e. between HIV/AIDS and certain other forms of sexually transmitted infection.

The second section, researched and written by a biomedical clinician with specialist experience of STD in Uganda (Dr Frank Kaharuza), is geographically and analytically more focused. It reviews the situation in the country as a whole, and then reports the results of detailed interviews with those who provide treatment for STD in Kamwokya. The respondents for this section were previously interviewed for the Treatment Sources Survey (described in Chapter 6), during which they identified themselves as 'regularly' or 'occasionally' treating STD patients.

The third section changes the perspective to treatment seekers rather than providers. It uses the results of interviews and group discussions, carried out with Kamwokya residents of various social and age/sex categories, to map laypersons' views of how STD is and/or should be managed in the local context. The distinction between ideal and normal strategies, which is referred to in other chapters on treatment seeking, is made especially sharp by the elements of shame and moral failure associated with these infections. It is emphasized that these social aspects, as much as any constraints of money, time or information, impede the sufferer from getting effective treatment; and that women, who are most strongly and most painfully stigmatized in this regard, are particularly prone to delay treatment.

Finally, an appendix to the chapter lists a glossary of local terms for STD, and the signs interpreted by local people as symptoms of venereal infection 'serious enough' to warrant treatment outside the home.

Links Between HIV and STD

Because in Africa the transmission of the HIV virus occurs primarily via heterosexual intercourse it has been classified as one of the 20 or more sexually transmitted diseases (STDs) currently known to be present there (Prual *et al.*, 1991). Beyond this bio-social classification, however, a number of linkages between HIV and other STDs are significant. Most important are the associations between STDs, primarily genital ulcer diseases (GUDs), and susceptibility to HIV infection, since they have serious implications for intervention. This brief review focuses on data collected in the eastern and southern regions of Africa where the STD and AIDS epidemics follow a pattern distinct from Europe and the USA on the one hand and from Asia on the other.

The literature concerned with the association between HIV and the other STDs is roughly divided into two types: studies and reviews focusing on issues of pathology – i.e. on ways in which GUDs and other STDs may facilitate the transmission of HIV – and a smaller body of data which considers the social and behavioural connections. Both aspects are relevant here.

By the mid-1980s researchers began to be aware of the association between current or past history of STD and infection with the virus that causes AIDs (e.g. Quinn *et al.*, 1986; Piot and Laga, 1988; Kreiss *et al.*, 1988). It is now generally agreed that STDs that cause ulceration of the genitals facilitate the transmission of HIV. The primary reasons for this are that GUDs disrupt the integrity of the genital mucosa, creating open lesions which permit the penetration of the virus (Chirgwin *et al.*, 1989).

Research has also been conducted exploring the associations between other types of STD and the transmission of HIV. One study found an *insignificant* correlation between gonorrhea and HIV transmission among Nairobi prostitutes (Kreiss *et al.*,1988); and another reported that men having GUD and recent prostitute contact were more likely to seroconvert (i.e. to become HIV+) than were men with urethritis, another common but non-ulcerative STD (Piot *et al.*, 1988). An earlier study, again with a population of Nairobi sex workers, showed a positive correlation between past history of GUD and/or a positive syphilis test and HIV (Piot *et al.*, 1987).

But because some degree of trauma to the genital tract is a common feature of most STDs, these other infections are also implicated in the transmission of HIV. The PANOS Dossier (1990) on women and AIDs, for example, affirms that a woman is *more* likely to be infected with HIV by a seropositive man with GUD than by one without; and that if she has GUD a woman is more likely to pass on her infection to her partner. But it asserts also that non-ulcerative STDs are important, especially for women. The Dossier contends that some studies found HIV+ women more likely to have had an STD without ulcers (e.g. cervical infections, gonorrhea or chlamydia) than with them. They stress the importance of acquiring a greater understanding of STDs likely to be more significant for women – i.e. those without ulcers and those that cause painless sores. The Dossier discusses the point that genital sores or discharge are more likely to be noticed in a man and unseen or unremarked in a woman. The biological/pathological links between HIV and other STDs illuminate social and behavioural issues that have yet to be as thoroughly studied. Much of the research that has been conducted in this arena indicates that lessons learned about the pathways of transmission of other STDs in Africa apply also to HIV, since they will all follow the same pathways of transmission and are spread by the same sexual behaviours (Klovdahl, 1985; Hunt, 1989). Because GUD may be antecedent or co-incident with HIV it is widely agreed that adequate treatment and diagnosis of GUD/STD should have a major impact on the spread of AIDS, and the control of GUD in particular could be an important focus for AIDS intervention. These writers warn that over-emphasis on AIDS has diverted resources from STD management which may, in fact, be more critical and more cost-effective in the long run (Lal and Kennedy, 1988). There is nonetheless widespread agreement that sexually transmitted diseases are a sign of unsafe sexual practice and a factor in vulnerability to HIV infection; and that prevention or reduced incidence of STD and effective early treatment of any infection will reduce the incidence of HIV.

The STD Situation in Uganda: Treatment Provision

Sexually transmitted diseases have long been common in Uganda (Lombolt and Nsibambi, 1972). As recently as 1988, STD, excluding AIDS, was the sixth commonest diagnosis in Ugandan hospitals and among adult male patients attending private clinics (Twa-Twa *et al.*, 1988). STD syndromes then identified were:

Genital discharge	40%
Genital Ulcer Disease	21%
Pelvic Inflammatory disease	15.4%
Bubo (*Lymphogranuloma venereum*)	0.9%
Genital Warts	0.53%
Others	2.16%

The most common presentations of STD that are taught to Ugandan health providers are:
(i)   discharge from the penis or vagina
(ii) sores or wounds on the genitals of men or women (genital ulcer diseases)
(iii) abnormal growth on the genitals in either sexes (genital warts)
(iv) abnormal swellings of lymph nodes in the groin (buboes)
(v)   AIDS (Kalibala *et al.*, 1992).

A treatment source survey was carried out as part of the ethnographic survey in Kamwokya II (Chapter 6). The specific objectives were:
(i)   to estimate the incidence of STDs treated by the informal health sector;

(ii) to identify diagnostic procedures and management of STDs being used in the informal health sector;

(iii) to identify the various treatment options for STDs being given by the informal health sector. The informal health sector was defined to include everything outside formal government facilities − i.e. all the health-care providers that practise traditional medicine (spiritual healers, diviners and herbalists), clinics and drug shops that all sell over-the-counter drugs.

Table 9.1 *STD management by different providers*

STD Treatment	Clinics n=14		Drug shops n=13		Healers n=9		Herbalists n=6	
Syphilis (Kabootongo)								
Regular	9	64%	3	23%	7	78%	1	17%
Occasional	1	7%	5	38%	–	–	1	17%
Never	2	14%	4	31%	2	22%	4	66%
Gonorrhoea (Enjoka ensajja; Enziku)								
Regular	6	43%	2	15%	2	22%	–	–
Occasional	4	29%	3	23%	2	22%	–	–
Never	2	14%	7	54%	4	44%	6	100%
Genital Ulcers (Amabwa)								
Regular	7	50%	1	8%	4	44%	–	–
Occasional	1	7%	2	15%	1	11%	1	17%
Never	3	21%	9	69%	4	44%	5	83%
Other STD								
Regular	1	7%	–	–	4	44%	1	17%
Occasional	–	–	3	23%	2	22%	–	–
Never	2	14%	–	–	2	22%	4	66%
Lymphogranuloma venereum (Lwekika)								
Regular	5	35%	–	–	2	22%	–	–
Occasional	2	14%	4	31%	1	11%	1	17%
Never	5	35%	8	62%	4	44%	5	83%
STDs Men								
Regular	3	21%	–	–	3	33%	1	17%
Occasional	–	–	–	–	–	–	1	17%
Never	3	21%	12	92%	5	56%	4	66%
STDs Women only								
Regular	3	21%	–	–	3	33%	1	17%
Occasional	–	–	–	–	–	–	1	17%
Never	4	28%	12	92%	5	56%	4	66

Selection criteria for the treatment providers interviewed were:

(i) those who reported treating STDs

(ii) those who expressed willingness to be involved in future studies

(iii) those who were available at the time of contact for this survey.

There were 27 traditional healers identified by the ethnographic survey research assistants; of these 8 were not interviewed in that survey. Thirteen of the remaining 19 reported occasionally or regularly treating STDs; 11 of these had expressed willingness to participate further in any related research. Six healers and herbalists were then selected from the eleven and interviewed. Three clinics out of the fourteen in the area were also to be visited and nurses or health-care providers interviewed. (An assumption was made that clinics relied on treatment guidelines set by the formal medical sector). A pre-visit was carried out to make appointments with the selected herbalists, healers and clinic managers and to secure their agreement to participate. Two invited the researcher to attend an STD healing session, but he could not do so as the patients were very few. For similar reasons, no drug shop operators were interviewed on the specific question of STD (but see Chapter 6). The National STD Control Programme clinic was also visited as it was situated only three kilometres from the target area.

Interviews were carried out by the present author in Luganda with the healers, and in English at the clinics. A topic guide was used, and the average duration of an interview was one hour.

STD is an illness It is not witchcraft.

Although a question on prevalence was asked, it was not well answered for lack of record-keeping. The STD patients were too few and far between. One healer had last treated a STD three years previously.

The commonest STD syndromes reported were syphilis, gonorrhoea, *Lyphogranuloma venereum*, and genital ulcers (see Appendix for glossary of local terms). Some of the local terminology is used interchangeably by the healers.

'Kabootongo' is the same as 'Ekiwo' – it does not allow sexual intercourse. The husband may even refuse the wife and it can lead to divorce.

Moreover, some herbalists believed that certain STDs occurred together or would lead to other STDs.

The healers/herbalists do not physically examine their patients but depend entirely on the history. The questions posed were similar by gender, except that the expected symptoms were delayed in women.

The social effects of STDs were marital instability, non-communication between husbands and wives and poor source and contact tracing.

They pretend to be very sick so they do not have sex with their partners.

Specific diseases

SYPHILIS (LOCAL NAME: *KABOOTONGO*)

The incidence of syphilis was the highest reported for any STD, with one healer reporting three patients a week and another two patients a month.

All the six healers knew something about 'syphilis'. Three of them relied on similar diagnostic symptoms. The four common themes to emerge as diagnostic features are:

(i) Skin rash (4 of the 6 healers)

The key idea was a skin rash that occurred both in women and neonates. The skin rash was described as 'similar to a measles rash or that of "*Ebisente*"' (local terminology for a common fungal infection of the skin – *Tinea corporis*).

(ii) 'Bone' infection (3 of 6)

Painful joints indicated 'syphilis of the bone'.

(iii) Genital ulcers (2 of 6)

The ulcer of syphilis was said to be red and dry and was different from *Ekiwo* which was red and discharging.

(iv) Neonatal infection (2 of 6).

The effect of syphilis on pregnancy was mentioned by two healers.

This is syphilis that is in the blood and affects women who deliver dead babies.

All those who treated syphilis did so for a prolonged period of time ranging from one month to three months. Herbal options ranged from three (from one healer) to six with another. Herbs were mixed and applied to the skin, while others were taken orally. One herbalist used herbs to determine clinical cure: a herb was given after treatment with a type of herbal mixture; cure was said to have occurred if there was no rash appearing on the body within four days of treatment.

GONORRHOEA (*'ENZIKU'*)

Four of the healers mentioned treating (or ever having treated) gonorrhoea. Such patients were very few; one reported only one a month. Female patients were commoner than male patients. Single women were more commonly seen by one healer. An important misperception was noted from one healer.

If you have Slim (HIV) you do not get gonorrhoea, if you have gonorrhoea you do not get Slim.

The key clinical features of gonorrhoea were dysuria and a pus-like discharge from the urethra or genital area. Some women presented with an associated lower abdominal pain.

All the herbalists had single, reportedly very potent, treatments; that 'never' failed. All treated their patients for only three days. Cure was said to have been achieved by one herbalist when the patients began passing thick yellow pus at the genital area.

'EKIWO' (PAINFUL GENITAL ULCERS)

The incidence was reported to be low, i.e., only about one person every 3-4 months. This condition was said to be infectious by two healers. It was also thought to be transmitted through water. One traditional healer believed it was not an STD but a 'blood-borne' disease that occurred in children who had a rash and vaginal discharge.

Four of the traditional healers each presented different symptomatology for this disease. The common themes that emerged as diagnostic parameters were:

(i) Genital ulcers (3 of 4)

(ii) Pruritus (itching) (2 of 4)

(iii) Pus discharge from the genital area (2 of 4)

Other presentations included dysuria, dyspareunia and a mass (or lump) in the perineum.

There were two treatment options reported, though one healer offered only one option.The herbs given to children for this condition were pre-chewed for the child by the parent or healer and administered directly to the child.

LYMPHOGRANULOMA VENEREUM (LWEKIKA)

All six healers had seen or treated this disease at some time. More patients were Kamwokya residents and about two per month were seen by one of the healers.

The commonest presentation was masses in the groin. Males were more commonly seen than females.Only one healer related the lumps to ulcers and two mentioned syphilis as an associated illness. One healer mentioned dysuria associated with the lump.

A herbal mixture was applied to the mass. They were expected to 'dissolve'. If they formed an abscess they were treated with a 'hot spoke' (a sharp metallic rod, usually made from a bicycle spoke heated in an open flame and introduced into the abscess).

Clinics

Of the three clinics visited, two were run by midwives. The other, run by a medical assistant, provided laboratory services as well as carrying out simple laboratory tests. The two midwives had attended sessions with STD programme doctors and were now allowed to treat STDs. Unfortunately, the information they had on STDs was rather scanty.

Although all three providers reportedly depend on a laboratory for STD diagnosis, a number of patients were treated without confirmatory tests being done, either by choice or because of lack of money for payment for these tests.

Some patients demand treatment without lab investigation. They know their symptoms so I give them treatment.

The health providers paid some attention to health education of the patients and emphasized partner treatment. It was more difficult to get partners treated where female clients were the ones who were diagnosed first. The health-care providers voiced their concern about the marital instability that could be caused by partner tracing and treatment.

Men do not agree to treatment. They go to other private clinics without their partners' knowledge.

Patients had a short waiting time in the clinics and could pay in installments.

Specific diseases

SYPHILIS

The reported incidence is high, between 3 patients a week and 3 a month. The diagnoses were made from: (i) previous clinical notes; (ii) laboratory diagnosis; (iii) clinical examination without laboratory confirmation.

Clinical features mentioned included: penile ulcers, genital ulcers, vulval itching and infection in the newborn.

Treatment followed a standard regimen, with a weekly injection of Benzathine Penicillin for three weeks. Some patients were advised on no treatment when they presented with a history of having had four injections for the same symptoms.

These patients are usually impatient. They have a tendency to move from clinic to clinic − sometimes not finishing the treatment.

A deliberate attempt to treat partners was made at one clinic. There were no records available as the midwives were previously not allowed by law to treat people with antibiotics, despite doing so in reality.

GONORRHOEA

The incidence ranged from 4 patients a week down to two a month. Most were, reportedly, Kamwokya residents.

Clinical features mentioned were a thick pus discharge, urethritis and bloody micturition. This was associated with extra-marital sex and 'party-goers' (merry-makers).

The diagnosis was supposedly made from a high vaginal swab in women and a urethral pus swab in men. The midwives had three options for referral of patients for laboratory investigation. These were suggested according to the patients' ability to pay (New Mulago, Dr Matovu's clinic, Muna's clinic) . This diagnostic procedure was carried out only when the patient could afford it.

Reported treatment options were those advocated by the STD programme, namely: Chloramphenicol, Tetracycline, Gentamicin, Erythromycin. Some patients, however, were given higher doses than those recommended.

OTHER STDS

The other STDs were mentioned only after probing. Genital ulcer disease was mentioned by two providers, one of whom simply referred such patients to Mulago Ward 12.

Genital ulcers are associated with HIV. They have tried many treatments and it simply does not go away − it simply increases, I normally send them to Ward 12 Old Mulago.

Other diseases mentioned included Trichomoniasis, Moniliasis and Buboes.

Mulago STD Clinic: Uganda STD Control Programme

The Mulago STD clinic is the main referral clinic for STD management for the Uganda STD Control Programme. Its main focus is the reduction of STD transmission through recognition and appropriate treatment of sexually transmitted diseases. The strategy of the national programme since January 1993 is to provide STD drugs and ensure their proper utilization in all health-care settings. A treatment regimen and patient management flow chart have been written and distributed to health-care workers, especially those in the formal sector.

The Mulago STD Clinic is run by two Medical Officers, three Medical Assistants, two enrolled nurses, two laboratory assistants, three registered nurses, one records officer and two STD counsellors. About ten to twenty new patients are seen every day in the clinic. A number of patients come back for follow-up and collection of results. Recently more women attend the clinic. Those from Kamwokya over the previous three months amounted to 16 out of 361 (about 4.5%). Patients are usually referred from: (i) the AIDS Information Centre; (ii) Old Mulago Outpatients Department; (iii) other hospitals; (iv) private clinics; and by (v) self-referral (usually advised by friends or relatives).

Patients are first seen and recorded by the records officer, then counselled by the counsellor and examined by the doctors or medical assistants who make a provisional diagnosis and prescribe treatment. They are sent to the laboratory for mandatory RPR (Rapid Plasma Reagin test) for syphilis and for an HIV test when requested. Simple investigations done in the lab include a wet preparation, and a Gram stain of the pus swab taken from the patients. They then go for treatment and the results are reviewed after two weeks. Confidentiality is maintained throughout all stages of the patient flow. Follow-up and contact tracing is attempted at the clinic but with rather poor results. The patients come back to the clinic or are encouraged to bring their partners to the clinic.

Sometimes when wives are brought here they are only informed (of their illness) in the counselling room (Counsellor STD clinic).

Overall, however, patients dislike attending the Mulago Clinic because of a delay in obtaining services. This delay is not in the clinic itself, but at the point of referral from the out-patient department.

Traditional healers by comparison are respected for their confidentiality and privacy.

Findings and recommendations

* The estimated reported incidence of STDs seen by each treatment provider in Kamwokya is quite significant. It varied from none to 20 a month. The commonest seen were syphilis, genital ulcer diseases, gonorrhea and buboes. STD patients were attended by all types of health providers in Kamwokya. But we know from other data (Chapter 7) that community members feel that self-treatment is the treatment of first choice, and this suggests that only complicated cases are seen by the providers.
* Despite the reported incidence of STD among hospital patients, very few actually went to the referral centre in Mulago. Community members relied on the full range of providers in Kamwokya and selected the provider according to their perception of the quality of service rendered.
* The National STD programme treatment guidelines are being used by

some of the non-government clinics. Although the diagnostic aloga-rithm is available to them, most local clinics and drug shops did not have or did not use this information.

- The traditional healers have an undefined syndrome approach to STDs which might be standardized so as to improve their diagnosis and management. Both diviners and herbalists have operated for so long that they have legitimized their service and the community respects them for it. The conspicuous absence of spiritual healing for STDs suggests their understanding of it as a biological disease.
- Treatment options should be evaluated socially as well as medically, but it is vital to determine those treatments which are beneficial and those which are harmful. Some herbs used are very effective in giving symptomatic relief, but their usefulness in disease cure requires a pharmacological study.
- Clinics and drug shops need stronger emphasis in the use of STD guidelines. Counselling should be emphasized and drugs made available in all clinics at affordable prices.
- Confidentiality and privacy should be assured by the 'modern' as they are by the traditional healers.
- Further exploratory discussions to formulate a diagnostic alogarithm for the traditional healers should be carried out. They see large numbers of patients and warrant being better informed about STD.
- Early diagnosis and referral of patients from traditional healers to formal practitioners should be encouraged, and each 'side' encouraged to co-operate more closely with the other.
- Record keeping at all levels should be facilitated so that case management, monitoring and supervision of STD might become more effective.

The STD situation in Kamwokya: Treatment Seeking

The content: summary of treatment seekers' views on STD

These brief remarks on STD treatment seekers/seeking introduce a report on the group discussions held in Kamwokya against background data from the surveys and from discussions during the course of fieldwork. It highlights the main points that local residents have made about STD and the implications of their views.

1. Residents on the whole are well-informed about STD symptomatology. With prompting they describe the various kinds of STD that are prevalent in Kamwokya, and the local names for these diseases. It is not surprising that, according to biomedical definitions, they were not 100 per cent correct all the time. They may be conflating symptoms of more than one STD in their descriptions. This may be due to the fact that it is not uncommon for someone to be infected with more than one disease at a time. It may also be that some of this information

does not come from first-hand experience but from second, or even third-hand anecdotes told by friends. Either way it is important to recognize that this is a well-informed community.

2. Each group, without prompting, expressed the conviction that 'other STDs disappeared when AIDS came'. This is clearly important to treatment seeking. The fact that AIDS is considered to be a more significant threat to health in Kamwokya is also demonstrated in the survey material. 71 per cent of those interviewed identified AIDS as a major health problem compared with 4 per cent who so identified STD.

3. Stigma – STD and the people who suffer from it are highly stigmatized in the community. Two (related) points:

(i) STDs are associated with immoral sexual behaviour. This means that a person who has an STD is seen as lacking discipline or *empisa*, a central social value in Kamwokya. This is a transgression against proper behaviour and against 'marriage', and carries heavy social penalties (or the fear of these penalties), perhaps the most severe of which for a woman is the loss of her sexual partner, especially if he is her 'husband' and therefore takes some kind of financial and emotional responsibility for her and the children he fathers with her (see Chapter 5). People feel strongly that a possible repercussion of getting an STD is public humiliation and the loss of your husband/wife.

(ii) STDs are closely associated with AIDS, itself a highly stigmatized disease for many of the same reasons, but also because of the death sentence that it carries with it. When someone gets an STD the fear that it is AIDS adds a new complication to sexual relationships.

4. Fear – This STD-AIDS association means that getting an STD is a frightening thing. Ironically, fear of AIDS is a major reason for *not* seeking treatment for a suspected STD.

Treatment and diagnosis

1. While all sources suggest that the 'big' hospitals should be the best for diagnosis and treatment, there is a general lack of confidence in them – both because of long (and public, exposed) queues and because they lack the necessary drugs. In addition, respondents complain that some doctors and nurses at Mulago demand bribes before treatment of any kind is given, and patients can end up spending more money (for inferior care) at these 'free' hospitals than at private hospitals or clinics where there are set fees for drugs and services.

2. Clinics were also favoured as places to go for diagnosis or treatment, especially a clinic that is not in the area. Most women would advise someone to go to a clinic in an area where they do not know anyone so that the fact that they have an STD does not get back to the community.

3. Most people felt that herbalists are no longer effective in the cure of STD. One of the participants in the young men's discussion, however,

said that he thought traditional healers kept confidentiality better than hospitals or clinics.

4. Self-diagnosis and self-treatment was generally felt to be the best solution (Chapter 7). If someone thinks that they have an STD they can go to a drug shop or pharmacy and get septrin or ampicillin tablets as they would if they or their child had any other kind of infection. They can then treat themselves from home privately. Only if the situation does not improve will the patient be forced to go outside the home for treatment. He/she may seek the advice of a good friend or close family member, or may just go to Mulago or any clinic outside of Kamwokya. The ideal form of treatment for STDs was generally said to be an injection (or series of injections) of antibiotics.

Why delay?

The reasons given for delaying seeking treatment outside the home were:

- fear of being told that one has AIDS
- lack of money
- inadequate services (at the 'free' hospitals)
- shyness/shame – in addition to the shame associated with these diseases, the young especially expressed a fear of mentioning 'those types of symptoms' to doctors
- the symptoms are not serious enough
- stigma – people are ashamed to be seen in the queue at an STD clinic, and are afraid that someone will tell their spouse
- ignorance/lack of education were both mentioned by young men
- some clinics insist that you bring your sexual partner(s) in for treatment and this can be a cause of embarrassment or marital difficulty for the patient.

Treatment seekers' views: notes from Focus Group Discussions

MAJOR HEALTH PROBLEMS IN KAMWOKYA

In each of the focus group discussions the moderator opened the proceedings by asking the participants to discuss the main health problems in Kamwokya. This was by way of a warm-up, and it got the participants thinking about health and illness in their community.

1. All but two of the groups identified lack of proper sanitation as being one of the more serious health problems in Kamwokya generally. The feeling was that poor drainage led to increased mosquito breeding and therefore malaria. The lack of a sewerage system was also thought to bring flies to the area which then contaminate food. Some participants also mentioned that there were too few latrines/urinals, relative to the excess of (alcohol) drinking that goes on. They said that 'drunkards' defecate and urinate anywhere, and children playing around the area get contaminated.

2. Diarrhoea and malaria (primarily in children) were also mentioned by

a majority of the groups (male youths and pregnant women did not mention these).

3. Fever was mentioned by one of the female youth groups, the pregnant women and the brewers.
4. Typhoid was mentioned by the pregnant women and the brewers.
5. The only illness mentioned by all the groups, and the one identified as the most serious in Kamwokya, was AIDS, which is seen by some as overshadowing all other diseases.

Other responses included measles (adult men), poverty (adult men and young women) and headaches (pregnant women).

PERCEPTIONS OF STDS

All groups stressed that AIDS has replaced other STDs. The following are some of their comments on this point:

Other STDs disappeared when AIDS came (young women I)

Other STDs are no longer heard of. When AIDS came, it swallowed all other STD (young women II)

Slim has replaced all other STDs and they are no longer common (pregnant women)

Since AIDS came, people no longer talk about other STDs. They just buy drugs from drug stores for self-treatment because people fear other STDs are associated with HIV (middle-aged men).

Six focus groups were identified and recruited: middle-aged men and women; young men and women; pregnant women; and local brewers.

The participants said that *other STDs like gonorrhea and syphilis used to exist but when AIDS came, those ones disappeared* (brewers);

AIDS has overshadowed other STDs (adult men);

AIDS has submerged all other diseases including STDs (young men).

Most groups remarked that there is a strong stigma now attached to STDs because of the connection between them and AIDS. It was said that whenever a person gets an STD he/she may then think that they have AIDS and will therefore 'keep quiet' about it. The association between STDs and AIDS, and the general feeling that AIDS is a much more important problem, was expressed also by the brewers who felt that there was no use in talking about other STDs because AIDS is the biggest threat of all.

This theme pervaded the discussions and is a significant factor in the treatment-seeking process.

SYMPTOMS AND SYMPTOMATOLOGY

The appendix to this chapter explores further the extent of fit between the symptoms identified by the participants of the focus group discussions for the various STDs and the biomedical definitions and symptomatology, and the nature of the common (vernacular) terms and their etiologies. Do they, for example, describe symptoms or sets of symptoms, or are they simply names given to the condition? The following note highlights similarities and differences in the responses of the various groups.

178

a) Young women's group I. Although these young women said that
'*all other STDs disappeared when AIDS came*' they conceded that '*other STDs
do exist but in a dormant manner*'. For example, one participant said:
 *Syphilis used to exist but now, even if someone has it, he will think that he has
AIDS.*
 Another remarked that
 Even gonorrhea is there but you can't know these days.
 There was some discussion about the existence and nature of the disease
called *Iwekiika (Lymphogranuloma Venereum)*. Some of the girls argued that it
is an STD that is common in the area. Others disagreed saying that it is
ania (hernia). Finally, they resolved the dispute by agreeing that if the boil
is located around the genitals, then it is sexually acquired, otherwise 'it is
something else'.
 The participants were then asked to list symptoms for each STD. They
listed symptoms for:
SYPHILIS: (rash around or on the genitals, mostly affecting women. Of two
types: one 'inborn' which is incurable, and one 'in blood' which is curable);
GONORRHEA: (difficult urination, pain in lower abdomen, genital itching,
often asymptomatic in women but easily detected by men);
IWEKIIKA (boils in the lower abdomen).

b) Young women II. The STDs identified by this group were:
GONORRHEA (skin rash, pus discharged through genitals, boils in the lower
abdomen);
SYPHILIS (two types, one that is in the bones and one that is in the blood).
The one in the blood is 'deadly' (incurable). Babies will be born deformed,
difficulty and pain in urination; and
AIDS (no symptoms listed in the transcript).

c) Pregnant women's group. Members of this group also said that
STDs other than AIDS no longer exist. Others insisted that they do exist,
but it is difficult to tell these days. They identified three STDs:
GONORRHEA (boils and pus in the genitals, pain in the lower abdomen and
when urinating);
SYPHILIS (skin rash, sores in the genitals, and genital itching);
AIDS (a person with AIDS will have all the symptoms of the other STDs
mentioned above, and that is why it is difficult to tell the difference between
a person with AIDS and someone with other STDs. But they did note
that people with AIDS always have fever, are cold in the evenings, have
headaches, diarrhoea and a cough).

d) Local brewers. This group was the most insistent that AIDS has
superseded all other STDs in the area. One participant said:
 Whoever dies, people say 'kekano' (it's the one that has killed him, meaning AIDS).
 Another participant said:
 Other STDs and other diseases have been swallowed up by AIDS. AIDS has made

people afraid to go for treatment even for other diseases. Whoever suffers from any disease is very sure that it is AIDS and therefore has no need of treatment.

In general the participants felt that because of the importance of AIDS in the community, and the fact that it has 'replaced' all other STDs, the discussion should be about AIDS alone. With some prompting, however, the discussants agreed to think about other types of STD. They too identified three types and discussed their symptoms:

SYPHILIS (if inherited, the following symptoms are found in children: difficulty in breathing, yellowish skin that tears off and itches, the umbilical cord will 'over bleed').

We are always told by the doctors that when any one delivers a baby with funny eyes (eyes with white substances or dripping eyes) 'You take that baby to hospital'.

In adults, especially men, it is not as easy to see the symptoms as it is in in children, but they do get a skin rash 'in some parts'. When asked by the moderator if there are many people in Kamwokya with the kind of skin rash described, one of the participants said: *they do exist but they are being mistaken as having AIDS.* Another said, *syphilis has existed, but when you get it now, people will say 'kamukaze' (he/she is finished).*

GONORRHEA (passing blood and pus in urine, pus and sores around the genitals). Some of the women insisted that the symptoms which used to be for gonorrhea are now symptoms for AIDS and therefore it is hard to tell whether a person is suffering from AIDS or gonorrhea.

AIDS (in addition to the symptoms mentioned above for gonorrhea and syphilis, an AIDS patient 'becomes very small' and gets diarrhoea, but some look healthy).

When you get boils that is one of the symptoms that you have AIDS.

One participant noted, *It is very difficult to tell that someone has an STD unless you are a close friend.*

e) Adult men. The men were far more graphic and detailed than the women in discussing the symptomatology of STDs. They also named several more than the women's group did, but did not discuss the symptoms of all of them. The common term used to describe STDs in general was *edwande yabuzila*, 'disease of the brave'.

GONORRHEA (*'One can find out that one has it by the time one takes when urinating. It can take the patient 40 minutes to urinate, and with much pain!* (laughter)); wounds develop in the urethra and block it. When a baby is born to parents with gonorrhea it will have pus (where?) and a child born with gonorrhea experiences problems when urinating, especially between the ages of one and three: *Such babies are always scratching their penises.* One becomes pale and loses most of the hair from one's head.

SYPHILIS (skin rash – like AIDS patients)

LWEEKIKA (boils around genitals)

They also mentioned and used the common term for non-gonococcal urethritis (*ekiwo*), and '*sores and boils in the genitals*' (herpes simplex?).

f) Younger men. The young men were also more descriptive in their discussion of STD symptoms than the women's group were. They also mentioned *Herpes zoster* (a common, though non-venereal opportunistic infection in those with HIV), and there was some disagreement as to whether or not it was an STD. One participant said that because it is a symptom of AIDS it must be an STD, but one of his colleagues pointed out that it is only a 'symptom' (of AIDS), and is not itself sexually transmitted.

GONORRHEA (difficulty in passing urine – *It can take up to 10 minutes! (laughter) One passes pus, has a nasty smell and even wets one's clothes. Urine just passes, doesn't have breaks.)*

SYPHILIS (multiple, painful and badly smelling wounds on genitals, skin rash). Two types of syphilis identified: one which is inherited – *enogga* – which new-born babies get from their infected parents. The other 'attacks the bones' and makes one extremely weak. It was said that some women who have syphilis become sterile.

LYMPHOGRANULOMA VENEREUM (difficulty in movement, frequent fevers, boils on either side of the inguinal ligament).

One participant said that some STDs cause people to look pale with a yellowish skin 'as if one has no blood', but did not specify which STD he was referring to.

WHERE SHOULD ONE GO FOR DIAGNOSIS?

A strong association between diagnosis and treatment is evident from the data. Obviously some level of self-diagnosis is the initial step in seeking treatment. Perceptions of causation are also important. Again it is evident that the connection between STDs and AIDS has an effect on how one pursues diagnosis, as does the shame and stigma attached to these illnesses.

Most of the participants felt that the 'big' hospitals should be the best place to be diagnosed because there are 'experts' there. Many felt that at clinics the doctors might not have specialized knowledge about STDs (they might, for example, be paediatricans).

The best place to go is the big hospitals like Mulago and Rubaga where you are examined thoroughly and given a prescription, though they may have no drugs, you can buy from other places (young women).

Lack of money is the other reason for choosing a big hospital:

Some people who are not able to raise money to meet the treatment bills in clinics go to hospitals because their services are supposed to be free. (young women).

Mulago Hospital, in particular, should be the best place to go because it is nearby, and the services are (at least ostensibly) free. Many participants, however, noted that there are 'no drugs' at Mulago. Patients are given a prescription or a referral which they then have to take to a pharmacy or clinic which, they said, is usually owned by the prescribing physician. Therefore, the fact that one often has to wait in long queues and will have to pay for treatment anyway once a diagnosis is made, led many to conclude that it is just as well to save yourself the time and go to a local private clinic.

The brewers mentioned herbalists as an option for diagnosis, but there was some disagreement among them on the effectiveness of 'Ganda herbs'. Most felt that these remedies used to be effective for curing STD but they no longer are. One woman said that they are effective if you believe in them. Another said that gonorrhea has no Ganda cure: '*If you try it you will die*'.

The pregnant women said that one could go to Mulago or to the AIDS Information Centre (AIC) for diagnosis, but stressed that people hide their STDs, thinking they have AIDS and therefore do not go for diagnosis. The men (both the youths and the adults) favoured self-diagnosis. The young also mentioned the big hospitals and the AIC, but said that some people go to traditional healers as well:

One can be afraid to go to a medical doctor or tell a friend, but with a traditional doctor you are not afraid to inform him/her since it is between you and the healer.

Another participant, however, said that only adults – primarily women – go to traditional healers, and that the young go to a friend or to a clinic. Others agreed that you go to a traditional healer only if you think the cause is bewitchment. If traditional cures fail, they said, most will go to hospital.

WHERE TO GO FOR TREATMENT?

The community held various views on the treatment providers. Treatment-seeking ranged from self-treatment and buying drugs from drug shops to attending traditional healers, clinics and hospitals.

Because there is a strong link between diagnosis and treatment, many initially stated that clinics were the preferred place for treatment because the necessary drugs are readily available there. The adult men mentioned that the clinics have the additional advantage of privacy. One, however, made a curious point about their costs:

Clinic owners are like traditional healers, they are interested in money – they give half the dose so that you go back again (men's group).

The young men said that Mulago is best because it is free and nearby, and because the doctors there are specialists in STD diagnosis and treatment. Some of the boys preferred clinics or traditional healers, and one mentioned the Kamwokya Catholic Church clinic where patients receive free treatment and/or a referral to Nsambya Hospital. Others in the group disagreed with this, asserting that the Church clinic has become stigmatized because it is associated with treating AIDS patients. The pregnant women said that for treating STDs one should go to a clinic or the hospital. But generally, they felt, people first self-treat with ampicillin or septrin: *It is after self-treatment has failed that people go to hospitals to seek treatment.*

The brewers were the most explicit about the treatment process. They also said that people who believe they have an STD will first self-treat (buying the drugs they think are appropriate from the drug shops or pharmacies). If that fails they will go to a clinic. Finally, if they fail to get cured at the clinic they will go to the hospital. They said, however, that most people only admit to having an STD when they are close to death. The adult men also mentioned that self-treatment might be preferred due to the STD/AIDS link, and associated stigma.

The stigma associated with STD – both in its connection with AIDS and in its own right – has an effect both on where and when treatment is sought. The brewers noted that some people are afraid to go to hospital because they may be seen queueing at the 'Skin Clinic' by friends. *It is shameful to get an STD*, said one of the women.

They said that some men will go for treatment without telling their wives that they have an STD, and fear that their wives will find out if they are seen queuing at Mulago.

People prefer clinics so as to keep their privacy and avoid stigmatization when they are found in Mulago Ward 12 (men's group).

When asked why someone should choose to self-treat, a participant in the pregnant women's group answered that there are two reasons: (i) money (she may not have the cash needed to seek treatment outside the home) and (ii) *Shyness … you feel good to treat it (the STD) from home before other people know.*

Other comments underline the same point:

These days, people go for diagnosis only as a last resort for fear of being diagnosed as having AIDS (women's group).

The best place for treatment of STD is either at home if facilities are available or at private clinics because in these places publicity is minimized (women's group).

When people see some signs of an STD like boils, they think they have AIDS and so they resort to drinking and avoid seeking treatment because they know AIDS has no cure (local brewers' group)

Even in nearby clinics, people are afraid to go there for treatment for fear of being known by friends as a person having an STD (female youth).

THE BEST FORM OF TREATMENT

Most of the participants in all the groups were agreed that injection is the best treatment for most STDs. The young men said that injections were better than tablets because they move more quickly 'through the circulatory system'. The adult men mentioned that if the STD is treated early 'tablets can be enough'

Although the possibility of treating with herbs was raised (by the adult men and the brewers) it was argued in both situations that herbs were no longer effective against STDs.

Herbs do not cure but still they temporarily kill the pain (men's group). One participant among the adult men even argued that herbs have made the diseases more resistant. The pregnant women, however, noted that there are those diseases which are curable in hospital but not by local herbs, and some are curable only by local herbs but not by Western medicine, although they did not elaborate on the specific types of disease they were referring to.

Private Disease

When you get boils now and then you know that it is AIDS. You either decide to go for treatment, knowing well that there is no cure or you do not go at all (brewers).
AIDS has made people afraid to go for treatment even for other diseases. Whoever suffers from any disease, is very sure that it is AIDS and therefore there is no need for treatment (brewers).
How can you get treatment when you don't even have money for aspirin? (brewers). *Why waste my time? Why should I go to hospital when I know I am going to get nothing* (brewers).

The discussions about where to seek diagnosis and treatment raised the point that people delay for varying periods of time before actually getting their STDs treated in some way – especially outside the home. The first young women's group again mentioned the problem of shyness and shame in response to this, as did the brewers. The young women said that people were afraid of going for treatment because they may see friends there. They are also shy about mentioning sexually related illness symptoms to medical doctors. These young women said that some people home-treat STDs because they do not consider the illness 'serious enough' to treat in hospital (to spend money on?). Others think that STDs are Ganda diseases and therefore they go first to a traditional healer. In these cases, the girls explained, the symptoms are not properly treated and the patient becomes seriously ill. By the time he/she decides to go to hospital for treatment the disease is quite advanced and is difficult to cure. The second group of young women also said that people are afraid to go to nearby clinics and hospitals lest they are seen. Some people, they said, do not get treatment because of ignorance. But the main reason for delay in treatment-seeking for STDs, they said, is lack of money.

The pregnant women's group also said that people delay because of both financial constraint and fear of being seen. The brewers and the young men said that delay is often a result of a lack of education. Other reasons mentioned by the brewers were (i) the 'character' of the person; (ii) the fear of being told that they have AIDS; (iii) lack of drugs in hospital ('...why waste my time?') and (iv) lack of money. The adult men said that one might delay because some hospitals require you to tell your partner and this is often difficult to do. They said that it is anyway possible that the patient had had 'sex for pleasure' and might not know who gave them the disease. It is not always easy to trace all your partners, another participant commented.

The young men mentioned that another reason for delay could be that the patient might not know the nature of the disease. They also said that young people find it difficult to tell their parents about their symptoms, and so might wait until the condition was serious before seeking treatment. Finally, they said that a young person might first consult a close friend who had had similar problems, and might even obtain drugs or herbs from them and wait to see if they did any good before going outside for treatment.

WHO DECIDES WHERE TO GO FOR TREATMENT?

All the young groups, both boys and girls, said that the parents or guardians (whichever adults the young person is living with) should decide on the treatment action. The second group of young women said that, even so, adolescents might not tell anyone that they had an STD, but would just go by themselves to get treated. This group also said that adults hide their STDs as well. The brewers and the pregnant women said that, if one is married, then the first person to detect the STD should start the treatment. They said that usually the men feel it first and that some tell their wives, but some do not. The husbands are afraid that they will be the ones accused of bringing the disease into the home. A participant in the pregnant women's groups said:

There is no way of running away from an STD if you are married. Even if you are faithful your partner may not be and therefore you will get it anyway.

The brewers noted that it is 'safer' for the woman if the man is the first to detect the STD because then she is less likely to be accused of introducing the STD. They also commented that sometimes an older person was able to help the woman to get her husband to agree to go for treatment. The adult men noted that the decision-maker in the situation depends on the severity of the problem. If one is extremely sick relatives can decide the course of treatment, but if possible it is better that one should decide for oneself. If you are not married, friends may decide for you. If you are employed, your employer may decide for you, in so far as most companies have arrangements with specific hospitals and will pay bills which come only from there. Women, they asserted when asked, are not counselled in these matters.

The young men said the decisions rest with those with whom you are living, if they have money. If one is not living with parents, then neighbours might take the decision about treatment seeking; otherwise close friends or someone who has experienced a similar problem can advise you on the best course of action. Others in this group said that it depends on your condition. For example, if you begin to lose weight your parents may think that you have been bewitched and may take you to a traditional healer.

It is clear that fear, shame and stigma dominate people's perceptions of sexually transmitted disease and decisions about appropriate treatment. Sexually transmitted diseases such as gonorrhea, syphilis and LGV, formerly known – at least to the men – as 'diseases of the brave' are now heavily stigmatized as being symptoms of AIDS. This seems to impact on how people go about treating their STDs in at least two ways. Firstly, a pervasive fear in obtaining treatment and/or diagnosis is that the sufferer will be told that he/she has AIDS, and this is information no one wants to receive. Secondly, sexually transmitted disease, including HIV, carries with it connotations of immoral, or at least inappropriate, sexual behaviour on the part of the patient. This is threatening to social status generally and puts any serious sexual partnership at risk:

Private Disease

I shall not be seen as a proper woman/man – wife/husband in sexual partnerships especially. They will say I lack discipline...

A few words about 'discipline'

One informant suggested that the only solution to the AIDS crisis is to create schools where people, old and young, learn 'discipline'. Families, she said, should take on that role, and what the children learn at home should be reinforced at school.

If we teach our children then they can teach theirs. But for us it is too late.

But families are not what they once were, and in town this may be especially so. Of course, as AIDS claims the lives of the parents who should be providing these examples, and children are increasingly being raised by grandparents or other already over-burdened relatives, the focus on this type of socialization is bound to decrease. This informant also talked of the problem of trust between spouses – another key factor inhibiting early and effective treatment for STDs. A woman, she said, needs to have a man. If you show discipline and are working hard people will be asking themselves why you are not married, what is wrong with you that no man wants you? So a woman wants a man, and at almost any price to herself in other respects. But men, in general, she said, lack discipline. They do not respect women, and this leads to many of the problems they face today. Men and women no longer have a mutual understanding. Men without discipline may antagonize their wives into quarrelling and creating problems. She says that a woman should 'at all times be cool, even when the man quarrels and mistreats her.' She should show him, by her example, the proper way to behave, otherwise they cannot go forward in their marriage. Once he realizes that she is not responding to his bad behaviour he may see that he was wrong. *'He may ask himself: 'Why am I always abusing my wife?' and he can give up and they can negotiate.'* If a woman behaves in the right way and he still does not change his behaviour, then she would be justified in leaving him. When a man behaves in that way he cannot expect to get a 'real woman' she said. *'Men like that will just be like that, and until their death they will be alone.'* After some reflection and further conversation, she noted that she had not seen a man with discipline around their area.

Another woman involved in the same conversation said that the problem with men was that they liked to go to prostitutes who know how to please them, *'make them fried eggs and what not'* so that he comes back home to you, the wife, and picks a quarrel with you so that he feels justified in going back to his prostitute. She said that when a man first brings a woman to his home, she is like his prostitute in that he wants to look after her and admires her. Over time, however, he wants to pick a quarrel with her so that he can go out again...

STDs present huge and complex problems for both women and men, but perhaps for women in particular (gonorrhoea, for example, was only called 'the disease of the brave' in reference to male, rather than female, sexual prowess and conquest).

People in Kamwokya regularly fail to get their STDs treated in a timely and effective manner – but not simply out of awkwardness, backwardness, laziness or ignorance. Similarly, the transmission of HIV is not wholly due to promiscuity, sexual permissiveness or immorality. The treatment seekers whose views have been summarized in this chapter are relatively well-informed individuals who find themselves in a no-win situation: they have both a stringent moral value system and a limited set of reasonable treatment options to choose from. The women in this community have aspirations to be decent, hard-working, disciplined mothers and wives, respected by their neighbours and above reproach. Getting an STD threatens the very basis of these achievements. And if having an STD means having AIDS the repercussions are even more devastating.

Appendix: Local glossary and symptomatology

Local terms

Amabwa: Ulcers. Any ulcer on any part of the body is called *ebwa*. They are identified by locating them on the part of the body affected.

Ekikuba–Insiko: This is a form of consultation fee demanded by the traditional medical sector – especially herbalists. It is related to going to the bush to collect the herbs for the clients' disease.

Ekiwo: This term is sometimes used for many diseases but relates to genital ulcers.

Enziku: This is a specific term for gonorrhoea.

Lwekika: These are lumps (usually lymphnodes) in the groin.

Kabootongo: This term refers to syphilis but is also used for a number of conditions, especially rashes.

Kisiipi: Herpes zoster rash.

Slim: AIDS.

Common local names and symptoms for various STDs in Kamwokya as mentioned in FGDs

Common terms for STD generally:

1. *Edwande yabuzila* (disease of the brave), mentioned by the men's group;
2. *banabagalye,* mentioned by the boys' group.

General symptoms of STD: one of the boys said that 'some sexually transmitted diseases cause people to look pale with a yellowish skin "as if one has no blood" '.

1. *Syphilis – kabootongo.* Symptoms: rash all over the body, watery blisters on the body, loss of hair, abortion in women, sores in private parts, private parts itch. One of the boys said that a person develops multiple wounds in the private parts which are painful and smell badly.

   Enogga, which newborns get from their infected parents, is also recognized, but not, apparently, as a *kabotongo* infection. Even among the young men it was known that 'some women get sterile when infected with STDs'.

2. *Gonorrhoea – Nziku/Enziku.* Used to be called *Kawala* but this has now become a common term for AIDS; according to the men, other names are *njoka ensuzza* and *bana bagalye.* Symptoms – 'queer walking styles' in men; pain and long time in urination (especially men); women get white, thick, smelly discharge from the vagina, and men exude pus from the penis. Other symptoms mentioned were boils and pus, pain in the lower abdomen. One becomes pale and loses most of the hair from one's head. The boys noted that 'one passes pus and has a nasty smell and even wets one's clothes'. Another boy said that 'urine just passes, has no breaks' (*talina kasiba*).

Both the women's and men's groups noted that gonorrhoea can be transmitted to children in childbirth, and identified the symptoms of gonorrhoea in children as pus in the eyes and difficulty in urination. One man noted that 'such babies are all the time scratching their penises'. The men's group also noted that gonorrhoea is a disease of the 60+ age group: 'that is their disease', it is rare to find anyone under 30 who 'has a blocked urethra'.

3. *Lymphogranuloma Venereum – Nalwekiika/lwekiika; baloon; ebizimba; basuka* (by boys' group). Symptoms: painful boils in the lower abdomen/genital area. One of the men noted that people with this problem find it difficult to move and are attacked by fever in the mornings and evenings. One of the young men said that it 'attacks on either side of the inguinal ligament', *embalakaso*' and others nodded in unison.

4. *Herpes zoster – Kisüpi.* Mentioned not as an STD *per se* but as a symptom, esp. of AIDS (see below); the boys' group, however, had some discussion of this, one saying that because it is a symptom of AIDS it also qualifies as an STD, another saying that it is only a symptom, not an STD.

5. *Non-gonococcal urethritis – ekiwo*

6. *AIDS – Silimu; slim; kaveera; kamuyola; yalugwamu; mukenenya.* Symptoms – skin rashes all over the body; recurrent illness, especially malaria; diarrhoea; vomiting; sores in mouth; *kisüpi*; coughing and a general emaciation. The men said that people with AIDS will have the same symptoms as for other STDs: fever, cold in the evenings, headache, diarrhoea and a cough.

Ten

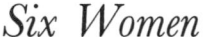

Six Women
Individual Women's Accounts
of Treatment Seeking

GRACE BANTEBYA-KYOMUHENDO & JESSICA OGDEN

This chapter changes the perspective on symptoms of illness and strategies for cure. It brings the issues raised in group discussions, interviews with practitioners, and general accounts of home treatment down to the level of individual practice. In an effort to understand which characteristics make the most difference to women's treatment seeking in Kamwokya, six case studies[1] were conducted. The case-study participants, all women, have small children in their household under their care, have lived in Kamwokya for at least six years and are of sexually active and reproductive age.

Given these basic criteria, the different case studies take up different emphases. The first set, selected by Bantebya-Kyomuhendo, reflect economic range and autonomy, with some of the women being supported financially by men and others with primary responsibility for themselves and their children; some with relatively secure economic resources and some with little reliable income of any sort; some with full autonomy in household decision-making, and some who share these responsibilities with a resident man.

The second set, selected by Ogden, explore how adherence to the local notion of the proper woman (omukyala omutufu) may affect treatment-seeking styles and choices. The interest in these cases was not economic standing as such, but social status of a different sort. These three women were selected with knowledge of the ways in which they define themselves within, and are regarded by, the community.

Each case comprises a brief biographical sketch and then an account of treatment seeking for children in general, covering the latest illness episode; and own illness in general, with an account of the latest own illness episode. Some also indicate the sums of money spent in each episode. The women's real names are not used. All six are referred to by pseudonyms.

---

[1] Mitchell (1983) writes that the case study is a 'detailed examination of an event (or series of related events) which the analyst believes exhibits the operation of some identified general theoretical principle'.

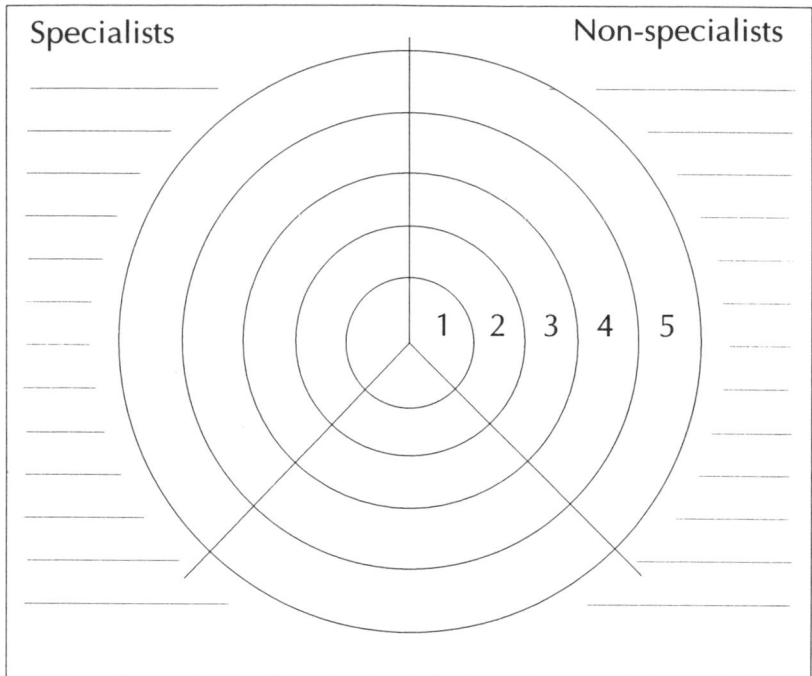

Figure 10.1 *Treatment-seeking diagram*
The diagram is based on those developed in a previous study to chart the networks and resources of case-study households (see Wallman, 1984). Two charts were used, one for general treatment-seeking choices/resources and the other documenting the treatments sought for two specific illness episodes: the most recent illnesses of the respondent and one of her children. Each ring of the diagram represents a general geographic area. The innermost ring represents the household itself and each successive ring moves farther away from the household in geographic distance, with the outer ring denoting rural home area. Should any of the respondents have sought treatment further afield a sixth ring could have been added for 'Outside Uganda'. We asked for both specialist and non-specialist treatment sources consulted in each 'ring' as well as any home treatment(s) administered. For each treatment source used, the respondent was asked its specific location; the characteristics of the treatment provider; how much she had to pay for the treatment; how long the treatment process took. For the specific episodes we also asked: whether she was given further information and/or a prescription to get filled elsewhere; how long it took for the patient to get well; and if she was satisfied with the outcome. We also asked how she came to know of that particular treatment source, and why that source was used. In addition, the respondents were asked to identify any of the noted sources that they felt uneasy about consulting and why.

Case Study 1: 'Betty'

Betty was born in Masaka district in 1955 of a poor peasant family as she describes it. Despite their poverty, however, Betty managed to get a considerable amount of formal education, being trained in ante-natal and infant care, elementary paediatrics, nutrition and family planning. When she finished training in 1970, Betty worked as a health worker at Kitovu Mission Hospital on the paediatric and maternity wards. In 1971, when she had a child she left this job and went to Kampala. The child's father helped with the move, even arranging for Betty to attend a commercial college where she studied elementary accounts. By 1974 Betty was employed as a kindergarten teacher, and lived on her own until she married. She and her husband moved to Kamwokya in 1984. She now runs her own nursery school in Kamwokya. Her husband has a taxi cab business which is not very successful, but the family have a poultry unit and keep some livestock on their compound in Kamwokya. By local standards Betty and her family are considered prosperous, living in a four-roomed permanent house. Betty has ten children, all of whom are living with her in Kamwokya. Although in the past she used contraceptive pills to help with birth spacing, she was unable to continue because of high blood pressure.

Children's illness in general

When a child falls ill, the first thing Betty does is to consult her husband about it. If the illness is not very serious she will then buy drugs or use whatever is available in the house to treat the child. The drugs are normally purchased from a nurse friend who lives in Kamwokya. The nurse operates from her home, treating and selling drugs to those who know her. She has children at Betty's school, and normally sells Betty drugs at reduced prices. Betty stressed, however, that because she herself has a background in child health she usually treats the children on her own. It is only when she cannot handle the situation that she seeks outside treatment. She said an illness is serious enough to require a doctor's attention when temperatures do not go down and when there is 'bad breathing'.

If the child exhibits these symptoms, Betty goes to the Kisenyi Valley Clinic located nearby in Kisenyi 1 zone, Kamwokya. She was introduced to the clinic by a friend. One does not just go to any clinic: it is more common for someone to introduce you, or people go where they have friends. The owner of the Kisenyi Valley Clinic, a doctor who also works at Mulago Hospital, has now become her friend, and his children go to her school. Betty noted that during the course of an illness episode she may see both the nurse/friend and the doctor frequently. When all attempts fail she will take her child to Mulago Hospital, usually on the doctor's referral.

If she has non-medical worries about her children, Betty's first step is to consult her mother-in-law who lives a few miles outside of Kampala. They have a very good relationship and visit each other regularly. Betty said the old woman is knowledgeable about problems that could affect a child. In case she fails to see the mother-in-law, the second step is to consult her sister-in-law in Makindye, Kampala. She is a *Nalongo* (mother of twins) who works in the Ministry of Works, and is also knowledgeable about children's problems.

Latest child's illness episode

The child who was most recently sick is a boy aged 4½. He had a high fever and cough. Betty first gave him some quinine she had in the house, but he did not get better. He was then taken to the Kisenyi Valley Clinic where he was given Camaquine. He still did not improve, and was then taken to the nurse/friend who gave him penicillin and chloroquine injections. In the evening of the same day he was given another chloroquine injection. This treatment cured him.

Total cost of treatment:

Kisenyi Valley Clinic	Ush. 3,000
Nurse (injection)	Ush. 2,000
Total	Ush. 5,000

Apparently Betty was charged less for what she considered superior treatment (injection) of her child at the nurse's home compared with the tablets (regarded as inferior) which the child was given at Kisenyi Valley Clinic.

Own illness in general

Generally when Betty herself feels ill, she first self-treats with medicinal herbs. If the illness symptoms persist, she visits her nurse/friend for a check-up and treatment. If there is still no improvement she visits Kisenyi Valley Clinic. The last step, if there is no positive response, is to visit Mulago Hospital and she says this is always on the doctor's advice. At Mulago the doctor helps her to get specialist attention.

Betty says that she seeks treatment in the above fashion mostly when she is suffering from hypertension, a chronic condition for her. Otherwise she successfully treats herself either by using home remedies (herbs and over-the-counter drugs) or by consulting a traditional healer in Kamwokya to whom she was introduced by a friend. At the time of the interview Betty had some burns on her arm and was treating herself by dressing them with a rabbit's skin. She also said that she had been immunized against HIV/AIDS by a certain traditional healer. Despite Betty's background of health training, she still firmly believes in the potency of traditional medicine especially in curing ailments afflicting herself. Later, when asked about the treatment of her skin burns, she said that she initially got treatment in the form of an antibiotic injection. Betty refused to disclose who did the HIV vaccination or where it was done but said that the vaccine (traditional medicine) is introduced to the body by means of a deep skin cut. The cuts on Betty's shoulders were still fresh and not properly callused. The implications for the spread of HIV infection can only be imagined if even people like Betty believe that they are immune to the disease.

Latest own illness episode

The last specific illness Betty suffered from was sharp pains in the ribs. Any movement of the body was a problem. Her first action was to treat herself with a concoction of herbs applied to the affected parts. The herbs included tomato leaves mixed with paraffin. She also applied Vick's Vaporub. When this treatment failed Betty went to the Kisenyi Valley Clinic and consulted the doctor who prescribed some tablets. After two days her condition worsened, and while working she 'became paralysed'. She sent for her friend the nurse who came and treated her on the spot. She was given three types of tablets and told to rest for two hours, after which she was given a penicillin injection.

Case Study 2: 'Rose'

Rose was born in 1972 in Kisenyi 1 zone, Kamwokya. When she was one year old, however, her mother died and she was taken to live with her grandmother in another Kampala suburb. When she was 11, Rose went back to Kamwokya to live with her father who had promised to send her to school. Unfortunately he never did so. At the age of 14, Rose began to make mats and tablecloths for sale to support herself and to help her family. At 15 she became pregnant, and went to live with the child's father. She has been living with him in Kamwokya ever since.

Rose's partner did not have steady work. Although he was temporarily hired as a truck driver, by the time they had their second child he had lost that job. Rose, therefore, had to intensify her income-generating activities to support him as well as herself and her children. She tried a number of business ventures, sadly failing each time. Currently Rose's husband is again out of work. Having borrowed some capital from a friend, Rose is cooking and selling *mulokoni* (a popular delicacy made of cow's hooves) at drinking parties in the evenings.[2] 'It is a taxing business', she says 'but then, do I have many other options?'

Rose has been pregnant four times, but has only two living children, having lost one child in infancy and one as a miscarriage. She has used modern contraception, pills and IUD, but not since her last pregnancy in 1990. She intends to start again with an IUD when her child stops breast-feeding.

Children's illness in general

When a child is sick Rose first contacts her husband because he is the one who provides the funds for treatment. Next she visits the Kisenyi Valley Clinic which is only a few metres away from her home. She was introduced to it by a friend. Sometimes Rose goes to Dr Matovu who has a clinic in

[2] In Kampala *mulokoni* is especially popular with people drinking locally brewed alcoholic beverages. Its thick glue-like soup is also believed to have medicinal qualities, especially in treating arthritis and rheumatism.

Market zone. He is a friend of her husband and will treat them on credit, but she generally prefers the Kisenyi Valley Clinic because it is so much nearer. If the child does not improve then she goes to Mulago Hospital, acute ward (Acute Care Unit).

If the child is suffering from a disease that needs a traditional healer, Rose consults her sister-in-law who lives nearby, and might also send for her maternal aunt who lives in Mityana. She might consult her younger sisters-in-law, one living in Kamwokya and the other in Bukoto (a neighbouring suburb), but they are not cooperative and she does not feel comfortable with them.

When she has worries about her children Rose usually consults her husband for advice. The next steps are the nearby sister-in-law, a friend in the neighbourhood who is an old woman, and the wives of her in-laws who live in Kamwokya. Lastly she consults her aunt in Mityana.

Latest child illness episode

Most recently, Rose's nine-month-old daughter developed laboured breathing, a high temperature and lack of appetite for food or breast milk. This indicated to Rose that the child had malaria. After a day, when the fever got serious, Rose began using a wet cloth to bring down the child's temperature, and bought Malaraquin, giving her daughter half a tablet. At the time of the interview, the child was in a critical condition, but Rose did not have the money to take her to the clinic. The researcher helped her get to the Kisenyi Valley Clinic where she found a nurse who knew them well. The nurse prescribed ampicillin syrup, linctus cough mixture, ventolin, junior aspirin and fansidar (half a tablet), and on each bottle or sachet wrote instructions as to how the drugs were to be used. She got a new syringe and injected the baby. She then got a stethoscope and put it on the baby's chest, but did not put it to her ears. The following day the child had improved significantly, and she was taken back to the clinic for a check-up.

Total Cost of Treatment – Ush. 3,300 (medicines and consultation)

Own illness in general

When Rose herself is sick she tells her husband and then treats herself. If the drugs she wants are not around the house she buys them. If she does not improve then she consults her neighbour. Depending on the advice, she normally goes for treatment to a nurse she met through a friend. Mulago Hospital would be the last step if she still has not improved. When Rose is worried about illness, she first consults two of her sisters who live in other parts of Kampala, then her aunt in Mityana, and a childhood friend who lives nearby. Finally she might consult another sister who is in the home village but she does not feel very comfortable with her.

Latest own illness episode

On Christmas Day 1991 Rose had a miscarriage. She was not expecting anything to happen but all of a sudden she had abdominal pain. She did not think it was serious until she began bleeding. In the morning she was taken to Mulago Hospital by her brother-in-law's wife's sister who was working there. All night in Mulago she suffered a lot of pain, but the next day she felt better. They did not have to pay for any medicine because they had been taken by their relative who worked there. Rose was not given any drugs after the initial treatment, but when she reached home she bought panadol from the shop because she had a headache from bleeding so much. After treatment she improved and it only took her a short time to recover completely. The panadol cost Ush. 1,000.

Case Study 3: 'May'

May was born in 1967 in Mulago parish, Kampala, but later moved to Kamwokya. Her father died in a motor accident, and so May and her five siblings were raised by their mother who sold food at Kampala City Council. May did not get much formal education. She was enrolled in school when she was 9, but her mother was unable to keep up the school fees and at 10, May went to live with her maternal aunt, also in Kamwokya, where she worked as an unpaid house-girl. May lived with her aunt until she was 16 when her mother coerced her into marrying a man who had been courting her. This man was employed as a watchman and had no accommodation of his own. They moved together to Kisenyi zone where they lived with friends.

May and her partner had three children together. When she was pregnant with their fourth, he enlisted in the army and disappeared until 1993 when he was demobilized. While he was away May had a child with another partner.

During her husband's absence May had a hard time, and had to do all types of work to survive. Eventually she started her current business selling cassava chips to passers-by near her home. She also continues to do odd jobs because what she earns from the cassava chips is not sufficient to sustain herself and her children. Life is so difficult that at times they go without meals and the children are severely malnourished. Her husband has been unemployed since he came back in 1993, and even when he gets odd jobs doing casual labour he does not contribute to the family.

May has had 7 pregnancies and one miscarriage. Five of her children are still alive, and she is currently expecting another child. She says that she has never used family planning because she is asthmatic.

Children's illness in general
Whenever a child is sick, May first treats it using medicines she has in the house or which she buys from the shops. The next step is always Mulago Hospital acute section (Acute Care Unit) or Mwana Mujimu (child nutrition clinic) where treatment apparently is free. She does not go to the clinics because of lack of money. Sometimes she consults her mother.

Latest child's illness episode

The child who was last sick is a 3½ year-old who is severely malnourished and had been attending the nutrition clinic at Mulago. May felt that the child had malaria symptoms and so treated it herself, using choloroquine tablets. When the symptoms persisted and the child developed a skin rash, it was taken to the Mwana Mujimu Clinic where measles was diagnosed. The child was admitted for one week, put on a course of injections and was cured. May was not asked to pay.

Own illness in general

May's main problem is pneumatic asthma. She normally treats herself if she has the drugs in the house. Otherwise the next step is to go to Mulago Hospital. If she has money she might go to Bukoto drug shop which is managed by a nurse May knows through a friend. This nurse knows May's problem and can treat her on credit.

Latest own illness episode

The last time May had an asthma attack she got medicine from the drug shop. It made her weak but she eventually improved.

Comparison and Analysis of Cases 1, 2 and 3

Comparing these three cases, it is evident that the women's decisions on treatment choices in the initial phases of illness episodes are influenced or limited by the level of money resources at their disposal. For example, Betty, who has comparatively more financial resources available to her, has a wider range of treatment options. When her children are ill, she can buy over-the-counter drugs, get advice from her nurse/friend at the latter's house (an unofficial clinic), go to Kisenyi Valley Clinic where a professional medical doctor is available, or be referred by the same doctor to Mulago Hospital where he officially works. The same pattern applies when she herself falls sick. Rose, on the other hand, does not have many options, especially among those which require money. Apart from a clinic close to her home where she has friends, and another further away where her husband knows a doctor and can get credit, she has no other possibilities. In fact she says that if a child's illness persists after exhausting these choices, the only next step is to wait until it is critically sick, whereupon she rushes it to Mulago Hospital Acute Care Unit where the child will be treated whether funds are available or not.

May, being poorer still, can only use home remedies (herbs), over-the-counter drugs in insufficient doses, or, if a child's symptoms are persistent and acute, she can take it to Mulago Hospital where she 'pays a little bribe' to get treatment. Alternatively, like Rose, she waits for the symptoms to worsen and then she rushes the child to the Acute Care Unit at Mulago where treatment is actually free and drugs readily available.

From these examples, it is apparent that in spite of limited financial resources at the women's disposal, and the exorbitant costs of treatment, mothers always prioritize their children's health care needs even at the expense of their own. All the women in the case studies, in spite of disparities in their money income, sought or attempted to get prompt treatment for their children. Because women do not prioritize their own health-care needs, more often than not they rely on self-treatment with home remedies and over-the-counter drugs, or they seek treatment from traditional healers. Thus an illness may reach a critical stage before treatment is sought.

Betty says that when she herself is ill, she does what she can herself so that money can be spent on more pressing household needs. Apart from hypertension, which is a chronic ailment, she treats herself with local herbs. In her latest illness episode, it was only when this and other remedies failed and she could not even move that she called in a nurse who treated her with modern drugs. She called for the nurse who is cheaper than the clinic, despite knowing that the doctor was better qualified to handle her situation.

Rose likewise went for professional help only when she was seriously ill with a miscarriage, and anyway the treatment was free in Mulago Hospital where a relative was working. For things like headaches and malaria, she treats herself. Many times during the research she was found ill in bed, but claimed either to have treated herself or that she had no money for treatment. Even when given money for it, she spent it on 'more pressing' needs at home, or on the young child who was chronically ill. This child is thought by neighbours to be HIV positive, not least because Rose's health is also deteriorating rapidily – but other factors such as malnutrition could account for both conditions.

Though May is asthmatic, she normally gets her treatment from the drug shops where she also has a friend who injects her if the situation worsens. During the interview period she was at one time found very ill but had not sought any treatment because she said she did not have any money. Even so, she had managed to buy cassava and was preparing cassava chips for the following day's business. She also mentioned that the friend who normally treats her had gone to her home village. Asked why she had not used that money for treatment she said that she had priorities other than her own health on which to spend money. Buying treatment would mean using her capital which is critical for the family's survival. Even the knowledge that her asthma might cause her to lose consciousness at any time did not override that priority.

The three women who make up the second set – Mary, Sally and Ann – live in the same RC1 zone. The following brief description highlights the differences between them in terms of their relation to the ideal of the 'proper woman' (*omukyala omutufu*).

Mary is unmarried (though co-habiting with a younger man) and though she is quite poor, she works to support herself and her two young children selling the popular alcoholic beverage *waragi*. Her previous partner died several years ago (of 'maybe AIDS') and since his death she has not become financially dependent on another man. This lack of male support makes it difficult for her to be seen as an *omukyala omutufu* according to the ideal. Sally, on the other hand, though also poor, is currently involved in a long-term monogamous relationship with a man she calls 'husband'. This union has not been formalized by an introduction ceremony in her father's village or a church wedding but her husband has fathered their three children and both families seem to accept that the couple are 'married'. He works as a casual labourer/handyman and she sells tomatoes, onions and charcoal from a small kiosk (*midalla*) outside their house. Although the family is poor, she is known by her neighbours as *omukyala omutufu*. Both Mary and Sally live in one of the most densely populated parts of the zone in rented accommodation that is in poor repair. In contrast to these two women, Ann has a husband by a 'proper' marriage. He was introduced in the traditional way to her family, and they also had a wedding in the Catholic Church. He has steady employment at the Uganda Commercial Bank, and she stays at home, looks after their large family, sometimes takes in sewing, and raises hens. Their large detached house is some distance away from the 'slum' area and is surrounded by a high security wall with a gate which can be locked. They own the house (though not the title to the land) and built it themselves with savings from a previous business venture. She too is *omukyala omutufu*.

Case Study 4: 'Mary'

Mary was born in the early 1960s in Masaka district. The family was well-off, but Mary never had any formal education. At fifteen she was married in the customary way, and moved in with her husband at his father's homestead. She worked tending the herd, cleaning the kraal and milking, but found her duties dirty and demeaning and was not happy. Mary gave birth to two children who died in infancy. By the time her third child was three she was fed up with her husband's philandering, so she left them both and went to live with her sister in Kamwokya.

After a few months she moved in with a friend in another Kampala suburb and they worked together brewing and selling *marua*, the local beer. Mary started a new relationship with a man and had another child. Not long after, however, the man left to fight in the 'bush war' and was gone for four years. She got tired of waiting for him, broke off the relationship, and sent their son to his father's village.

Mary went back to her sister's in Kamwokya, and began brewing and selling *marua* in the main market. One of her customers became her 'husband' when they had a child and moved in together. He worked as a hawker in the city centre, and she began selling *waragi* from home. After a few years, however, her husband died. Before his death Mary had another child, who died 18 months later, some months after its father. Mary stayed on in the same house after these sad events and continued to sell *waragi*. She conceived another baby who also died, this time at eight months old.

Mary's current partner, a man several years her junior, has another family in his village, and although he bases himself at Mary's house when he is in town he makes no financial contribution to her household, and she is unquestionably the household head. Mary's eighth child, a healthy daughter born just prior to the interview period, was conceived by this man.

Illness in general

Mary explained that when one of her children is sick, or if she herself is unwell, she will usually go to the Muna Clinic and see the doctor there.[3] If the illness persists she goes to a doctor she knows at Mulago Hospital. If there is still no improvement she might consult her neighbour and friend, Mama Beth, the woman who delivered two of her children. Mary treats certain conditions at home with medicines bought from a nearby drug shop, but only if she knows exactly what and how much to buy (she does not trust drug shop attendants and will not consult them). If she does not know how to treat an illness she will ask her friends for advice, and if she is really desperate for help, especially if she needs money for treatment, she can go to her sister in the home village. Mary explained that when she is suffering from 'certain kinds of diseases' (those caused by 'witchcraft' or 'charms') she has gone to a traditional healer in a neighbouring township. There is another healer in Kamwokya that she has used as well, but she still owes her for services and feels uneasy about going back.

Latest child's illness episode

Mary's six-year-old son had a skin rash and a heavy cough. A friend came to visit and found that the boy was ill. Because Mary was herself unwell, the friend took him to Bwaise (a neighbouring suburb) to get treatment from a paediatrician at a clinic run by the Kampala City Council. The boy stayed with this friend in Bwaise for a week and went to the clinic daily for a course of five injections. They were told to buy an ointment for his skin infection, but were never given a diagnosis or a treatment schedule. The clinic charged Ush.5,000 for the injections and wanted more money for the ointment. Mary could not afford the ointment. After returning from Bwaise the child's condition did not improve so Mary took him to Muna Clinic where he was given two more injections and received a tube of ointment for Ush 2,500. A few days later he was well again.

Total cost of treatment: Ush.7,500

---

[3] This clinic is popular throughout Kamwokya both for its reputation for effective treatment and because Dr Muna extends credit to patients who are known to him and to those in great need.

Latest own illness episode

Mary has been chronically ill since September 1992. The illness manifested itself first as a pain in her hand and she went to Muna Clinic where she was given four injections and some tablets, costing her Ush.2,000. This treatment gave her no relief. She then went to a herbalist who gave her various local medicines, including a bar of clay infused with herbs which is normally given to pregnant women. She was told to apply the medicines directly onto the painful hand, and mix the clay with water and drink that. She was charged Ush.3,000. Again, she got no relief. In fact the pain increased and started to affect her legs.

Mary then consulted a friend who said that she knew of a traditional healer in Bwaise who might be able to help. When she arrived she was told that she would be charged one hen and 10,000/- and that she would have to stay there to be treated. The healer divined the cause of the illness, telling Mary that she had been 'charmed' by a woman who was also in the *waragi* business. He then told her that he would draw all the 'things' that were causing the pain in her legs to one place and that they would then burst out. Over a five-day period he rubbed medicine on her legs. After realizing that she was not improving Mary asked the healer if she could go home and send someone every day to get the medicine from him. He agreed if they would give him another 10,000/. This made them realize that they were 'wasting their time with him'. She concluded by saying that this man was a good diviner because he gave a plausible explanation for her illness, but not a proper healer. She regrets that so much money was spent 'for nothing'. Mary's suspicion that this man was not a proper healer was finally confirmed when he continued to demand money from them, despite the fact that his medicines were ineffectual. Other healers, she explained, would wait until there was some evidence of a cure before requiring further payment.

Mary continued to live with the pain which seemed to increase daily. A customer told her about a woman friend of his who was a healer. This healer then came to see Mary and told her very simply, and without the help of spirits, what was causing her illness, divining the same cause as the Bwaise healer. The healer then asked for enough money to buy some paraffin (about Ush. 500) some of which she took home to 'cook' the medicine. She advised Mary to rub the remaining paraffin on her legs for four days. When the four days had passed all the 'charms' had come to one place. The healer then brought a *ekiwubilo* (cow's horn) and put it against the place which was now a swollen boil. She sucked through the horn and rubbed the leg vigorously. A number of objects emerged from Mary's leg through the horn. The healer then told Mary that she had done all that she could do, and that she should now go to Mulago Hospital. Mary reports that she got relief from this treatment almost immediately. The healer charged her 30,000/- after the treatment had proved relatively successful. Mary was only able to raise 10,000/-, and has not yet fully repaid the debt.

Soon afterwards the pain returned and she went to Mulago, where she was admitted for several weeks. A doctor from Kamwokya gave her a diagnosis although he was not the doctor treating her. He told her that she was suffering from a 'problem of the joints'. Mary is not sure of the cost of the treatment because the brother of her late 'husband' paid most of the bills. She does know, however, that they gave the admitting doctor Ush. 2,000 and that they paid Ush. 1,000 for each of the three X-rays. By the time she left the hospital in March 1993 she had been suffering for six months.

Mary continues to suffer pain and swelling in her legs. She manages the pain today with painkillers (usually aspirin or panadol) which she buys at local drug shops when she has the money. When the pain gets too serious for aspirin she goes to see her doctor at Mulago who prescribes something stronger, but she depends on the researcher to pay for prescriptions made up in town.

Total cost of treatment: Approx. Ush. 28,500 so far.

Case Study 5: 'Sally'

Sally was born in 1968 in Luwero. When she was five years old her father 'went mad' and her mother took the children to live with her parents. There Sally attended school through to Primary 7. She finished school at the age of 15 and stayed at home to help her mother cultivate food crops.

At 17 Sally was sent to Kamwokya to help her sister through a difficult pregnancy. She soon got a job in a 'hotel' in Kamwokya's main market, but lived at her sister's until she moved out with the man she loved, into the place they have shared ever since.

In two years Sally had 2 children. Her husband was selling milk but their resources were strained and Sally started a business with the help of a neighbour. She later expanded from selling only charcoal to selling tomatoes, onions, and other necessities such as pounded groundnuts and curry powder. Sally's husband eventually started to get regular work painting houses. Their third baby was born in March 1994.

Illness in general

When Sally is concerned about her health or the health of her children the first person she turns to for help and advice is a neighbour and friend. If one of her children is sick, Sally will treat them at home with drugs purchased from her husband's relative who runs a nearby drug shop. For certain conditions she collects and prepares herbs. If the child does not respond to home treatment, she will take it to the Muna Clinic.

When the child is seriously sick – defined by her as having no energy, vomiting, with diarrhoea and/or fever (see Chapter 8) – Sally will take it to Mulago Hospital. She knows no particular doctor there, so will just take the child to the appropriate ward or clinic. Sally also goes to Mulago when she herself is very ill. A friend of Sally's who works in a pharmacy is another source of treatment. She sometimes gives advice about treating a sick child. If the friend has the required medicines to hand, she will give them to Sally free of charge. If she does not she will direct Sally to a pharmacy.

Latest child's illness episode

Sally's one-year-old daughter had all the symptoms that she recognizes as 'serious'. When the child was first unwell Sally bought some tablets (septrin and panadol) and some syrup for worms. The medicines cost her Ush. 1,500, all she could afford that day. When she got home she went into the bushy area around her home and picked a herb she knows (*mululuza*) that brings down a fever when used to bathe the patient. She administered the pill and the herbal bath twice a day for two days. On the third day she saw that the child was not improving and took it to Muna Clinic. The doctor listened to the baby's chest and the nurse gave it two injections and told Sally to bring her back in the evening for a third. They gave her aspirin, Piriton, and a red syrup for her cough. Sally was not told what her child was suffering from and no one explained the course of treatment they were giving. They went back for injections that evening and every day for the following three days. By the time they finished the child was well.

Total cost of the treatment: 2,500/−.

Latest own illness episode

Sally's last serious illness, when her first born was only three months old, was an acutely painful headache that went on for a month. Neighbours told her that she had been 'charmed' because her husband was having an affair with another woman, and that she should go to a traditional healer. Sally refused. Within a week of her falling ill her husband bought her some tablets, and later a friend brought her some local herbs to pour over her head. Both remedies were ineffective.

When she realized that she was not getting better Sally went to Mulago and was admitted. The consulting doctor was a specialist in 'head problems'. He examined her chest, head and ears and gave her four types of tablets which included septrin and panadol. She stayed at the hospital for a week without any change in her condition, leaving only when her brother came from the village, bringing some medicine that their father had sent her. When they reached home her brother put three drops of their father's medicine in her nose. Upon the application of the third drop she was cured. 'It was as if I had never had a headache!' she told us. She did not have to give her brother or father anything for this treatment. Her father had made the medicine himself, having been taught by his own grandfather. She is not sure how much the treatment at Mulago cost because her husband paid the bill.

Case Study 6: 'Ann'

Ann was born in 1963 in Mawokota to a fairly prosperous family. She went to school for seven years, but did not attend regularly. When she was fifteen she was married, and she and her husband moved to a village where he had a job as a secondary school teacher. The school was closed after four months, however, because of the growing instability in the country. After a short period back at his home, Ann's-husband got a job at the Uganda Commercial Bank and he moved to Kamwokya, Central Zone. Ann soon joined him, and had her first baby at the age of 16.

Two years later they got a house and shop in Kamwokya, Kifumbira I zone and Ann delivered her second child. Her husband continued to work at UCB while she worked in their shop selling sugar cane, onions, tomatoes, potatoes and banana leaves. They stayed in that house and shop for ten years. During that period they built up the business and their family. Ann got a sewing machine and began to sew for extra income. Five children were born during those years.

In 1988–89, when Ann was 27 years old, they moved into their own, five-bedroomed, permanent home which they had built themselves. Their compound is surrounded by a high security wall and a heavy iron gate with a chain and padlock. A seventh healthy child was born in 1992, and their eighth, another healthy girl, was born in March 1994. Ann is no longer taking in sewing, but she now raises chickens and her husband continues to work at UCB.

Illness in general

Relative to the other women Ann has fewer 'non-specialist' resources, her illness episodes are less dramatic, and she does not report using traditional healers or herbalists. When the children are sick Ann goes to the Muna Clinic and buys any necessary tablets. She says that she knows the medicines and doses to ask for and does not seek the advice of the drug shop attendant. If she finds that this treatment does not cure the child, she goes straight to Rubaga Hospital (a private Catholic mission hospital in Kampala). She does not have a particular doctor there, but sees whoever is on duty. When she herself is sick, Ann says that she just goes straight to Rubaga Hospital. She does not try to self-treat. She says that she used to go to Father Anatole, a Catholic herbalist located in Bugolobi (another Kampala suburb), but no longer goes there because he has become too expensive.

When worried about the health of her children, Ann will first seek advice from her husband about where to take them for treatment. She also has a friend who lives nearby with whom she can discuss her worries. When she is concerned about her own health, however, Ann said she 'just goes to the church and kneels down to pray'.

Latest child's illness episode

Her two-year-old daughter was last ill in October 1993. After the child had spent a day with fever, Ann took her to the paediatric clinic in Bwaise. They tested the child's blood and gave her a general examination. They administered one injection and also gave her tablets. Because her temperature was high they said that she was suffering from *omosuga*, a generalized term for fever which can also mean malaria. Ann thinks that the injection was chloroquine but she was not told. There was no need for a follow-up visit because the baby was fine within about five days. *Total cost of treatment:* Ush. 3,500.

Latest own illness episode

The last time Ann was ill was one and a half years ago. She had a very high fever with no other symptoms. She went alone straight to Rubaga Hospital where she saw a doctor who checked her blood and urine. She was then told that she had malaria. They gave her a chloroquine injection and some tablets. *Total cost of treatment:* Ush. 4,700.

For the specific episodes described, Ann's chart is again different from those of the other women. Here she lists no non-specialists, and only one treatment source for each episode.

Comparison and Analysis of Cases 4, 5 and 6

The lives of these three women thus emerge as both similar and richly different. Marrying young and well, Ann's later life reflects her relatively affluent up bringing. It is not insignificant that Ann arrived in Kampala a married woman, and did not have to support herself or make her own way as Mary and to a lesser extent Sally had to do. Though by no means simple, her life course has not been marred by the difficulty and tragedy that Mary has had to contend with, or by the relative poverty and uncertainty of Sally's life. These differences are apparent in their treatment-seeking styles.

The most outstanding difference between the three women is their different use of personal networks, or 'non-specialists'. They operate their lives within two distinct parts of the community. Mary and Sally need to maintain acceptance amongst their neighbours more than Ann does, and this entails a specific set of behaviours and actions. Their 'proper woman-ness', and the extent to which they are able to achieve that status, depends upon the skill with which they manage, negotiate, define and redefine themselves within a tight and densely populated physical and moral space; both have extensive networks which they can mobilize in an illness crisis (see further, 'Neighbouring', Chapter 4).

Ann, being physically and morally separate, manages her life and her family under different circumstances, and is subject to a different aspect of the normative code. She is seen most often by her neighbours at church and other social functions, and the church community is the moral community to which she must respond. She and her husband aspire to a social status that the women in the 'slum' do not bother to dream about. The disadvantage of her social and geographic position is that it more tightly constrains the nature of her social networks and the treatment options available to her. She has less room to manoeuvre in this regard. Her social and economic status make it much more difficult for her to solicit help from her neighbours. She is also prevented from using traditional healing options by her status and religious orientations.

Conclusions

These six case studies bring another perspective to the treatment options in Kamwokya (Chapter 6): the ways in which women use the system available to them, and the sorts of factors which can affect treatment choice. Two general conclusions can be usefully drawn:

(i) *Women's treatment choices will reflect the types of resources available to them.*
Those with less access to cash will necessarily rely more heavily upon resources such as personal networks, informal connections and their own health-care knowledge. Those, like Ann, with relatively easier access to cash can side-step the informal economy of health, and have less immediate need for close-knit networks. Women such as Betty, Sally and Mary who are economically constrained but are seen to be good neighbours and/or proper women, use that status to forge networks which can be mobilized in times of illness. Treatment options are most severely constrained for those women who, like May and Rose, have been less successful in both dimensions – who have very little financial or social security, and whose resource base is very limited.

(ii) *Women consistently give their children's health preference over their own and are normally reluctant to spend time or money treating their own illnesses.*
This point is most clearly demonstrated by May who, despite the serious nature of her condition, will choose to invest her small daily accumulation of cash in cassava for the next day's work or in medicines for her sick children rather than on medicines for herself. The risk of losing the income which goes towards household survival is deemed greater than the health risks posed to herself. In the longer term this might not seem the best choice, but the short-term realities of having to provide food and shelter for her family are more pressing, and these are also health-producing activities in a more general sense. At the other extreme, Ann felt that she 'could not afford' to get seriously sick, and sought immediate attention for her symptoms. But she likewise wasted little time in getting her children treated when they became ill. No mother wants to see her children sick and will use any resources available to relieve their suffering.

Eleven

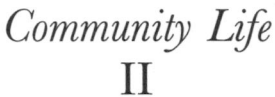

Community Life
II

Participants' Views
(The video project)

SOLVEIG FREUDENTHAL

This chapter's most obvious purpose is to show Kamwokya as the people who live there see it. In this sense it adds a dimension to the story accumulated so far, and serves as a direct complement to Chapter 4. But other things are happening here at the same time. First, in documenting the production of a video film of, by, and for the people of Kamwokya (as well as for the health research project), this piece also shows the community deciding which image of itself is best suited to which audience – demonstrating both its familiarity with 'development rhetoric', and the double bind of aid supplicants who must show the right balance of need and independence of need in order to be 'worthy of aid'.

Second, the process of visualizing events and items necessary before and (repeatedly) after videotaping re-presents everyday realities in non-normal ways. It alters the perspective on the subjects in view willy-nilly, shifting them from back to front stage (or vice versa), and not always in line with the intensions or explicit purposes of those directing the film.

Third, in this chapter these processes combine to reveal local attitudes to responsibility for local problems – notably for the very poor quality of environmental 'wellbeing' which would not otherwise have been articulated. In effect, the making of the video produced new data on Kamwokya which are not recorded in the video film itself.

Introduction

The recent development of low-cost, portable, user-friendly video equipment has made it possible for ordinary people to produce and view their own video films. They now have a chance to tell their stories the way they want to tell them, for whatever purpose and for whatever audience they want. The ethnographic filmmaker, Jean Rouch, envisaged this development in the early 1970s:

And tomorrow? Tomorrow will be the day of the self-regulating colour videotape, of automatic video editing, of 'instant replay' of the recorded picture ... a mechanical 'cine-

eye-ear' which is such 'participant' camera that it will pass automatically into the hands of those who were, up to now, always in front of it. The anthropologist will no longer monopolize the observation of things. (1975: 102)

In order not to monopolize the 'observation of things', we invited people in Kamwokya to make a video film about the community as they saw it. We wanted views of participants on the 'inside', to add to those of observers from outside, on the grounds that the two together would both expand and clarify perspectives on wellbeing.

The 'self-regulating' qualities of the colour videotape and the 'instant replay' of the recorded picture are especially relevant here. Video cameras are easy to handle, for the most part fully automatic, and they can be operated after minimum training. And videotape does not have to be sent away to be developed before it can be watched; it can be instantly replayed and viewed by the people in front of the camera as well as those behind it. This gives the subjects a unique opportunity to see themselves, and more important, it gives them the chance to react, to change, to add things they feel are missing and to take away the parts they do not like.

How did the residents of Kamwokya present and re-present themselves and their neighbours when given the chance? What images and voices did they choose? Who made the decisions during the recording of the film, and later in the editing process when residents had to decide which scenes to use in the final film and which to remove? And what is the practical effect of people seeing themselves and their problems on the TV screen?

Videomaking is a process. This chapter describes the whole process of making and viewing the video film *Kamwokya 1994*. Different issues came into focus at different stages, and insights were triggered by the viewing of the film which were not articulated at the planning stage. The discussion around responsibility for the public health environment is a striking case in point.

The Ethnography of the Video Production

Video and film production can be divided into four main stages: planning, shooting, editing and viewing. This chapter gives an account of the whole sequence; which local residents were involved in the planning. shooting, editing and viewing of the film, in what way they were involved, and who they were representing. It includes observations on the research team's role in the production; the types of issue and concern that were brought up at the different stages; the negotiation and decision-making processes which took place.

Stage 1: Planning

The video project began when the fieldwork period was more than half over. Many of the sub-studies within the larger project had been completed and preliminary results from these studies were available. The research team was by then integrated and respected in Kamwokya and personally known by many residents, so it was easy to introduce a new component to the project. The thirty local residents who were trained as interviewers for the Ethnographic Survey (ES) had been encouraged by their experience to set up an organization called 'Friends of Kamwokya' (FOKA) to promote health issues in the area. The video project was introduced at a FOKA meeting. Some of the speeches given there were videotaped and played back after the meeting: everybody was very pleased to see themselves. This served to introduce the idea of making a video film about Kamwokya to them.

This idea was well received and 10 people (6 men and 4 women) were chosen by the others or volunteered themselves to work with the video production. As it turned out, all the people who were involved at the various stages of the video process were RC officials at RC 1 or RC 2 level. However, they did not all represent the same point of view. On the contrary, there were many heated discussions, showing diverging interests and ideas. And even in this small group there were several religions represented: Catholic, Protestant, 'born again' and Muslim, as well as many different ways of earning a living, from selling charcoal to working for the Catholic church on its 'development projects'.

At the following day's meeting. after the inevitable opening remarks, the filmmaker (SF) was asked to talk: *What would you like to present about Kamwokya on video? What kind of place is Kamwokya to you? How do you 'get by' here? I have put flip charts on the wall and invite you to come up and write down anything that comes to your mind that you think would be interesting or important to film in Kamwokya.* At first the group was rather puzzled and hesitant and the RC 2 Chairman, Mr Ssenoga, suggested that the filmmaker should decide since she knew how to make films. She professed herself willing to explain the basics of video recording, but said they should discuss amongst themselves and then tell us what kind of issues and topics they wanted filmed. At this point, Charles, an RC 2 councillor, walked up to the flip chart and wrote these words: *Development projects. Problem areas. Activities.*

Now the discussion took off and both men and women (although mainly the men) offered their suggestions and ideas. They started by thinking of activities which should be filmed. Charles stood at the flip chart writing down whatever the people said: 'nursery schools like this one' (the meeting was in an old nursery school), 'markets', 'carpentry workshops', 'brick layers', 'car washers', 'health centres' (suggestion by a woman), 'family planning' (another woman), 'video shops', 'traditional healers', 'churches and mosques'. The list became longer and longer. After a while the other researcher present (SW), asked about toilets: *Don't you want to have toilets in your film, pit latrines?*

One man said: *Why latrines? Are they activities?* A second man said: *No. no, no, but it's OK because those are the problems, and we should also take up our problem areas.* This was the trigger to talk about garbage heaps, dumping areas, drainage, swamps, unprotected springs. Everybody came up with suggestions. All the problems mentioned were related entirely to the environment, to water and sanitation issues.

Coming to the last headline, *development projects*, the group was confused until Charles referred to projects in Kamwokya 'trying to alleviate poverty and sickness': the brick-making project for young people; the many activities of the Catholic Church, from teaching young women 'at risk'[1] to cook, make shoes, and sew in order to keep them off the streets, to anti-AIDS education clubs (called Youth Alive): there is an outreach programme for AIDS patients and an orphanage for children whose parents have died of AIDS.

Asking the group to try to identify common concerns gave rise to an animated discussion about the aim and purpose of the film. One man said: '*I would like to have a film about all the problems in Kamwokya which could be shown to donors so that they might fund development projects in the area.*' Another did not agree: '*I would like to have a film for the people of Kamwokya about what we think is important. For example, our religious lives are very important to us and that would never appear in a film only for funders. We need a film about Kamwokya which shows both the good and the bad things, so that we can show it both to funders and to residents in our area.*' A third man said: '*Now, how can we show other people that this is Kamwokya? What are the achievements we can show others?*' The group finally agreed that the film should show the good and the bad parts of ordinary life in Kamwokya, and that it was to be shown both to the residents of Kamwokya and interested outsiders (*'like donors and funders'*).

At this meeting as well as in many later conversations it was quite clear that the group were choosing a development discourse when they were talking to us – the others – the outsiders.[2] The topic was first raised by mentioning projects 'to alleviate poverty and sickness in the area.' But we can also wonder whether the list of problems identified by the group was itself part of this discourse and an effect of the health research project.

In all types of fieldwork the anthropologist may be conceptualized as a resource, but especially when associated with 'development' – in this instance with a large health research programme. Either way we are all outsiders with money, maybe with jobs to dispense, and – here – also with video equipment. It therefore becomes important for the insiders to show that they know the development jargon and can act as people who need help from the outside and furthermore are worthy of this help. The question: 'What are the achievements we can show others?' shows that the

---

[1] 'Women at risk' in this context are women who have been involved in commercial sex or are at risk of becoming involved. The Catholic Church has a vocational programme to teach these women a skill like sewing, shoemaking, cooking, etc. to be used as an alternative means of support.

[2] According to Escobar, countries in Asia, Africa and Latin America started after World War II to be seen, and to see themselves, as 'underdeveloped' and to be treated accordingly. 'To develop' became a fundamental problem for them, they thus embarked upon the task of un-underdeveloping themselves by subjecting their societies to systematic and minute observations and interventions that would let them discover and eventually eradicate their problems once and for all (1991: 675–6). This is a huge topic, only touched on here, to show the sophistication of local residents and their acquaintance with the 'development discourse'.

speaker realizes that, in order to receive help, he has to show himself worthy of it, prove that he is himself trying to achieve something and not just sitting back and waiting for things to happen.

After having decided the purpose and audience of the film, the group went back to discuss how to group the activities and problems around certain themes. After a number of false starts ten themes were identified – *Shelter; Food; Clothing; Spiritual Life; Health; Children; Administration of Kamwokya; Earning a Living; Development Projects* (those already identified); and *Leisure*. The group became very enthusiastic about this last topic, talked all at the same time, and had suggestions to make about leisure activities in Kamwokya: playing games, draughts, drinking beer, *malwa*, playing soccer, etc.

Most of these topics seemed to derive from a development discourse – what is relevant to the development of the area – and so are of interest to donors and funders. But it also gives 'us' an insight into how 'they' view donors and funders – donors and funders are people who are not interested in their spiritual life. Probably not in leisure either. It was the 'spiritual aspects' which had begun the debate about the purpose and target audience of the film and the topic came up again at the editing stage. On the whole, the planning reflected a development discourse with some other local culture priorities added to it.

Finally, the film needed a title. 'This is Kamwokya' was one suggestion, 'Kamwokya 1994' was another. It was a group decision that the film was to be called 'Kamwokya 1994' on the grounds that *this film is going to show Kamwokya in 1994, but not what it might look like in 1995. So if the film is shown in 1995 or later, Kamwokya will probably look very different. When people see it in the future, they will not know when it was made. That is why 'Kamwokya 1994' is better.*

Stage II: Shooting

The following day, Charles (the same RC 2 councillor) and Margaret (the recent widow of a respected senior RC councillor) appeared with a long list of things to be filmed. Under each of the ten themes they wrote *what* should be video recorded and *where* to find these places, activities or issues in Kamwokya. For some they had even written *when* they should be recorded: churches on Sunday, the mosque on Friday.

Charles was most keen to learn how to use the camera, Margaret seemed happier to work with the microphone. Nothing they said was decided before recording or was rehearsed in front of the camera. Margaret began: *This is Kamwokya today 1994. It has ten zones* [she reeled them off]. *These are the zones we have in our area, Kamwokya II.*

Charles then took the microphone and said:

Kamwokya as you see it, has a very busy centre. We are viewing the heart of Kamwokya which is the market area which has a lot of activities. Kamwokya in this year is developing a bit faster and has so many activities, including the market, the shops as you may see them and it has very busy, smart, enthusiastic and happy people.

Again, Charles seems to want to present Kamwokya people as 'worthy help objects'; they are 'very busy, smart, enthusiastic and happy people'.

We proceeded to film the large, very busy market area (see Chapter 4). When stall attendants noticed us, they called out: 'What are you going to do with the film you are taking?' 'Do you have permission to film here?' 'Why are you filming?' 'Who is the film for?' Charles and Margaret explained to everyone who wanted to hear that the film was going to be a film about Kamwokya for the residents of Kamwokya, and that all RC leaders were behind it and involved in it.

When filming in the covered market area, the butchers selling meat quickly put on their white coats when they saw the camera. (Did the video camera bring out the ideal way of living, the 'proper' way of behaving as a butcher in Kamwokya? Or were they perhaps afraid of the health authorities?) In an area attached to the back of the market, there were small eating rooms or 'restaurants' where men who have no women at home to cook for them come to have lunch. The women working there were busy preparing the food for their customers and did not pay much attention to the camera.

After the filming in the market area, we began recording different types of houses: permanent, semi-permanent, and temporary (Chapter 2). Charles and Margaret indicated the houses we should record and the two of them took turns 'narrating' the scenes.

This shows one of the semi-permanent structures, of house and family life. You can see them cooking, washing their utensils, they have washed their clothes and they have hung them up to dry. (At this point the people who are being filmed are giggling and laughing towards the camera). *This is another structure we have in Kamwokya. It is privately owned and belongs to one of the permanent residents. This is where Hassan lives, this is the toilet he uses and his coffee plantation, and in the plantation is the graveyard of his forefathers.* And so on.

The unit on health included two interviews with nurses who were running private clinics. When we approached one of them and asked if we could interview her, she agreed but first she had to put on her uniform (like the butcher). She felt it important to present herself as a 'proper' person on film. We never warned people that we were coming with our camera, or made appointments to come back and video record some time later, so nobody was prepared for our visits. In Goffman's (1959) terms we could say that the butcher and the nurse were putting on uniforms to 'stage a character': the nurse character or the butcher character.

Malaria is a big problem in the area, and it was a topic on many people's minds. We went to visit a woman who was the head of a nursery school. She was also a good business woman; she reared chickens (to sell eggs and chickens) and she had some cows, a goat, a pig and some rabbits. Asked about Kamwokya she replied: *The place is OK except that these days we have the problem of malaria. Here we have a lot of malaria because of the water. The water is not flowing well, we have a lot of stagnant water. We don't know if anybody is coming to help us because it is terrible. Last year the City Council used to come and pour some medicine in the water. But these days they don't come. I don't know why.*

These topics came up several times during the recording – the problem with malaria, stagnant water, open sewers and who was to *blame*. The question of *responsibility* was implicit in every reference to the public health environment. It came into focus in the editing process and became a big issue at the viewing of the video (Stages III and IV).

Responsibility, or the lack of it, also featured in the unit on children. It included some lovely footage in a nursery school where the children were being taught mathematics and were singing songs, and an interview with the headmaster of the primary school, Kamwokya Education Centre.[3]

The problem we have at the school currently is firstly with our neighbours. People surrounding the school keep on making disturbances, breaking the fences and sometime misusing school property. This week we faced a big problem when a mad man came and broke a side of the house. In the school we have some orphans who are being sponsored by the community from Kamwokya church and the children are doing very well since they got that assistance. In addition, we have some children who are sponsored by the Ugandan Red Cross, those whose parents have died from AIDS.

... We also have some problems with children who live round about. They have started to practise sexual intercourse at a very early stage and currently we have been inviting some people to come and educate them right from nursery up to Primary 6. In fact this is not a new thing because even the young ones are doing the same. We have been trying to discourage them and educate them. That is the major problem we are facing here, because the parents leave their children to hang around over the weekends and even after school. They go to the drinking places and it is very tough for us to bring them into line. Secondly, another problem we are facing is people who come here at night and try to remove some of our benches and other things from the school. We are trying to work hand in hand with the RCs to settle all these problems, but all the same we are still facing them. In the future we are planning to put up a permanent fence so that we may not have the same problems with our neighbours. And as for those children who are misbehaving, I would like to call the parents and other officials from the RCs to educate the parents so that they can teach their children how to behave. As we also do the work here from the school we would like to call upon the parents to join hands with us to educate their children on how to behave in the community rather than misbehaving as they are still very young. I think that is all.

Again it is a matter of who to blame when things go wrong. The headmaster is blaming the neighbours, the thieves, the children and the parents. He is at the same time, of course, presenting himself and his school as 'worthy' of help.

The headmaster became very formal when he spoke in front of the camera. He was clearly addressing it, making a speech. The question is to whom: was it to 'the people of Kamwokya', to the parents who should recognize their responsibility and look after and advise their children, or was it the *muzungu* (white person) he wanted to impress? Maybe it was both. The fact that this video-recording was going to be shown in Kamwokya gave him an opportunity to address the parents. Equally he knew that the video was going to be shown outside Kamwokya and his speech made him look

---

[3] There is no public primary school in Kamwokya.

like a proper headmaster (he was 'staging the Headmaster character'). The camera crew as well as the camera and microphone provided him with an *occasion to perform* (Fabian, 1990:6–7), and almost certainly his performance would have been different if we had not had the camera. People familiar with video and TV address the camera and not the other person standing in front of them; the presentation of self is different when people address a camera instead of talking directly to other people. The camera provides an occasion to perform: it transforms the action into a performance, the participants into actors, and the arena into a stage. And in doing so it encourages the now-actor to articulate a 'frontstage' persona.

The 'worthiness' of Kamwokya's residents tended throughout to be presented as a function of how positive they felt about its future. This too was a responsibility. All through the video recording Charles seemed anxious to show that people were 'busy, smart, enthusiastic and happy'. Almost every interview began with one or other commentator asking: 'How do you like it here in Kamwokya?' and leading their interviewee towards an enthusiastic answer. And just as there was a standard way to begin a conversation, there was a standard way to end: 'What advice do you have for the people of Kamwokya?' The interviewer's mother and grandmother each came through appropriately:

Mother: *I advise people in Kamwokya to work harder to fight poverty and illiteracy.*
Grandmother: *People should cooperate and work together and live in harmony.*

An R.C. official ended with: *I advise the youth to work hard and avoid looking for quick money and projects. As a Defence Secretary in this area I advise the youth to work hard and avoid getting involved in bad practices like stealing or armed robbery. Personally 1 don't like free things. That is why I have worked very hard to build myself a house and another for renting out.*

What happened at the shooting of the video? The camera clearly provided an occasion to perform: it transformed the action into a performance, and the arena into a stage. But the people played out their roles in many different ways. The people who were 'staging a professional character', like the butchers, nurses and headmaster, were addressing the camera much more formally (even putting on white coats and uniforms) than the mother and the grandmother. But the camera seemed to encourage all of them to articulate the 'frontstage' with ideal versions of behaviour and social value. (The emergent theme of responsibility and moral blame is an obvious case in point.) At the same time, however, it recorded 'backstage' behaviour and 'backstage' scenes – people who were not being interviewed but just appeared in the frame, or people who did not say what the interviewers wanted to hear. And the less than ideal side of Kamwokya – the garbage heaps, the dirt and filth at the market, the open sewers – was there on the film for all to see.

The editing process provided another forum for the local video-makers to negotiate and decide what information should be pushed frontstage for 'them' and what should stay hidden, 'ours', backstage.

Stage III: Editing

The editing task was to convert 12 hours of videotape into a proper film about Kamwokya. Four local residents (2 women and 2 men) were informally nominated for the task: Charles and Margaret who had done most of the camera work and interviewing during the recording, and two other senior community members, Judith and Badru, both RC officials at RC 1 level, and, like Charles and Margaret, members of the original (ES) interviewing team. The principal researcher (SW) and the filmmaker (SF) were to be present as resource persons.

Before we could start to edit, we had to discuss the content of the video film, review the videotapes, decide how to shorten the 12 hours to a 'proper' length film (and how long that should be) and decide in which order the sequences were to appear in the final product.[4] The group agreed that our conversations should be recorded on an audio cassette in order to remember what had been said. We put our old list of ten themes on the wall and began to discuss what to remove and what to shorten, given the objectives of the research programme, i.e. How do people manage health in Kamwokya?

We had not recorded anything about 'Administration of Kamwokya' so that could be taken off the list right away. The next theme to discuss was 'Spiritual aspects'. What is the relation between spiritual life and health?

Judith: *Somehow our spiritual beliefs determine our physical health! Because if I believe in God I have a different world view which affects my way of living.*

Charles: *We have also recorded AIDS counselling in the Catholic Church on the videotape. Someone could comment on how faith has an impact on people's health...* So there should be a few minutes about worship as well as AIDS counselling in the video.

'Clothing', it was decided, was not to be a topic on its own in the video: it would anyway be possible to see how different people belonging to different tribes were dressed in the different scenes. But it was important to have 'shelter', 'food' and 'clothing' in the video to show what kind of place Kamwokya is.

Judith: *The houses are big health problems; lack of ventilation, water, sanitation.*

Charles: *... and congested. We can look at shelter, food and clothing as some of the factors establishing health in Kamwokya.*

Judith: *We can explain why we have those types of shelter in Kamwokya, why we take that kind of food and why we dress the way we dress.*

Concerning 'development projects', Badru suggested that part of that topic could come in as 'earning a living', because many projects are 'income-generating', like brick-making and other such things. Charles did not agree: *The projects are there as a solution to the problems in Kamwokya so they*

---

[4] To edit video requires copying shots from the original tapes onto a new tape. No material is ever physically cut away. This means that one has to decide beforehand the order in which the sequences are to appear in the finished film. We were fortunate to be able to borrow two VHS video machines and one monitor from UNICEF, so we could do a simple form of editing, with clear cuts, i.e. we could not do any inserts or overlapping of sounds.

can be seen as social activity more to improve life and health in Kamwokya. For example, the 'women at risk project' is an answer to the AIDS scare. Badru was outvoted, but everyone agreed that 'earning a living' was an important topic which should be a big chunk in the film. Since there was a good 4 hours of recorded material on 'earning a living', it was thought best to include all the different activities which had been recorded, but not more than one representative of each type of work.

Judith wanted to talk about 'Children' and she asked: *Is it possible to film another bit about immunization so that we bring in the health aspect in the section on children? As it is we only have children and education but nothing on children and health.* It would technically have been possible, but the feeling was that we should try to put together a video with what we had. Charles therefore suggested that the children could be part of the introduction to Kamwokya. This gave rise to a discussion about what the introduction to the video should look like.

Badru: *I think the introduction should be someone talking about Kamwokya: 'This is Kamwokya. It looks like this. These are the type of houses. This is the type of market they use. Kamwokya is in a certain area of Kampala, like what and what'. I think this should be the introduction. I think we should begin with an overview of Kamwokya, then we take them for a minute in the Mosque, in the Church, in the Pentecostal Church, then people moving in the market. I think we can be finished within 5 minutes. Then we start the real film.*

SF: *I think in an introduction that could be effective, then you go into longer sequences. In the West, we have a lot of action films, with only a few seconds between the cuts. But what is your own comment on this?*

Badru: *I have just seen another film about Uganda. In the beginning you see the president who says that 'I want Uganda to be self-reliant'. Then they put other things, and other things. Yes, it was a good film. It showed the mountains, the lakes, the hotels, just small portions of everything in the introduction, then larger portions later.*

Charles: *I saw a film with a very exciting start. It starts with an overview, a street scene with many people moving around and a song.*

SF: *If we start with a song, what song should we start with?*

Badru: *I think we can put on the children.*

Judith: *Then on what note should we end the film?*

Badru: *If we start with children singing we can end with the man rapping.*

Margaret: *We can have the children coming out of school, enjoying the view, laughing and that is the end of the film.* (Margaret looks very happy and laughs when she talks.)

Charles: *We could have people coming out of the churches, hugging each other, children singing. So that we end upbeat.*

We looked at our papers on the wall and roughly divided the video into six parts:

1 *Introduction* (around 5 minutes: physical overview of Kamwokya, children singing, churches, mosque, leisure, market, people milling around in the streets)

2 *Shelter* (different types of houses)

3 *Water and sanitation*
4 *Other health issues* (nurses, drug shops, traditional healers and AIDS patients, counselling, etc.)
5 *Earning a living*
6 *Concluding scene* (people coming out of churches hugging each other, children singing, man rapping – upbeat)

We then viewed each tape to decide which parts should be in the final version of the video. In which order should the different pieces come?

Judith: *I think the overview should come first, then the taxi bit, then other activities, then the song comes in between the other shop activities and the market place activities. Maybe the places of worship come in there and a portion of leisure activities... From the market I like the view when someone was pushing a cart with charcoal and you see a little of the restaurants and when a hawker comes through the market with his load...*

Badru: *We should have the part when this man is eating. The woman selling charcoal should come under earning a living.*

Margaret: *The selling of tomatoes and onions should also be there.*

At this point the video tape showed different types of houses and then the camera focused on some cows grazing outside a house.

Judith: *I think this too is income-generating, earning a living.*

Badru: *We shall take this one out, this is useless in the film.*

SF: *Why?*

Badru: *Because it is only this man in the whole parish who has cattle, so it is useless to have this in. He cannot represent Kamwokya. I think we should leave this picture out. Let's move on.*

Next on the tape Charles was interviewing a resident of Kamwokya who is also an RC leader, Kayongo Robert.

Charles: *This is one of the RCs: vice chairman of Contafrica, Mr Kayongo Robert. Mr Kayongo Robert, how do you find Kamwokya? The life, how do you enjoy it, the activities?*

K. Robert: *The life is OK. The bad thing is that the majority of the people are poor. They don't have jobs, there are many children like these ones* [pointing to some children] *who don't have money to go to school. Most of the time they stay at home.*

Charles: *What have you done to alleviate some of your problems?*

K. Robert: *We have done almost nothing because we don't have any assistance. In a developing country like this one, we have no assistance, unless somebody will assist us.*

Charles: *Why do you think assistance is the only form, don't you have any prospects, any efforts at what to alleviate?*

K. Robert: *We don't have any income-generating projects from which we can get money to pay the school fees for our children.*

Charles: *So what future do you have in Kamwokya? What do you feel? Is the future bright? What hope do you have?*

K. Robert: *The future is with Sister Duggan, because ...* [he stops abruptly].

We stopped the videotape and discussed this interview. Judith felt that this interview was very important for the film. Badru did not want to have it in.

Judith: *First, we all agree we are poor, and then we say we have not done anything about it and need outside assistance. Then a member from our committee is trying to*

put into our minds that we can still do something for ourselves before other people come in. I think we can develop this idea.
SF: *Badru, why don't you want to have it in?*
Badru: *Well it's OK to put in.*
SF: *But you said you did not want it in. Please try to explain.*
Judith: *He does not want us to expose all our weaknesses!*

This is an example of the kind of dialectic process that went on during the editing. It provided another forum for reflecting on frontstage and backstage, on what kind of behaviour they wanted to show others, and what should stay hidden. In the interview on the videotape we hear Charles again pushing his positive view of life in Kamwokya frontstage and showing competence in the development jargon: 'What have you done to alleviate some of your problems?' He wants the other man, Kayongo Robert, to answer in such a way that demonstrates he is a 'worthy' help object – that he is trying hard to do something himself, but might also need a little support. But Kayongo Robert does not answer according to Charles' script. He gives us an answer which belongs backstage: 'People are poor, there are no jobs, we have not done anything because we do not have any assistance'. This was not the answer Charles wanted when he did the interview, but it did not become problematic until we were doing the editing. It is at the editing stage that the decision has to be made. Shall we have this piece in the film or not? How much of our backstage do we want to show? How much of our weakness do we want to expose? What happens in the editing is that every scene – frontstage or backstage – is pushed frontstage the moment it is decided that this scene is going to appear in the final film. The group therefore has to decide what they want to push frontstage (to make public), and what they want left backstage (private). We can also see that Judith and Badru might have different audiences in mind. When Judith says she wants the piece in the film, it seems that local residents are her audience: *Somebody is trying to put into our minds... Listen, people of Kamwokya, we can do things ourselves.* Badru (as Judith interprets him) is afraid of exposing our weakness. But afraid of exposing it to whom? It could be the funders, the donors and other outsiders, but it could also be the residents of Kamwokya. As the executive video-makers the RC leaders might want to show only a good frontstage to their constituents to avoid being blamed for not making Kamwokya a better place to live in.

One of the tapes contains a long interview with the RC Chairman of Green Valley zone. He talks about problems in his zone, mainly with malaria, stagnant water, poor drainage, garbage and poverty in general. People are so poor that they cannot afford health care. He says: *People go to the hospital and then they get prescriptions for medicines but they have no money to buy the medicine so they go home and die.* After the interview we see the Chairman on camera, pointing to the garbage heaps and filth outside his house.

The group started an animated discussion about what of all this should be in the video. Margaret wanted the first part where the Chairman talks about problems and Badru wanted the last part where he says that people in Kamwokya are hard-working people but that they might need some support from outside.

Reflecting on the images of garbage, SW asked if there were any groups of people in Kamwokya who had organized themselves to collect garbage. Charles answers: *None at all. Why? Well, in Kamwokya people still have the feeling that the garbage issue is a City Council issue and the same goes for the drains. Because once the City Council helped us with spraying the drains against malaria, people expect them still to do it. Then there is another problem. The majority of people living in Kamwokya are not landlords, they are tenants, who know that if conditions get pressing they can just move out. They are migrants, they come, find a house, spend some time, but the community spirit is not in them.*

Judith: *The drainage problem also has to do with the way we build our houses. They are not planned at all. You can't have any drainage planned because there is not enough room between the houses, or the houses are built in such a way that the water from one house flows straight to another house. We need to restructure the area and plan it properly.*

Charles: *It is also the nature of the slope which makes it hard to find a permanent solution. Even if people try to fix things, what happens when it rains is that the water gushes down the slope and destroys all our effort. Perhaps some people are also reluctant because they feel that the effort they have invested will not lead to a solution to the problem.*

SW: *So it is not something which an individual or even a small group can do?*

Charles: *It would be a lot easier if Kamwokya was a permanent community.*

Badru: *There are only 4 landlords in Kamwokya. Most of the people are tenants.*

SW: *If you are a tenant, are you automatically temporary?*

Charles: *OK there are lots of people who have lived in Kamwokya for more than 10 years, but they have not stayed in any one area for more than 1–2 years. They stay in Church area for 1 year, in Kifumbira for 1 year and so on.*

SF: *So what of all this should we have in the film?*

Charles: *Well, for the purpose of our film I don't think it will be good to point fingers at the City Council.*

Badru: *We might decide to take the film to UTV [Uganda television]. But they first ask you what is inside it. They first watch it and if they see that we are condemning the City Council, they might refuse even to put it on the television.*

Judith: *Now, why should we be afraid to tell them that they are not providing the service which they owe us. They should be serving us, even if they are not serving us we should still demand their service.*

Badru: [To Charles] *How do you see it?*

Charles: *Well, just showing them what exists without telling them who should do the work is enough.*

Judith: *Why are you so afraid? Is it breaking the law to state a fact?*

Charles: *It is not breaking the law, it is a question of respect.*

Judith: *Do you mean we are illegal?*

Charles: *No, we are legal but that is not showing respect in someone's presence.*

Judith: *If I put it like that, that the City Council is not providing the service they should provide, would I expect to be prosecuted?*

Charles: *OK what I want to tell you, one thing they told us when we visited the*

218

City Council was that according to the plans they are offering services to already planned and developed areas. So to areas which are not planned like Kamwokya they are not supposed to offer anything.

Judith: *So they are helping those who can help themselves, that is what they are saying.*

Charles: *That is what they told us.*

Judith: *In other words, we should continue to plan for ourselves.*

Charles: *We should look for self-help projects.*

SF: *How can we have this kind of discussion with other people in Kamwokya – so that people can begin to raise these questions about what can be done by ourselves and where do we need outside support? By leaving this piece in or taking it out?*

SW: *Charles, would you worry if this piece with the City Council was in the film next week when we are showing it to the different groups in Kamwokya?*

Charles: *I am not worried, but it does not help us, because the City Council will not come to help because Kamwokya is not on their plan.*

SF: *What kind of conclusion can we come to? Should we leave this piece out when we talk about the City Council or what?*

Charles: *Perhaps for the purpose of the group viewing we can leave it in. People are not aware of the duties of the City Council.*

The sequence with the Chairman of Green Valley and all the garbage and poor drainage in his area had given rise to fierce debate in the group. But the discussion was also a result of the questions posed by the outsiders. Having to explain to us how the system works made the insiders more reflective and self-conscious about issues which until then they had taken for granted. It also provided the group with an occasion to perform around the editing table – like giving Judith an opportunity to push Charles to answer her questions about the City Council – and to decide what should be in the edited video. Charles does not want to 'point a finger at the City Council'. He can have had many reasons for wanting to keep out the criticism. He might have aspirations to move up in the political system to RC3 and RC 4 and have felt that 'pointing a finger at the City Council' might just not be a good thing to do.

We went through all the 16 tapes together, discussing what should be in and where it should go. Here and there the discussion was heated as in the last example, but most of the time the group quite quickly reached consensus about how they wanted to present Kamwokya and what kind of images they wanted in the video.

Time and technical constraints meant that the version shown in Kamwokya the following week was only a rough cut. The sequences were put together and in the order decided upon, but not necessarily even having the right length. The total length of this version was 45 minutes. Showing it to different groups of people in Kamwokya provided feedback on the content of the film, but also on the lengths of the different sequences.

Stage IV: Viewing of Kamwokya 1994
The video *Kamwokya 1994* was shown to five audiences, all residents of

Kamwokya invited to a particular session on the basis of social criteria decided upon by the editing team. The invitation was open to anyone matching those criteria. Rather small numbers in some groups were explained by people not knowing about it or 'being too busy'. The viewing groups were:

(i) Elderly people, both women and men: about 25

(ii) Women (not RC leaders): about 10

(iii) Women (RC leaders): about 20

(iv) Men (both RC leaders and others. The original idea was to have two groups here as well but it did not work out): about 15

(v) Youth, both boys and girls: around 25

The idea was that each viewing of the video should take the form of a 'focus group discussion'.[5] The questions addressed followed the flow of the video:

1. Who is responsible for water, sanitation and environmental health in Kamwokya?
2. What are the treatment options in Kamwokya? When do people go where and for what diseases?
3. What ways can people survive in Kamwokya?
4. What is the relationship between economic activities and health in Kamwokya?
5. Changes in Kamwokya? For better or worse?

It was explained first in English and then in Luganda, how the video film was made that it was a collaborative effort of some of the people of Kamwokya and that we now wanted to hear the audience's reactions. Each audience was also told that we would stop the video at different points to discuss the five questions prepared, but that we were interested in their spontaneous reactions and opinions as well. Each question was discussed for about 10 minutes and then we went on to the next part of the video and the next question. Somewhere in the middle of each session soft drinks were served to everybody. The discussions were by and large held in Luganda.

When the video started the audience reacted almost immediately to what they saw – laughing, pointing at the monitor, exclaiming that they knew the person on the screen or that they themselves were there. But as soon as the heaps of garbage appeared the viewers became serious. The women especially reacted loudly: *'This is too much!'* and *'This is really bad'.* After all the water and sanitation problems had been shown on the video, we stopped the VCR and the facilitator asked the first question.

Only key aspects of the discussions that went on in all five groups can be summarized here.

The first group of 'elderly' women and men were quite lively. When they saw themselves on the screen they fell about laughing and pointed at the monitor. They were a very active audience and nodded or commented loudly at what people in the video said: *'Yes, he is right'* or *'Yes, that's the way*

[5] For the video viewings the facilitators were local residents who had been working with the project. Judith acted as recorder. Some of the questions addressed were decided beforehand.

it is'. At one point a drug attendant in the video says that she has no drugs below the price of Ush.1,000, but she was of the opinion that the people in Kamwokya could afford these prices. At that point the audience was outraged and disagreed strongly and loudly. When we stopped the video to ask 'Who is responsible for water and sanitation in Kamwokya?', Mr Ssenoga, the RC2 Chairman, said:

The film can assist us to really see our situation and see how we can rectify the situation ourselves, before we seek outside intervention.

A man in the audience continued:

We have problems with unemployment and we are therefore poor. We should appeal for projects to assist us to alleviate poverty and thereby also reduce health risks.

Another man said:

We tenants feel that the landlords are responsible. They have not built good houses or planned the area properly, so that it is impossible to have proper drains.

A woman complained:

We have so many tribes and cultures here in Kamwokya and it is therefore difficult to control the community. This film should be viewed by the RCs with an aim to using their powers to direct the community towards better living conditions.

Mr Ssenoga then replied:

Poverty is only an excuse for irresponsibility and undisciplined disposal of garbage everywhere. The residents in the area should take responsibility for their environment right from their homes.

In this discussion Mr. Ssenoga presents himself as a very 'development-minded' person. He uses this opportunity to address the outsiders by telling his people, the residents of Kamwokya, that they should make themselves worthy of help by *'rectifying the situation ourselves, before we seek outside intervention'*, and he blames them for not behaving the way they should; they are irresponsible, undisciplined and lazy. According to Mr Ssenoga, the local residents are the ones responsible for the environment. His views are not shared by the others watching the video. One man blames the situation on unemployment and poverty, another blames the landlords, the woman blames the RCs.

In this context, as in the editing, the question of responsibility for Kamwokya's poor conditions provoked intense discussion in every audience. Here are some of the points made by the other groups: The 'ordinary women' (not RC leaders) felt that the responsibility for water and sanitation rested with the RCs and that the RCs together with the landlords should contact the City Council in order to get garbage containers. Then the residents should work on the drainage. They also said that the residents would be prepared to work on their environment if they had facilities like dumping containers and hoes. Communal efforts should be encouraged because people cannot afford to do it individually. The City Council should distribute dumping containers in all zones. Landlords should recognize their responsibility and provide toilets for their tenants...

The RC women's group blamed the landlords and the City Council for being irresponsible – not the RCs. It was the City Council's responsibility to provide garbage containers. They did not blame the local people who they said were too poor to 'alleviate these problems themselves' but some of the women did feel that the main responsibility lay with the local residents. These RC women appealed to a non-governmental organization well known in the area to come and help them solve their drainage problem. Some of the women also mentioned that many people lack proper housing and that many semi-permanent houses were health hazards. They also felt that the City Council officers had been very irresponsible, that, instead of enforcing proper building plans, they take bribes and let people put up illegal structures.

The 'mixed group of men' also complained about the unplanned houses which had greatly contributed to the poor standard of health in the area. They expressed the need for proper roads in Kamwokya, so that the place could be accessible for garbage trucks and ambulances. The men felt that the RCs were irresponsible because they saw people puting up illegal houses without toilets and did not interfere. But they also said that the residents themselves were partly responsible, because if people dump rubbish all over the place there is no way that the City Council can collect it. People should approach the town engineers to assist them in proper planning of the area. The general feeling was that the community was ignorant of who is responsible for what in community health.

The last 'young people' group, mainly boys, did not say much. They commented only that 'developers' should plan for roads in Kamwokya to make all corners accessible for City Council vehicles to collect garbage. At present the City Council containers are situated in only one zone and so the rest of the people cannot use them. One of the young boys said: '*People need to be educated and know that they are responsible for their own sanitation.*'

In all five group discussions the word 'responsibility' was used to mean both structural position and moral blame. The video had pushed the 'backstage' – the garbage heaps, dirt, filth – to the 'frontstage'. In this way the video shone the spotlight on issues normally taken for granted. The special occasion and the structured discussion enabled or 'forced' people to reflect on them. Having done so, all five groups tended to allocate responsibility to others and to deny that any moral blame rested with themselves.

The questions 'What are the treatment options in Kamwokya? Where do people go when they are sick and for what diseases?' gave rise to quite lively interventions in all the groups, but it was hard to notice any specific differences of view from one to another. All seemed to agree that traditional healers and traditional medicine were used much more in the past and in the rural areas, and/but they were still used for specific illnesses.

Discussions centred to a large extent on the differences between the traditional and modern sectors, and comments largely confirmed the findings reported in Chapter 6. Among them: *It is only in towns among the elite that you find people who despise local herbs. If people cannot afford modern drugs they go to healers ... Our forefathers used herbs so they must be good. but we should combine the efforts of both medical and traditional treatment ... chronic diseases compel one to seek assistance from traditional healers ... many people also try self-treatment through praying ... people will go to healers if modern medical treatment fails ... traditional herbs are better than syrups for coughs ... spirit-related diseases are to be cured by traditional healers ... where you go depends also on distance and the money you have ... drugs are expensive so people only buy half doses and end up even worse off than before ...*

In the mixed group's viewing of the 'earning a living' section, a woman remarked that all food business, apart from butchery, is done by women so that they can support their husbands and rear their families: husbands earn so little and school fees are so high. One man agreed and said that men generally appreciate women's contribution to family welfare, but another complained that women's extravagance forces men to hide their actual income. The women protested loudly and argued that men have a habit of trying to spend all their wives' incomes before they touch their own.

One woman commented that the video shows how people combine activities to survive. Women mainly work within Kamwokya, while men often work outside of the settlement – again confirming other findings (see Chapter 2, 'The Urban System' and Chapter 3). All the groups saw a clear relationship between health and economic activities. Many observed that no one could afford medicine, or at least not enough of it, nor could they afford proper treatment. Somebody also suggested that people have to work so hard to survive that they ignore their health (see Chapters 7 and 10 re women's priorities).

At the end of each session changes in Kamwokya were considered. Different opinions emerged: *It is a problem that there are so many tribes mixed together in Kamwokya ... the population explosion has caused many health problems... Kamwokya is not properly planned: Kamwokya used to be a village, then it started to develop and now it is underdeveloping ... stop here and start restructuring Kamwokya ... there is a lack of cooperative spirit ... most residents are tenants and therefore not so interested in putting any effort into changing the place...*

At the very end of almost all the sessions someone in the audience would say something like: *We have seen the film and realize the problems: How would you [film people] advise us?*

Why were there such strong reactions to the pictures of garbage heaps, stagnant water, and dirt everywhere in Kamwokya? Did the video help people to see things in their environment which they pass by everyday but do not really 'see'? Do living conditions become visible when the video camera sheds the spotlight on them? Parallels between the written word and video recordings are suggestive. Both put a filter between 'reality' and a person's own experience of reality which makes it possible to agree or disagree, add or take away. A text can be read over and over and a video film can be looked at over and over, each time revealing new meanings or things not noticed at first.

One woman said, for example, that the film made her aware that the market place was in very bad shape, filthy dirty, and had to be cleaned up and fixed. When asked if she had been aware of this before she saw the film, she answered that she had, but it became very much clearer on film: *Now we have really seen how bad it is and we can do something about it. The film should be seen by many people.*

The viewing itself provided a forum in which individuals could reflect and express their views on these topics. The decisions that the editing team had made about what to present and not present on video had consequences for everybody: the discussions around who was responsible and who was to blame in Kamwokya for garbage disposal, etc. would not have occurred had the topics not been put on video in the first place. And it might have consequences for the people being blamed and for those who gave the residents an opportunity to 'point fingers at the City Council' for not doing its job.

The Making of a Commentary

After the viewings were completed the editing team felt that the video needed a commentary in order for it to be a 'proper film'. They decided that there should be two versions, one in Luganda and one in English. Because some residents spoke in Luganda and others in English, the edited version contained sequences in both languages. It was therefore decided that there should be voice-overs translating the 'wrong' language sequences of each version. Finally, the RC 2 chairman Mr Ssenoga wanted to say a few things – as a commentary at the beginning and at the end of the film.

Mr Ssenoga at the beginning of the film: *The aim of the film is to show us life in Kamwokya the way we see it. Economic activities, water and sanitation, drainage system, garbage disposal, housing conditions and where people go when they are sick – the purpose of the film is to begin to act on the problems we are facing in our area.*

Mr Ssenoga at the end of the film: *We have seen Kamwokya 1994, we have seen the way we build our houses, the way we are living, how garbage disposal is done in the area, the poor sanitation. Now the question is who is responsible? Is it the area's RCs, the Kampala City Council, or some assistance from somewhere else? How prepared are you to improve this kind of situation in Kamwokya? The challenge is yours! Thank you.*

Once more, Mr Ssenoga makes plain that it is the ordinary residents of Kamwokya who should take up their responsibilities with regard to poor sanitation and garbage – and who would challenge him?

Concluding Remarks

What happened at the different stages of the video production process?

At the planning stage, themes and audience for the final product were discussed. This makes the whole exercise a very different endeavour from ordinary fieldwork. The product is also different in that it is meant for the local public – the people in the area – and not exclusively for researchers or TV audiences in the West.

During the shooting of the video, the camera provided people with an occasion to perform, turned the arena into a stage, and transformed people into actors. In doing so it encouraged them to articulate the 'frontstage' and give the onlooker a view of normative or ideal behaviour in that cultural context. In one sense therefore the camera promotes the wish to show how things ought to be. But the same camera picks up parts of the private 'backstage' which people might not want to show others. People's behaviour in front of a camera is also affected by their knowledge of the video media: we have mentioned the 'butcher syndrome' – how the butchers put on their white coats when the camera was on. In general, people in Kamwokya seemed very knowledgeable about TV and video.

At the editing stage a tension between the backstage and the frontstage came to the surface and the editing team had to make decisions as to which sequences to use in the edited version. When they decided to use some of the 'backstage' material, it was converted into 'frontstage' stuff for everybody to see and discuss.

A final note: The choice of the title of the film *Kamwokya 1994* indicates that its people experience Kamwokya as a place of change. However, the video itself cannot show process and change: it is a limitation of video and film that, despite moving images, they give a fixed impression. But the video does offer a portrait of the place and its people at a certain point in time, and with it later changes will be more readily recorded.[6] A woman remarked after seeing the video: *10 years after showing this film to all of Kamwokya's residents, we shall see marked change in the area.*

Only time will tell.

Epilogue

Did we learn/ will we learn anything about Kamwokya and its people from the video that would not otherwise be known? Certainly both the residents (as insiders) and the researchers (as outsiders) have gained an extra perspective – the former seeing themselves and their lives on screen; the latter being privileged to watch them do so.

Replay of the recorded scenes amongst the people filmed and in a public arena objectifies Kamwokya and allows them to interact with it as well as with each other about it. These interactions in turn seem to trigger a special kind of reflexivity, notching up the community's awareness of itself and so enhancing its capacity to define and deal with 'development' (cf. Freudenthal, 1990; AMREF et al., 1986; Wallman et al., 1990).

As for the research project, at the very least it can begin to spell out mental and moral processes which prevent private citizens from taking responsibility for public health. The extent to which these same factors may get in the way of treatment for private infection is a theme taken up in the concluding chapter.

---

[6] The final edition of *Kamwokya 1994* is available to the parish as well as to health authorities and potential donors in Kampala and elsewhere. It can be purchased from FFF Baldersgaten 10B, Stockholm 11427, Sweden.

Twelve

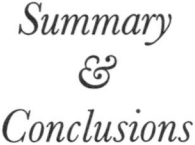

Summary
&
Conclusions

The perspective of this study is holistic: our strategy has been to define and describe dimensions of the local setting and the social context most relevant to treatment seeking in one Kampala neighbourhood. The focus of the narrative is on the options that women have for managing health and dealing with illness. It takes particular account of the bases for, and constraints on, their decisions to treat or not to treat, and how and when to treat, STD infection in themselves or acute sickness in a young child.

Each piece of the research exercise and, to a lesser extent, each chapter of the book has a separate bearing on the problem. For analytical purposes it is right for them to be distinct. But these distinctions are necessarily arbitrary: they do not and are not intended to match the experience of actors on the scene who must cope with all the dimensions at once. On this reasoning, the function of previous chapters has been to tease out and clarify the working of the various elements; and the function of the final chapter must be to bring the pieces back together in ways that highlight the links between them.

The rest of this chapter restates the original aims of the project (now put in the present tense) and then summarizes its main findings. The final paragraphs, returning to matters of personal risk and public responsibility, draw some general inferences for health policy and disease management in Kamwokya and settings like it.

Scientific and Technical Objectives

The general aim of the project is to contribute to AIDS control by specifying the factors preventing early and effective treatment of STD among 'ordinary' women in low-income urban Africa. Specifically it examines and seeks to explain evidence suggesting that relatively few such women use government hospitals/clinics for STD treatment.

The research is centred in social anthropology, but is multi-disciplinary, involving medical and social researchers and practitioners, and the active

226

participation of residents of the field area. It compares the management of STD and crisis illness in children under the age of five. The comparison is designed to assess the effect on STD treatment-seeking of stigma and the moral judgements excited by it.

The study notes which venereal or paediatric symptoms are regarded as traditional disease, appropriately dealt with by traditional (rather than biomedic) means, and how far the practical problems of resource scarcity and poor formal services account for treatment choices. Evidence for the match/mismatch of folk and biomedical symptomatology/aetiology is noted wherever it occurs.

The project encompasses township (parish), neighbourhood, household and individual contexts of treatment and treatment-seeking. It shows inter-relations among the separate elements being monitored, and the interaction of the urban system and the informal economy of health.

It covers formal and informal institutions as a single system of options, as do the people seeking treatment, but addresses the urgent need for data on the unenumerated ('informal') economy of STD and HIV. Most directly, the aim is to further STD/HIV prevention in three ways:

- By identifying the dimensions of context which make STD/HIV prevention inappropriate, or which impede early and effective treatment of STD, it may promote more cost-effective targeting of national or other intervention efforts to control the HIV/AIDS epidemic;
- By addressing the question 'What most needs doing?', i.e. does it make better economic/medical/social sense to prioritize transport, clinic management, drug supply, support for women, the integration of traditional healers, or to spend scarce resources on STD information and more extensive health education? At the very least the problem will be clarified by a full and 'thick' description of its constituent elements;
- By bringing medical and social perspectives to bear on a full range of 'informal' STD treatment options, and documenting the extent to which they are merged with the biomedical system, the project enables assessment of their actual or potential contribution to disease management.

Results and Interpretation of Findings

The findings, which are explored at length in each of the topic chapters, are summarized here under six headings: *urban setting; treatment options; gender balance/position of women; household resources and their control; private risk;* and *public responsibility.*

Urban setting

- Kamwokya II is vibrant, crowded, mixed, 'open'. These features are the bones of it as an urban system and have important implications for identity and the way resources are managed (Chapter 1 and below).

Systematic comparison with a similar but different area would allow more powerful generalization about the relative significance of each variable to the issues in focus.

- There is severe crowding in some parts. Density is 26,500 per sq. km., giving a resident population of about 14,000 in the one by one-half km area of the settlement. Both these are official calculations made in 1991 and are probably an underestimate. The terrain is uneven, well-drained at the top (along Kira Road), sloping to swamp in the lower part.
- The profile of Kamwokya's population mirrors that of Kampala as a whole. Its people are mixed by ethnicity and economic status, clustered in different parts of the parish, and associated with different lifestyles in the five 'cityscapes' defined.
- Outsiders are attracted by its accessibility, roadside market, churches, mosque, bars, entertainments, etc. Residents value its mixed housing options and therefore the possibility for improving without moving. Movement in, out and within is linked to opportunities in the vibrant informal economy.

Treatment options

- Treatment providers are many and various. There is a wide range of private clinics, drug shops, herbalists and other traditional healers. Home treatment is commonly the first resort.
- Mulago (the government hospital) STD and paediatric clinics are known and near, so they are not less accessible than other options. Distance is not the factor pushing people to use alternatives.
- Impediments to and choice of effective treatment vary with resource implications as well as the type/definition of symptoms and person sick. Not even 'free' government provision is without cost.

Gender balance/position of women

- Men and women have a different relation to the local area: women are more likely 'never' to leave Kamwokya II; men come and go daytime and evening; also male outsiders come for business, for the candlelight market and for entertainment.
- 25 per cent of households contain only female adults and/or are headed by a woman.
- Formal marriage is 'rare'. It remains the ideal for some, but single mother status is preferred by others because few men can/do take economic responsibility for children '*as a good man should*'.
- The age:sex ratios of men and women are very different. There is a striking and important surplus of girls/young women in the 10–20 year-old bracket. Men aged 25–40 are still in excess. The implications for sexual behaviour, patterns of STD/HIV transmission and the risk of infection should be noted.

Household resources and their control

- Access to and management of social capital and non-material resources affect a woman's capacity to seek and get treatment at least as importantly as money.

- Resources are different and/or are deployed in different ways according to whether it is the woman or her child who is sick; and according to whether the symptoms are secret/shameful/stigmatized/morally tainted or not. These assessments necessarily get in the way of early and effective treatment of STDs.

- Control over resources was greater, certainly for economically independent women and possibly for any woman living alone, than for women who must defer to a resident partner or his patrikin. This logic applies whatever the level of resources. Even if her man makes contributions of food or money such that a woman is materially better-off than she would be living alone, she will not expect to control the resources he brings. In this sense she has less autonomous scope than lone women who may be among the poorest Kamwokya residents.

- Women prioritize children's health and treatment for children's illnesses, and they delay spending time or money on their own symptoms unless or until they are *in extremis*. Given the crucial role of women in health care and treatment-seeking, their tendency to self-neglect may ultimately jeopardize the wellbeing of all members of the household.

- This is not the only context in which what looks like irresponsible behaviour in respect of one kind of risk may be understood as responsible judgement in respect of another. The tragic circumstance in which commercializing her sex is the only option available to a woman who needs to pay school fees or funeral expenses, who must find the money for medical treatment, or who has no other means of securing the family's basic sustenance demonstrates the same dilemma.

Personal risk

- STD/HIV risk is never the only thing women (or men) have to worry about. Reputation as a proper and reproductive woman must be protected if status in the community is to be maintained.

- The risk of offending or losing a male partner by suggesting a checkup or a condom may be more significant than the risk of one more infection in an infectious environment.

- Ordinary people are generally well informed about the vectors of STD and HIV infection, and know the risks of unprotected sex, etc. Continued emphasis on prevention information, however cleverly it is targeted, is not the most efficient use of scarce local/national/international resources.

- To the extent that tendencies to deny risk and/or to feel fatalistic/helpless/not in control are aggravated by fear, hectoring repetition of 'Stop AIDS' or 'safe sex' messages may actually be counter-productive at this stage of the epidemic in Kampala.

- There is a provocative link between lack of control over the risk of infection generated in the public arena (from sewage, unclean water, garbage, mosquitoes, etc.) and the general sense of non-control over 'private' infection.

Public responsibility

- The public health environment is very poor overall. Even the better areas suffer the effects of the unplanned slums: no overall drainage, open sewers, chaotic garbage disposal. The water supply has recently been improved by the efforts of Catholic NGOs, but many households are without access to good water. The majority anyway spend substantial time and energy (even if not money) to get it.
- Responsibility for public health is not taken by the Kampala City Council. Its resources are limited, but the crucial impediment is the fact that most habitations are unplanned, built temporarily and without official permission. The same is true of Kamwokya II as a whole, and is in sharp contrast to Kamwokya I across the highway.
- Responsibility is not taken by residents because they are mostly tenants ('this is not our place') and mobile ('soon we shall move'), even though they are committed to staying in Kamwokya. They are aware that environmental health problems cannot be solved by households as individual units, and the wellbeing of their own separate household in many cases leaves no surplus resources for the public sphere. The discussion of this issue in the video viewing (Chapter 11), however, suggests that the separation of public and private spheres is not immutable.

Last Words

Assessments of risk and of responsibility are functions of two kinds of control: on the one hand there are the facts of power and authority; and on the other, the sense of being – or not being – able or entitled to act. Just as the Kampala concept of wellbeing conflates the facts and the experience of livelihood, so the capability of a person, a household or a community to initiate or change health-related behaviour is misconstrued if only half the story is taken into account.

Capability notions of one kind or another were not always fashionable (Wallman, 1996b). They reflect the political ideals which Western governments now espouse in their relations with the so-called Third World and, maybe coincidentally, provide the rhetoric to justify leaner aid and development packages. Gradually it began to be clear that the hapless frame did not fit the reality very often, and that it was resented by those whose autonomy it denied. One good effect is that the habit of social scientists and liberal politicians to blame the world system and/or the rich for the poverty of the poor has been reversed: the unfortunate, in whatever sense of the word, are no longer visualized as passive, not responsible, without capacity to take charge of their lives (as e.g. by Valentine, 1968; Frank, 1969; Rodney, 1972). Much less good are the twin tendencies to depend too heavily on local capacity to go it alone, and to exaggerate an individual's power to alter risky behaviour, decrease the risk of infection, respond to directives from health authorities − i.e. to act on what she knows.

A note from an earlier urban study treads between the two extremes in the way we intend here:

> ... Although the subjects of this book are typical inner city residents their collective story is not a bleak tale of deprivation and disadvantage. It is not that they want for nothing: all of them work hard to make ends meet and can remember times when everyday life was too much to cope with. But most of them get by well enough, and as they see it, the inner city setting offers as full a range of possibilities for a decent life as any other... (Wallman, 1984: 3).

In even the most dire circumstances these 'best view' representations are entirely realistic, based on the assumption that every setting, every person, etc. has capabilities, however limited. It rests on the definition of social structure as a more or less fixed framework of options within which the process of social life is organized (Chapter 1, p. 13, quoting Firth, 1951, 1954). The aim of this book has been to give evidence of 'all' the elements affecting the options available, the choices made among them, the constraints on and the reasons for those choices being made by various categories of Kamwokya resident.

Each piece of evidence pertains to one or other level of the local scene, and makes sense only in one or other context of its happening. And because every event, attitude, action, etc. *could* be interpreted in any number of ways, we have tried throughout to pay deliberate attention to the difference that context can make.

This effort confirms the primacy of anthropological perspectives in this research: the discipline is distinguished from other social sciences by a quiver of analytical tools in which the notion of context is essential. It shows in the way we tend to 'explain' the item in question by looking for its connections with other-things-happening. And because neither the dynamic nor the scope of the system in which those other things are happening is empirically given (Gellner, 1973), it is inevitably necessary to decide which kind and which level of context is most relevant to making sense of the matter in hand.

There is an extra difficulty when a work sets out (also) to be useful to praxis and planning. These days to say that 'social context counts' is only to state the obvious. The real world now expects to be told how it counts. Which aspects count? Do they count equally in every situation? What are the key elements needed to understand that piece of behaviour? To solve this problem? To ameliorate this or that crisis? And, hardest of all, what specific interventions are demanded or justified by the findings?

Given the aims of the project (Chapter 1, pp. 3−4 and above), it may be useful, in the light of this discussion, to reprise two particular 'capability' concerns. One relates to personal risk and to the offensive and dubious notion that STD/HIV transmission is 'caused by' risky sexual behaviour and would stop if that behaviour were simply to be changed. The other relates to public responsibility and an explanation for the lack of effort put, by an otherwise energetic community, into dealing with the open sewers and festering latrines which are also characteristic of Kamwokya.

Private risk and STD

At first sight, the focus or research into STD might seem to belong in the area narrowly defined as sexual behaviour. Much of it does. Investigations into demographic and behavioural risk factors have concentrated on quantifiable elements such as numbers of partners or contacts with 'high risk' groups. Significant prevention of STD and HIV, however, depends on understanding, and ultimately dealing with, 'risky sexual behaviour' in its context. Without context it has no social meaning, and without knowing what it means, we cannot presume even to know which aspects of life are or should be included under the 'sexual behaviour' or even 'sexual attitudes and behaviour' rubric.

In terms of STD/HIV narrowly (clinically?) defined, the significance of people's sexual behaviour lies in the body contact, physical stress, skin abrasions and exchange of fluids that it entails. In terms of the realities of prevention and treatment, it is about family life, local organization, morality, cosmology, opportunity, economics, mobility, self-esteem – most, if not all, the elements of livelihood described for Kamwokya in the preceding chapters. However clinically sound the understanding of the 'risky sex' practices of individuals, without reference to other-things-happening, it is not an appropriate basis for health interventions.

Since risky sexual behaviour cannot be addressed without reference to context, any approach to STD prevention must do more than acknowledge that context counts. The capability question may help: *In these circumstances, given this knowledge, these constraints, what scope do these women have for avoiding infection, or for diagnosing/ acknowledging/ treating infection once it occurs?* Identifying the impediments to their doing so is prerequisite to knowing where and how best to intervene.

It is to be noted in the international AIDS literature that specific reference to risk groups is no longer made, and that concepts of risky behaviour, risky sex, etc. are increasingly less current. The first change was politically inspired, but the others, though perhaps also guided by heightened sensitivity, reflect the greater context-awareness of professionals in the field: sexual practices which are 'risky' where STD or HIV prevalence is high, general health is poor and the population is disrupted by war, might, in a different context, be so much more safe as to constitute quite different behaviours (compare Barnett and Blaikie, 1992: 68–85 with Wellings *et al.*, 1994, p 356–801).

Similarly, references to *vulnerability* in recent medical and epidemiological discourse imply (also) the social factors which incline categories of people to infection (Mann *et al.*, 1992). This at once demedicalizes the term and brings context into play. More interesting, it is similar to, although opposite from, the *capability* notion: both disallow emphasis on the individual as a strategizing or psychologically prone risk-taker (Adams, 1985) who is in control, should be responsible, and can be 'blamed' for not acting to avoid the risk that experts have identified (Paine, 1992b).

Public responsibility and the urban system

The reasoning of the last paragraph points to the conclusion that direct intervention at the level of individuals is probably unuseful and certainly uneconomic. In medical terms it is neither effective nor efficient. The indications are, on the contrary, that change will be brought about by 'community' response. However specific the objectives of an intervention therefore, its success will depend on some prior understanding of the scope, style, dynamics and general *capability* of the community in question.

In this final section, given our concern with the health environment, the emphasis falls back on the question of responsibility for private and public health-relevant decisions. In Kamwokya, where 'health' and 'well-being' are conflated, residents are already wise to the fact that any decision about the use of resources of any kind is health-related. Underlining the point, evidence for and explanations of who takes or refuses that responsibility in a variety of contexts is spread throughout the book.

Two important features of the evidence, both having special relevance to the practical issues, are the degree to which resource decisions are negotiable, and how much scope there is for people to agree to differ. The inference is not that there are no constraints on choice or outcome (see the *structure:organization* distinction above and in Chapter 1), but that the style of resource management in Kamwokya is only rarely homogeneous. For some people in some circumstances, as the materials show, this constitutes a widening of their options. In the local area as a whole, it accounts both for the diversity and individualism of the economic scene, and for the absence of firm boundaries of responsibility for – in terms of our particular interest – the public health environment.

Our argument has been that the homogeneity: heterogeneity distinction is a characteristic of urban systems. The main points of it, and its basis in previous studies, are indicated in Chapter 1 (pp. 13–15). Here it brings the focus back to the question: *What are the capabilities of this urban system?* It is addressed by asking again: *What difference makes most difference to the way life and livelihood are organized in Kamwokya?*

The discussion reflects on an ideal type model developed from the comparative study of two similarly low-income, multi-ethnic areas (Wallman, 1982, 1984, 1985). By virtue of different industrial structures and patterns of work, the two areas function as quite different urban systems. In one the various boundaries of difference do not overlap, the structure is relatively open, and the organization of identity and other resources is heterogeneous. The other is consistently opposite: tightly bounded, relatively closed, consistently homogeneous. Moreover, in the matter of identity options at every level, the preferred style of the first area ('Type A') is *localist*, and of the second ('Type B') *ethnic*.[1] By this token, when two areas of similarly mixed population – one heterogeneous, the other homogeneous – are compared, ethnic difference will count less in the first than in the second.

When the evidence for Kamwokya is measured against this model, it fails immediately for lack of consistency. It is not one thing or the other, not Type A *or* Type B throughout the system. Nor does it fit some inter-mediate position on a continuum between them.

But the A:B contrast does hold for sub-systems within the whole. For some people in some contexts, ethnicity counts (whether or not to their advantage); in other contexts, for them as well as for other people, localism has more cogency. Some occupations and activities sustain ethnic net-works, but on the whole they are loosely bounded and it is not unusual for their members to exchange resources and form friendships without reference to origin. These observations apply to women as well as men.

With one exception, the classification of each sub-system as *either* open/heterogeneous/localist *or* closed/homogeneous/ethnic is not prob-lematic. The anomaly is women's networks at the neighbourhood level (see particularly Chapter 10). They are exclusive and tightly bounded in ways that suggest a closed, ethnicity-driven, Type B system – but belonging in this case is *achieved* by locally appropriate behaviour, as it is in the localist (Type A) prototype, not *ascribed* by the immutable characteristics of origin. When it comes to resource access, exclusion and responsibility in this context, ethnicity does not count.[2]

In effect, Kamwokya differs from Type A *and* Type B urban systems in two ways: first, its boundary principles are not consistent; and second, there is a gender difference – women's identification with the micro-local area is stronger and tighter than men's (to a degree that did not show up in the London cases).[3] But consonant with the A:B model both these special features follow from the structure and organization of work.

The consistency of boundary style in the two Londons is an effect of local structures which are heavily industrial and of very long standing. The options for organization which they offer are fixed by time and

---

[1] This typology should not be confused with that of Southall (1961), which was prepared for a different purpose. He distinguishes established and homogeneous *cities* (called Type A) from new and heterogeneous (called Type B). The heterogeneous/homogeneous contrast holds in the version proposed here (although the A:B labels are reversed), but for us the essential difference is held neither to be a matter of age nor to apply to whole cities as in Southall's model. Our point is that urban *systems* may be quite small parts of the urban whole and that the structure of options (and the social style) characteristic of each of them can be independent of how long they have been established (Wallman, 1985).

[2] The point above (Southall, 1961) is confirmed by the fact that not all parts of Kampala are or have been a-ethnic in this sense – as Grillo (1974) shows in a study of Nsambya.

[3] It is often noted in London and other industrial cities, however, that women with children 'choose' to work close to home and/or part-time for the sake of their normal or crisis child-care responsibilities.

infrastructure, echoed in political tradition, and sustained by the work cultures of in-migrants in both areas. Public responsibility is clearly allocated (which is not to say that it is always fulfilled), and the division between public and private spheres is not expected to be a matter for personal negotiation.

The structure and infrastructure of Kampala is entirely different. It has never been an industrialized city, and many of the formal institutions which began to thrive after independence did not survive the disruptions of Amin and Obote. Options for steady employment are now rare, and the informal economy makes the running. In this context, wellbeing depends on seizing every opportunity, using every contact, organizing in whatever way it takes. Too consistent a boundary style just gets in the way of getting by.

The structure of options in the informal economy also accounts for the peculiar localism of women. Relative to men, custom and responsibility give women extra incentive to take up even the smallest chance of earning a living close to home. And – again relative to men – there is currently more work that women are expected to do or prepared to do in the local economy.

This local focus is key. Above the age of twelve, male residents are twice as likely to go out of Kamwokya 'regularly', and the 'main occupation' of close to 90 per cent of the women surveyed (in the WS) is carried out within the parish. These findings begin to explain the observation that there are more women than men 'around' in Kamwokya. They also confirm the prior importance of *local* reputation which cannot, in a multi-ethnic and heterogeneous environment, be left to depend on ethnic resources.

At this level of the system and in the core area of Kamwokya, it looks as though men and women are operating in different kinds of urban system. Women live and work and socialize in one place with one set of people; men, by contrast, spread themselves about.

Our final inference has to be that to assume that similar options are open to men and women, to people of the same ethnic or social standing, or to residents of the different cityscapes in the settlement is to discredit the resource value of difference in Kamwokya. This has profound practical implications. While it is widely agreed that interventions designed to improve local wellbeing cannot usefully be targeted at individual persons or households, the Kamwokya case demonstrates that it may be folly to target groups fixed by any criteria. The apparent untidiness of the system gives it a distinctive kind of capability for getting by.

References

Adams, J. (1985), *Risk and Freedom: An Analysis of Road Safety Legislation*, Cardiff, UK: TPP.

Akhtar, R. (ed.) (1987), *The Geography of Health and Disease in Tropical Africa*, Chur, Switzerland: Harwood.

AMREF, UNICEF and WIF (1986), *Video for Development: Why and How?* Workshop report, Nairobi: AMREF (March).

Anguyo, G. (1993), 'Paediatric Oral Surgical Practices, especially treatment of "false teeth" in Arua District', *Child Health and Development Centre Report*, Makerere University.

Ari News (1989), No. 14, Lead Article, August.

Bantebya-Kyomuhendo, G. (1994), *The Health Care Provider Woman Client Relationship: Health Workers Perspectives*. Geneva: WHO/TDR.

Barnett, A. and Blaikie, P. (1992), *AIDS in Africa: Its Present and Future Impact*, London: Belhaven.

Barton, T. and Wamai, G. (1994), *Equity and Vulnerability: A Situation Analysis of Women, Adolescents and Children in Uganda*, Kampala: CHDC/UNICEF.

Belshaw, D. (1988), 'Agriculture-led Recovery in post-Amin Uganda', in Hansen and Twaddle.

Berman, P., Kendall, C. and Bhattacharyya, K. (1994), 'The Household Production of Health: Integrating Social Science Perspectives as Micro-level Health Determinants', *Soc. Sci. and Med.* 38 (2): 205–15.

Blaxter, M. (1983), 'The Causes of Disease: Women Talking', *Soc. Sci. Med.* 17 (2): 59–69.

Browner, C.H. (1989), 'Women, Household and Health in Latin America', *Soc. Sci. Med.* 28 (5): 461–73.

Bushkens, W.F.L. and Slikkerveer, L.J. (1982), *Healthcare in East Africa. Illness Behaviour of the Eastern Oromo in Haraqhe* (Ethiopia). Assen: Van Gorcum.

Busuulwa, J., Konings, E. and Wallman, S. (1994), *Report on the Ethnographic and Women's Surveys, Kamwokya II Parish, Kampala*, CHDC, Makerere University and Dept. of Sociology and Anthropology, University of Hull.

Bwengye, E.L. (1992), 'Uganda: Newborns, False Teeth and Diarrhoea', *Dialogue on Diarrhoea*, 48: 2.

Castle, Sarah (1994), 'The (Re)negotiation of Illness Diagnosis and Responsibility for Child Death in Mali', *Medical Anthropology Q.* 8 (3): 314–35.

CHDC (1994), *Health Workers' Report*, Kampala: CHDC, Makerere University.

Chirgwin, K., Dillon, S., Dettovitz, J., Landsman, S.H. and McCormack, W. (1989), 'Genital Ulcers and HIV Infection in an Urban Sexually Transmitted Disease Clinic'. Paper given at V International Conference on AIDS, Montreal, 4–9 June.

Dodge, C.P. and Wiebe, P.H. (1985), *Crisis in Uganda. The Breakdown of Health Services*, OUP.

Economist, The (1994), *(Pocket) World in Figures: 1995 Edition*, London: The Economist Books Ltd.

Edmonds, K. (1988), 'Crisis Management: the Lessons for Africa from Obote's Second Term', in Hansen and Twaddle.

Eisenberg, L. (1977), 'Disease and Illness: Distinctions between Professional and Popular Ideas of Sickness', *Culture, Med. and Society*, 1: 9–23.

Escobar, A. (1991), 'Anthropology and the Development Encounter: the Making and Marketing of Development Anthropology', *American Ethnologist*, 18 (4).

Fabian, J. (1990), *Power and Performance. Ethnographic Explorations through Proverbial Wisdom and Theatre in Chaba, Zaire*. Madison, WI: University of Wisconsin Press.

Firth, R. (1951), *Elements of Social Organisation*, London: Watts.

Firth, R. (1954), 'Social Organisation and Social Change', *J. Royal Anthropological Institute*, 84.

Frank, A.G. (1969), *Latin America: Under-development or Revolution?* New York: Monthly Review Press.

Freudenthal, S. (1988), 'What to Tell and How to Show it: Issues in Anthropological Filmmaking', in J. Rollwagen (ed.) *Anthropological Filmmaking*, New York: Harwood Academic Publishers.

Freudenthal, S. (1990), 'Video: A Means to Hear Vox Populi. A Participatory Evaluation

References

Exercise of the FTP Project in Babati, Tanzania', *FTP Newsletter*, Uppsala: SUAS.

Gellner, E.A. (1973), 'Concepts and Society' in I.C. Jarvie and J. Agassi (eds), *Cause and Meaning in the Social Sciences*, London: Routledge & Kegan Paul.

Gershuny, J.I. (1983), *Social Innovation and the Division of Labour*, Oxford: OUP.

Gluckman, M. (1982), 'The Logic of African Science and Witchcraft', in M. Marwick (ed.), *Witchcraft and Sorcery*, Harmondsworth: Penguin Books, 2nd edn.

Goffman, E (1959), *The Presentation of Self in Everyday Life*, New York: Doubleday Anchor Books.

Graham, H. (1984), *Women, Health and the Family*, Brighton, UK: Wheatsheaf Harvester.

Graham, H. (1985), 'Providers, Negotiators, and Mediators: Women as the Hidden Carers', in E. Lewin and V. Olesen (eds), *Women, Health and Healing: Towards a New Perspective*. London: Tavistock.

Green, E.C. (1992), 'Sexually Transmitted Disease, Ethnomedicine and Health Policy in Africa', *Soc. Sci. Med.* 35(2): 121–30.

Gregory, C.A. and Altman, J.C. (1989) *Observing the Economy*, (ASA Research Methods No. 3), London: Routledge.

Grillo, R.D. (1974), 'Ethnic Identity and Social Stratification of a Kampala Housing Estate', in A. Cohen (ed.) *Urban Ethnicity*, London: Tavistock.

Grosskurth, H. *et al.* (1995), 'Impact of Improved Treatment of STD on HIV Infection in Rural Tanzania: randomised controlled trials', *The Lancet*, 346, 26 August.

Gutkind, C.W. (1973), 'Bibliography on Urban Anthropology', in A.W. Southall (ed.) *Urban Anthropology: Cross-Cultural Studies of Urbanization*, New York: OUP.

Hakansson, N.T. (1988), *Bridewealth, Women and Land*, Uppsala: Studies in Cultural Anthropology.

Hannerz, Ulf (1993), 'The Cultural Role of World Cities' in A.P. Cohen and K. Fukui (eds) *Humanizing the City? Social Contexts of Urban Life at the Turn of the Millennium*, Edinburgh: Edinburgh University Press.

Hansen, H.B. and Twaddle, M. (eds) (1988), *Uganda Now: Between Decay and Development*, London: James Currey.

Hansen, H.B. and Twaddle, M. (eds) (1991), *Changing Uganda: the Dilemmas of Structural Adjustment and Revolutionary Change*, London: James Currey.

Harding, P. and Jenkins, R. (1989), *The Myth of the Hidden Economy: Towards a New Understanding of Informal Economic Activity*, Milton Keynes, UK: Open University Press.

Hoffman, S. (1987), 'Women's Activities and Impacts on Child Nutrition', in W. Gittinger *et al.* (eds), *Food Policy*, Washington DC: World Bank.

Hogle, J., Lwanga, J., Kisamba-Mugetwa, C. and Musonge, D.L. (1991), 'Uganda Traditional Healer Study: Indigenous Knowledge and Management of Childhood Diarrhoeal Disease'. Working paper, CHDC, Kampala: PRITECH/USAID/UNICEF.

Horton, R. (1973), 'Levy-Bruhl, Durkheim and the Scientific Revolution?' in R. Horton and R. Finnegan (eds), *Modes of Thought*, London: Faber.

Hunt, C.W. (1989), 'Migrant Labour and STD: AIDS in Africa', *J. Health and Social Behaviour* 30: 353–73.

International Labour Office (1991), *The Urban Informal Sector in Africa*, Geneva; ILO.

Jamal, V. (1991), 'The Agrarian Context of the Uganda Crisis' in Hansen and Twaddle.

Jamal, V. and Weeks, J. (1988), 'The Vanishing Rural–Urban Gap in Sub-Saharan Africa', *International Labour Review*, 127 (3).

Janzen, J. M. (1978), *The Quest for Therapy in Lower Zaire*, Berkeley, CA: University of California Press.

Jonker, C. (1988), 'Health Care Utilization in an African Township: a Case Study from Lusaka, Zambia', M.A. Thesis, University of Zambia.

Kalibala, S., Nsubuga, P. and Kabaksi, D. (1992), *Sexually Transmitted Diseases: Training Manual for Primary Health Workers*, Kampala.

Kalumba, K. (with P. Freund) (1982), *Evaluating Health and Nutrition Services under the GR7/ UNICEF Program of Co-operation: The Nawinda Luampungu Survey*, Report No. 2, Lusaka: Institute for African Studies.

Kapoor, K. *et al.* (1993), *Uganda Growing Out of Poverty*, Washington, DC: World Bank.

Kellock, S. and Agunda, K.O. (1985), 'The Roles and Situation of Women', *Situation Analysis of Children and Women in Kenya*, (Section 3). Nairobi: Government of Kenya, Central Bureau of Statistics, Ministry of Finance and Planning, with UNICEF.

References

Klovdahl, A.S. (1985), 'Social Networks and the Spread of Infectious Diseases: the AIDS example' *Soc. Sci. Med.* 21: 1203–16.

Kreiss, J. K., Koech, D., Plummer, F.A. *et al.* (1986) 'AIDS Virus Infection in Nairobi Institutes: Spread of the Epidemic in East Africa', *New England J. Med.*

Krueger, R. A. (1989), *Focus Groups: A Practical Guide for Applied Research*, Newbury Park, CA: Sage Publications.

Laga, M., Nzilambi, Nzila and Goeman, J. (1991), 'The Interrelationship of STD and HIV Infection: Implications for the Control of Both Epidemics in Africa', *AIDS*, 5, Supp.I: 955–63.

Lal, D. and Kennedy, C. (1988), 'AIDS, Heterosexuals and Africa', *Papers in Economics* No. 88, University College London.

Last, M. (1992), 'The Importance of Knowing about Not Knowing: Observations from Hausaland', in S. Feireman and J.M. Janzen, (eds), *The Social Basis of Healing Health and Healing in Africa*, Berkeley, CA: University of California Press.

Lateef, K.S. (1991), 'Structural Adjustment in Uganda: The Initial Experience' in Hansen and Twaddle.

Leach, E. (1967), 'An Anthropologist's Reflections on a Social Survey', in O. Jongmans and P. Gutkind (eds), *Anthropologists in the Field*, Assen: Van Gorcum.

Levine, N.E. (1992), 'When Do People Seek Help and From Whom?', *Dialogue on Diarrhoea*, 48.

Litman, T. (1974), 'The Family as a Basic Unit in Health and Medical Care', *Soc. Sci. and Med.* 8: 495–519.

Lombolt, G. and Nsibambi, J. (1972), 'Venereal Diseases', *The Uganda Journal 1*: 105–13.

Maclean, C.M.U. (1966), 'Hospitals or Healers? An Attitude Survey in Ibadan', *Human Organisation*, 25 (2): 131–9.

Macrae, J. and Zwi, A. (1993), *Health and Health Policy in Post-Conflict Societies; A Review of the Literature*, Health Policy Unit, London School of Hygiene and Tropical Medicine.

Macrae, J., Zwi, A. and Birungi , H. (1993), 'Healthy Peace? Rehabilitation and Development of the Health Sector in a Post-Conflict Situation – the Case of Uganda.' Report of a pilot study, Health Economics and Financing Programme, Health Policy Unit, London School of Hygiene and Tropical Medicine.

Maliyamkono, T.L. and Bagachwa, M. (1990), *The Second Economy in Tanzania*, London: James Currey.

Mann, J., Tarantola, D.J.M. and Netter, T.W. (eds) (1992), *AIDS in the World*, Cambridge, MA: Harvard University Press.

Marwick, M.(1982), 'Witchcraft and the Epistemology of Science', in M. Marwick (ed.) *Witchcraft and Sorcery*, Harmondsworth: Penguin Books, 2nd edn.

Mbiti, J.S. (1969), *African Philosophy and Religions*, London: Heinemann.

McGee, T.G. (1973), 'Peasants in the Cities: a Paradox, a Paradox, a Most Ingenious Paradox', *Human Organization*, 32 (2): 135–42.

Mettelin, P., (1987), 'Activités informelles en Afrique Noire: les réalités urbaines', *Canadian J. Development Studies*, 8 (1).

Mitchell, J.C. (1983), 'Case and Situation Analysis', *Sociological Review* 31 (2): 187–211.

Moses, S. *et al.* (1991), 'Controlling HIV in Africa: Effectiveness and Cost of an Intervention in a High-Frequency STD Transmitter Core Group', *AIDS*, 5: 407–11.

Namboze, J.M. (1983), 'Health and Culture in an African Society', *Soc. Sci. Med.* 17 (24): 2041–3.

Nanchengwa, V.M. (1984), 'People's Beliefs about the Causation of Disease and Implications for Choice of Healthcare in Lusaka', M.A. Thesis, University of Zambia.

National Resistance Movement (1986) *Ten Point Programme*, Kampala: Directorate of Information, NRM Secretariat.

Nelson, N. (1978), 'Women Must Help Each Other. The Operation of Personal Networks among *buzza* Beer Brewers in Mathare Valley, Kenya', in J. Bujra and P. Caplan, (eds), *Women United: Women Divided*, London: Tavistock.

Nelson, N. (1987), 'Selling Her Kiosk: Kikuyu Notions of Sexuality and Sex for Sale in Mathare Valley, Kenya', in P. Caplan (ed.) *The Cultural Construction of Sexuality*, London: Tavistock.

Nelson, N. (1988), 'How Women and Men Get by: The Sexual Division of Labour in the Informal Sector of a Nairobi Squatter Settlement', in J. Gugler, (ed.) *The Urbanization of the Third World*, Oxford: OUP.

Nsibambi, A.R. (1991), 'Resistance Councils and Committees: a Case Study from Makere'

References

in Hansen and Twaddle.

Nyamwaya, D. (1992), *African Indigenous Medicine: An Anthropological Perspective for Policy Makers and Primary Health Care Managers*, Nairobi: AMREF.

Obbo, C. (1980), *African Women and their Struggle for Independence*, London: Zed Books.

Obbo, C. (1991), 'Women, Children and a Living Wage', in Hansen and Twaddle.

O'Connor, A. (1988), 'Uganda: the Spatial Dimension', in Hansen and Twaddle.

Ogden, J.A. (1991), 'Autonomy and Interdependence in two Kenya Societies: A Challenge to the Universal Domination of Women', MA (Econ.) Thesis, University of Manchester.

Packard, R., Wisner, B., and Bossert, T. (1989), 'Introduction: the Political Economy of Health and Disease in Africa and Latin America', *Soc. Sci. Med.* 28 (5): 405–44.

Paine, R. (1989), 'Making the Invisible Visible: Coming to terms with Chernobyl and its Experts (a Saami illustration)', *Int. J. Moral & Social Studies* 4(2).

Paine, R. (1992a), 'The Marabar Caves, 1920–2020', in S. Wallman (ed.), *Contemporary Futures: Perspectives from Social Anthropology*, London: Routledge.

Paine, R. (1992b), 'Chernobyl reaches Norway: the Accident, Science, and the Threat to Cultural Knowledge', *Public Understanding of Sci.* 1: 261–80.

PANOS Dossier: (1990), *Triple Jeopardy: Women and AIDS*, London: Panos Publications Ltd.

Parkin, D. (1969) *Neighbours and Nationals in an African City Ward*, London: Routledge & Kegan Paul.

Piot, P., Kreiss, J., Ndinya-Achola, J. *et al.* (1987), 'Heterosexual Transmission of HIV: Editorial Review', *AIDS* 1: 199–206.

Piot, P. and Laga, M. (1988), 'Genital Ulcers, Other STDs and the Sexual Transmission of AIDS', *British Medical Journal*, 298: 623–4.

Piot, P., Plummer, F. A., Mhalu, F . S., Lambouray, J . L., Chin, J. and Mann, J.A. (1988), 'AIDS: An International Perspective', *Science* 239: 573–9.

Pons, V. (1969), *Stanleyville*, Oxford: Oxford University Press.

Pons, V. (1993/4a), *Broad Brush Survey of Kamwokya II*, CHDC, Makerere University and Dept. of Sociology and Anthropology, University of Hull.

Pons, V. (1993/4b), *File on the Context and Socio-demographic Characteristics of Kamwokya II (Based on the 1991 Census)*, CHDC, Makerere University and Dept of Sociology and Anthropology, University of Hull.

Preston, S.H. (1988), 'Urban Growth in Developing Countries: a Demographic Reappraisal', in J. Gugler (ed.) *The Urbanization of the Third World*. Oxford: Oxford University Press.

Prual, A., Chacko, S. and Koch-Weser, D. (1991), 'Sexual Behaviour, AIDS and Poverty in Sub-Saharan Africa', *International J. of STDs and AIDS* 2: 1–9.

Quinn, T.C., Mann, J.M., Curran, J. W., and Piot, P. (1986), 'AIDS in Africa: an Epidemiological Paradigm', *Science* 234: 955–63.

Radoki, C . (1991), 'Women's Work or Household Strategies?', *Environment and Urbanisation* 3 (2): 39–45.

Raikes, A. (1989), 'Women's Health in East Africa', *Soc. Sci. Med.* 28 (5): 447–59.

Rodney, W. (1972), *How Europe Underdeveloped Africa*, London: Bogle l'Ouverture.

Rogers, E.V. and Shoemaker, F.F. (1971), *Communication of Innovations*, New York: The Free Press, 2nd edn.

Rouch, J. (1975), 'The Camera and Man', in P. Hockings (ed.), *Principles of Visual Anthropology*, The Hague: Mouton.

Sargent, C.F., (1982), *The Cultural Context of Therapeutic Choice: Obstetrical Care Decisions among the Bariba of Benin*, Dordrecht, Netherlands: D. Reidel.

Smock, A. (1981), 'Women's Economic Roles', in T . Killick (ed.), *Papers on the Kenyan Economy*, Nairobi: Heinemann.

Southall, A.W. (1961), *Social Change in Modern Africa*, London: OUP for International African Institute.

Southall, A.W. (1988), 'The Recent Political Economy of Uganda', in Hansen and Twaddle.

Southall, A. and Gutkind, P. (1957), *Townsmen in the Making*, E.A. Studies No. 9, Kampala: East African Institute of Social Research.

Stack, C. (1976), *All Our Kin: Strategies for Survival In a Black Community*, New York: Harper Row.

Staugard, F. (1985a), *Traditional Healers*, Gaborone: Ipelegang Publishers.

Staugard, F. (1985b), *Traditional Midwives*, Gaborone: Ipelegang Publishers.

Steptoe, A. (1989), 'The Significance of Personal Control in Health and Disease', in A. Steptoe and A. Appells (eds) *Stress, Personal Control and Health*, Brussels/Luxembourg: John Wiley.

References

Stren, R. and White, R. (eds) (1989), *African Cities in Crisis*, Boulder, CO: Westview Press.

Swantz, M.L. (1985), *Women in Development: A Creative Role Denied*, London: C . Hurst & Co.

Talle, A. (1988), *Women at a Loss*, University of Stockholm: Studies in Social Anthropology.

Turnham, D. *et al.* (eds) (1990), *The Informal Sector Revisited*, Paris: OECD Development Centre.

Twa-Twa, J.M., Waibale, P., Mpeka, B. and Kengyeya, J. (1988). 'Impact of AIDS Control Strategies on Other STDs', *AIDS Control Programme*, Kampala: Ministry of Health.

UNICEF (1989), *Children and Women in Uganda: A Situation Analysis*, Kampala: UNICEF.

UNICEF (1993), *Annual Report*. New York: UNICEF.

United Nations (1989), *Prospects of World Urbanisation*, New York; UN.

Valentine, C. (1968), *The Culture of Poverty: Critique and Counter Proposals*, Chicago University Press.

Wadel, C. (1969) *Marginal Adaptation and Modernisation in Newfoundland*, St John's, Newfoundland: ISER, Memorial University.

Wallman, S., Dhooge, Y., Goldman, A. and Kosmin, B.A., (1980), 'Ethnography by Proxy: Strategies for Research in the Inner City', *Ethnos* 45 (1-2): 5-38.

Wallman, S. (in association with I. Buchanan, Y. Dhooge, J.I. Gershuny, B.A. Kosmin, M. Wann) (1982), *Living in South London: Perspectives on Battersea 1871-1981*, London: Gower Press/London School of Economics.

Wallman, S. (1984), *Eight London Households*, London: Tavistock.

Wallman, S. (1985), 'Success and Failure in the Inner City', *Town and Country Planning* 54 (12), December.

Wallman, S. (1996a), 'Ethnicity, Work and Localism: Narratives of Difference in London and Kampala', *Ethnic and Racial Studies* 19 (1).

Wallman S. (1996b), 'Appropriate Anthropology and the Risky Inspiration of "Capability" Brown', in A. Dawson, J. Hockey and A. James (eds) *Anthropology and Representation*, A.S.A. Monograph No. 3, London: Routledge.

Wallman, S., Kalumba, K., Krantz, I. and Sachs, L. (1990), *Community Capacity to Prevent, Manage and Survive HIV/AIDS*, Working Paper No. 1, 'Plan for Field Research in Rural Zambia', Stockholm: IHCAR, Karolinska Institute; Dept. Sociology and Anthropology, University of Hull and Lusaka: Institute of African Studies, University of Zambia.

Wallman, S. and Baker, M. (1996), 'Which Resources Pay for Treatment? − A Model for Estimating the Informal Economy of Health', *Soc. Sci. Med.*, 42 (5).

Watts, T., Ngandu, N. and Wray, J. (1990), 'Children in an Urban Township in Zambia: A Prospective Study of Children during the First Year of Life', *J. Tropical Paediatrics* 36: 287.

Wellings, K., Field, J., Johnson, A.M. and Wadsworth, J. (1994), *Sexual Behaviour in Britain: the National Survey of Sexual Attitudes and Lifestyles*, Harmondsworth: Penguin.

Whyte, S.R. (1991), 'Medicines and Self-help: the Privatization of Health Care in Eastern Uganda', in Hansen and Twaddle.

Williams, G. and Tamale, N. (1991), *The Caring Community: Coping with AIDS in Uganda*, Strategies for Hope No. 6, London and Nairobi: ActionAid, AMREF.

World Bank (1993a), *World Development Report: Investing in Health*, New York: Oxford University Press for World Bank.

World Bank (1993b), *Uganda Growing out of Poverty: A World Bank Country Study*, Washington DC.

World Bank (1993c), *Uganda Social Sector Strategy Vol I. and II*, Washington DC: World Bank.

World Bank (1994), *Adjustment in Africa: Reforms, Results and the Road Ahead*, Washington DC.

Wrigley, C.C. (1988), 'Four Steps Towards Disaster', in Hansen and Twaddle.

Yoder, P.S. (1989), 'What People Think and Do about Diarrhoea', *Dialogue on Diarrhoea* 39: 6.

Zirabamuzaale, C. and Jitta, J.N.S. (1989), *Baseline Survey on Health Status of Children in Mulago Village II Parish*, Child Health and Development Centre Report, Makerere University.

Index

accidents, 99, 101
'activity status', 63-6 *see also* occupations
Adams, J., 233
advice, 106-8, 157, 161, 196, 199, 201-2
age, 47, 50, 52, 55-60, 68, 70, 100-3, 105, 117, 118, 159, 228
Agunda, K.O., 11, 11n7, 13
aid, 146, 230
AIDS, 3, 71, 98-102 *passim*, 121, 129-41, 166-88 *passim*, 209, 214, 226, 227
Information Centre, 182
Akhtar, R., 153
Altman, J.C., 3, 10n6
Amin, Idi, 6, 23, 49, 63, 235
AMREF, 225
anaemia, 99, 121, 152
Anguyo, G., 154, 155
'Ann', 198, 203-5
ante-natal care, 105
antibiotics, 114, 126, 142, 144, 146, 147, 149, 151, 157, 158, 173, 177, 192
ARI News, 161
Asia/Asians, 6, 21, 209n2
assistants, drug shop, 115, 118, 119, 125, 135, 146-7, 157
asthma, 99, 101, 159, 196, 197
attendants, clinic, 119, 123-5, 128, 146, 148, 199, 203, 221

Bagachwa, M., 10
Baker, M., 12, 93
Bantebya-Kyomuhendo, G., 6-7, 11, 102, 142-51, 189-205
Barasa, Catherine, 114n2
Barnett, A., 232
bars, 20, 21, 24, 74, 83-5
barter payment, 119, 131, 133
Barton, T., 7
bathrooms, 25-7 *passim*, 42, 43, 96
Bavidi, 139-41
belonging, 14, 88, 89, 91, 109, 234
Belshaw, D.,
Berman, P., 143-5 *passim*, 151
Beth, Mama, 89, 199
'Betty', 190-3, 196, 197, 205
biomedicine, 4, 8, 112, 144 *see also* health sector
birth attendants, traditional, 93, 103, 105-7 *passim*, 129, 130, 137, 138
birthplaces, 58-61

Blaikie, P., 232
Blaxter, M., 11, 151
'Born Again' church, 81-2, 208
'brewers/brewing, 13, 22, 26, 93, 178-85 *passim*, 198
Browner, C.H., 11n7, 12, 143
bubo, 168-70 *passim*, 173, 174
buildings, 24-5 *see also* houses
Busuulwa, J., 4
Bwengye, E.L., 154

capability, 3, 230-5 *passim*
Catholics, 27, 62, 79-80, 208, 209, 209n1
CHDC, 96, 104
chest complaints, 99, 100, 152
childbirth, 91, 105-6, 121, 137
childcare, 11, 91, 104, 155, 156, 164, 165, 234n3
children, 11, 27, 35, 36, 50, 75-6, 78, 104-5, 212, 215, 229
sick, 11, 103, 107, 149, 152-65, 191-6, 199, 201-2, 204, 226 *see also* illnesses
under-fives, 2, 3, 104, 152-65, 227
Chirgwin, K., 167
chlamydia, 167
Church of Uganda, 20, 27, 62, 80-1
churches, 24, 27, 74, 80-2
clinics, 103, 104, 107, 114-25, 146-8, 169-70, 172-7 *passim*, 182, 204, 228
Catholic Church, 21n1, 182
Family Doctor's, 124
Kamwokya General, 123
Kisenyi Valley, 191-4 *passim*, 196
Kololo Polyclinic, 124
Mulago, 173-4, 228
Muna, 199-203 *passim*
Mwana Mujimu, 195-6
private, 7, 162, 172, 181, 183, 211, 228
'Silent', 123-4
clubs, 74, 84-5, 94
colonial period, 9, 50, 112
confidentiality, 143, 148-9, 151, 174, 175
consultations, 119-20
context, 231-3
contraception, use of, 191, 193, 195
convulsions, 121, 149, 154, 156, 158, 160, 162-5 *passim*
corruption, 6, 25

cost of living, 91
cough, 102, 103, 115, 120, 121, 147, 148,
    152-65 *passim*, 192, 199
courts, 85-8
credit, 76, 119, 120, 131, 133, 134, 147,
    196, 199n3
crowding, 25, 91, 96, 214, 228

deaths, 100-2
demography, 9, 45-57
development, 209-10, 221, 225
    projects, 209-10, 214
diagnosis, 8, 145-6, 161, 169, 172, 173,
    176-7, 181-2, *see also* symptoms
    self-, 181, 182
diarrhoea, 7, 11, 98-100, 103, 115, 120,
    121, 129, 135, 148, 149, 152, 154-61
    passim, 164, 165, 178
diet, 164, 165
disabled, 64, 100
'discipline', 186-7
disease, 90, 98-102, 113, 115-16 *see also*
    individual headings
    sexually transmitted, 2-4 *passim*, 92, 99,
    100, 107, 108, 116, 120, 121, 126,
    133, 138, 143, 148-51 *passim*, 166-88,
    226, 227, 229, 232-3
diviners, 107, 114-22, 129-31, 134-41
    passim, 169, 175, 200
divorce, 108, 170
doctors, 102-7 *passim*, 114, 115, 118, 142,
    145, 146, 174, 191-3 *passim*, 196, 197,
    199, 201, 202
Dodge, C.P., 146
donors, 7, 146, 209, 210, 217
drainage, 21, 26, 74, 177, 208, 217, 218,
    221, 222, 224, 230
drinking, 83-5
drug shops, 7, 102, 107, 114-22, 125-9,
    145-8 *passim*, 157, 165, 169, 175, 196,
    197, 201
    Bukoto, 196
    Frank and May, 128-9
    Jolly and Sons, 126-7
    Jukira Nsubuga, 125
    licensing, 115, 125, 146
    P and N, 127
    Patience, 127-8
    Semakula and Bros, 128
drugs, 114, 115, 125-9 *passim*, 142, 144,
    146, 147, 151, 156-8 *passim*, 169, 175,
    176, 182, 192, 196, 201-2, 221, 223,
    228
dysentery, 98-100 *passim*

earning a living, 11, 13, 71, 72, 214-16,

223, 235
Economist, The, 4
economy, 5-6, 20, 220, 223, 224
    magendo, 6, 71
Edmonds, K., 5, 6
education, 63, 66, 68-70 *passim*, 104-5,
    115, 118, 212, 215
Eisenberg, L., 112
electricity, 20, 24, 25, 95, 96
employment, 6, 10, 235
Escobar, A., 209n2
ethnicity, 14, 28-9, 33, 34, 62-3, 72, 84,
    117, 118, 228, 234
Europe/Europeans, 6, 9, 167
expenditure, social, 6-7

Fabian, J., 213
facilities, housing, 24-7 *passim*
    treatment, 119, 123
'false teeth', 103, 118, 121, 148, 149, 154-
    5, 157, 159, 162, 163
family size, 104-5
fees, consultation, 120, 187
    drinking club, 84-5
    market, 75
    school, 66, 70, 216
    treatment, 7, 119, 120, 131-8 *passim*,
    141, 176
    water, 26, 77, 77n2
fertility, 9, 105
fever, 102, 103, 115, 120, 121, 148, 152,
    154, 156-60 *passim*, 164, 165, 178, 192,
    194, 202, 204
Firth, R., 13, 231
flu, 98, 100, 102, 103
focus groups, 15, 153-4, 175-87, 220-4
football, 82-3, 210
Frank, A.G., 230
'Friends of Kamwokya', 208
Freudenthal, Solveig, 206-25

garbage, 25, 26, 208, 213, 217, 218, 220-4
    passim, 230
Gellner, E.A., 231
gender issues, 2, 3, 17, 130, 228, 234
Gershuny, J.I., 10
Gluckman, M., 112
Goffman, E., 211
gonorrhea/gonorrhoea (*enziku/nziku*), 129,
    131, 167, 169-71 *passim*, 173, 174, 178-
    82, 185-7 *passim*
Graham, H., 11-13 *passim*, 143, 148, 150,
    151
Green, E.C., 3
Gregory, C.A., 3, 10n6
greeting, 89

Index

Grillo, R.D., 234n2
Grosskurth, H., 3
growth monitoring, 11
Gutkind, C.W., 10n6
Gutkind, P., 10n6, 50

Hakansson, N.T., 12
Hannerz, Ulf, 10n6, 14
Hansen, H.B., 5, 6
Harding, P., 10, 10n6
headaches, 99, 101, 102, 120, 121, 132,
    134, 148, 178, 195, 197, 202
healers, traditional, 12, 107, 111-22, 129-
    41, 149, 161-5, 169-72, 174-7 *passim*,
    182, 184, 192, 197, 199, 205, 216,
    222-3, 227, 228 *see also individual
    headings*
    spiritual, 107, 129, 134-5, 175
health sector, 2-4, 6-7, 11-13, 90-1, 107,
    108, 111-13, 142-4, 161-5 *passim*, 211-
    12, 215, 220, 222, 223, 233 *see also
    individual headings*
    education, 3, 153, 155, 161, 164, 172,
        227, 229
    personnel, 7, 107, 153, 154, 164, 172
        see also doctors, nurses 'privatiza-
        tion', 146
herbalists, 93, 107, 111, 114-22, 129-34
    passim, 138-9, 169-72, 175, 176, 182,
    187, 200, 203, 228
    Association, 136, 139
herbs, 108, 115, 116, 129, 131-5 *passim*,
    157, 158, 171-2, 175, 182, 183, 192,
    193, 196, 197, 201, 222, 223
Herpes zoster, 129, 181, 187, 188
HIV, 3, 4, 132, 133, 151, 166-8 *passim*,
    171, 174, 178, 187, 192,197, 227, 229,
    232
Hoffman, S., 12
Hogle, J., 12, 149
homophily, 113-14
Horton, R., 112
hospitals, 7, 102-8 *passim*, 116, 162, 163,
    176, 181-8 *passim*, 226
    Mulago, 104, 114, 115, 130, 147, 162,
        176, 181, 182, 192-202 *passim*, 228
    Nsambya, 182 private, 162, 163, 203
    Rubaga, 203
houses, 1, 22-7 *passim*, 33, 37-41, 91, 94-8,
    211, 214, 218, 221, 222, 224, 228
    number of rooms in, 25, 96, 97
    semi-permanent, 25-7 *passim*, 39
Hunt, C.W., 168
hygiene, 25, 91, 94-8, 155, 164, 165
hypertension, 192

identity, 8, 12-14 *passim*, 227, 233-4
illnesses, 90, 91, 98-108, 111-51, 166-88,
    192-6, 199-202, 204
    children's, 103, 107, 133, 149, 152-65,
        191-6, 199, 201-4, 226, 227;
        mother's perceptions of, 153-7
    kiganda, 148-9, 154
    women's, 102-4, 150, 190-205 *see also*
        diseases, sexually transmitted
ILO, 10
immunization, 11, 91, 104, 155, 164, 165,
    192, 215
income, 10-13 *passim*, 33, 91-4 *see also*
    money, lack of
infections, paediatric, 145, 148, 149
    sexual, 145, 148, 149, 151 *see also*
        disease
infertility, 107, 121, 133-4, 140, 148
inflation, 5, 6'
informal sector, 1-3 *passim*, 6, 10, 13, 20,
    71, 113, 145, 146, 151, 168-9, 205,
    227, 228, 235
injections, 103, 104, 124, 158, 173, 177,
    183, 192-6 *passim*, 199, 200, 202, 204
interventions, health, 3, 231-3 *passim*
investment, 6, 13

Jamal, V., 5, 6, 10, 49
Janzen, J.M., 11, 113
Jenkins, R., 10, 10n6
Jitta, Jessica, 103, 149, 152-65
Jonker, C., 11, 113

Kabaka, 22, 23
Kafeero, Abraham, 25n2
Kaharuza, Frank, 168-75
Kalibala, S., 168
Kalumba, K., 112
Kampala, 9, 48-66, 68-72 *passim*, 106, 107,
    228, 235
Kamwokya I, 8, 21, 25
Kananembo, Miriel, 132-3
Kapoor, K., 7
Kazada, Abdul Zake, 135-6
Kellock, S., 11, 11n7, 13
Kennedy, C., 3, 168
Kenya, 4, 9, 167
Klovdahl, A.S., 168
Kokulowoza, Joyce Teddy, 133-4
Kosomo, 134-5
Kreiss, J.K., 167
Krueger, R.A., 154

labour, division of, 5-6
Laga, M., 3, 167
Lal, D., 3, 168

land, 21-3
  prices, 21-3
  reform, 23
landlords, 22-3, 218, 221
Last, M., 145
Lateef, K.S., 5
Latin America, 12, 143, 209n2
latrines, 25-7 *passim*, 46, 74, 96, 97, 177, 208, 232
Leach, E., 47
leisure pursuits, 74, 210
Levi-Bruhl, 112
Levine, N.E., 157
life expectancy, 9
lighting, 96 *see also* electricity
Litman, T., 11, 13
local government, 7-8
localism, 17, 36, 234, 235
Lombolt, G., 168
London, 13, 234-5, 234n3
Lymphogranuloma venereum (bubo/kwekika), 168-72 *passim*, 179, 181, 185, 188

Maclean, C.M.U., 11
Macrae, J., 7
malaria, 98, 100-2 *passim*, 152, 156, 177, 178, 194, 197, 204 211, 212, 217
Maliyamkono, T.L., 10
malnutrition, 98-100 *passim*, 152, 195, 197
malwa, 84-5, 210
Mann, J., 232
markets, 20-2 *passim*, 28, 73-7, 211, 223-4
  candlelight, 76, 228
Marwick, M., 112
'Mary', 197-201, 204, 205
'May', 195-7, 205
Mbiti, J.S., 114n1
McGee, T.G., 28
measles, 99, 101, 121, 154-60, 163-5 *passim*, 178, 196
men, 3, 13, 71, 74, 82-5, 101, 121, 167, 168, 172, 180-6 *passim*, 228, 235 *see also* partners; sex ratios
meningitis, 99, 101
Mettelin, P., 10
midwives, 105-6, 147, 172, 173
migration, 6, 9, 14, 28-9, 58-61, 71, 72, 108-9, 218, 235
miscarriages, 105, 193, 194, 197
Mitchell, J.C., 189n1
mobility, 34-6, 101, 228, 235
models, theoretical, 150
modernization, 112
money, control over, 12-13, 205
  lack of, 91, 102, 103, 177, 181, 184, 195, 196

moniliasis, 173
morbidity, 3, 144, 152, 165
mortality, 9, 100, 101, 105, 152-3, 165
Moses, S., 3
mosques, 20, 27, 74
Mukuuma, 137-8
Murramer, Olive, 138-9
Musawo, Asuman Matoyu (Jajja), 136-7
Museveni, President, 6, 7, 17
Muslims, 62, 118, 130-1, 208

Naduma, Kavina, 131-2
Namboze, J.M., 156, 158
Nanchengwa, D., 112
Ndagire, Gertrude (Mama Khadijah), 139
neighbouring, 88-9
Nelson, N., 9, 13
networks, 10, 94, 143, 204-5, 234
newborn, 159-62 *passim*, 165, 170, 171, 181, 188
NGOs, 7, 230
NRA, 7, 17
NRM, 6-7, 17
Nsibambi, A.R., 7
Nsibambi, J., 168
nurses, 102-6 *passim*, 115, 126, 147, 170, 191-7 *passim*, 211, 216
nutrition, 12, 91, 156, 161, 163, 164
Nyamwaya, D., 112, 114n1, 115, 129

Obbo, C., 6, 71, 115, 147
Obote regime, 5, 6, 22, 63, 235
occupations, 63-7, 91-3 *passim*, 110
O'Connor, A., 6, 49
Ogden, Jessica, 8n5, 12, 88n5, 92, 142-51, 189-205
origin, regions of, 29, 34 *see also* tribal factors

Packard, R., 12
Paine, R., 14, 233
PANOS, 3, 167-8
Parkin, D., 28, 83n3
partners, 2, 92, 102, 144, 170, 172, 173, 176, 184-6 *passim*, 189, 193, 195, 198, 199, 229, 232
payment, for treatment, 119, 120, 131-8 *passim*, 141, 147, 192, 194, 196 *see also* fees
pharmacies, 7, 102, 103, 107, 122, 146-8, 202
Piot, P., 167
planning, lack of, 1, 17, 25, 218-19, 222, 223, 230
plants, medicinal, 12 *see also* herbs
pneumonia, 98-100 *passim*, 121, 161

politics, 5-7, 17, 20
Pons, Valdo, 8n5, 10n6, 34n4, 35, 47-72
population, 1, 8, 9, 17, 20, 21, 48-57, 69-71, 228
  density, 8, 21, 21n1, 48-9, 228
  growth, 9, 17, 48-50, 152, 223
  Kampala, 49-52, 228
post-natal care, 106
poverty, 151, 217, 221, 230
  alleviation, 209, 216, 221
pregnancy, 105, 121, 131, 148, 156, 179, 182-5 *passim*
Preston, S.H., 9
professionals, 10, 154, 159
'proper' women, 92, 143, 150, 185, 197-8, 204, 205, 229
prostitution, 13, 70, 209n1, 229
Protestants, 27, 62, 80-1, 208
Prual, A., 167

Quinn, T.C., 167

Radoki, C., 11n7
Raikes, A., 11n7, 143
religion, 27, 62, 74, 79-82, 118, 130-1, 205, 214 *see also individual headings*
rents/renting, 23, 94, 95, 218
reputation, 15, 88, 92, 111, 143, 185-6, 197, 198, 229, 235
Resistance Councils, 7-8, 17, 20, 74
responsibility, 11-13, 15, 221-2, 229, 230, 233-5
'restaurants', 73, 211, 216
returnees, to villages, 70
risk, personal 229-33 *passim*
roads, 6, 20, 23-4, 222
Robert, Kayongo, 216-17
Rodney, W., 230
Rogers, E.V., 113
'Rose', 193-7 *passim*, 205
Rouch, Jean, 206-7

'Sally', 198, 201-2, 204, 205
sanitation, 11, 26-7, 88, 91, 94-8, 155, 177, 209, 214, 216, 220, 221, 224
Sargent, C.F., 113
schools, 27, 212 attendance, 27, 35, 63, 66, 68-9
security, 22, 24, 25
sewers/sewerage, 26, 27, 74, 88, 177, 212, 213, 229, 230, 232
sex ratio, 2, 9, 17, 35, 36, 47, 49-58, 63-8, 70-2 *passim*, 100, 130, 228, 235
sexual behaviour, 232-3
Shoemaker, F.F., 113
shops/shopping, 24, 28, 35-6, 39, 74-7

sickle cell, 101, 159
skills, 13, 91-3, 209, 209n1
slums, 25, 40, 74, 88-9, 152
Smock, A., 11, 11n7
soak pits, 24, 26, 27
Southall, A.W., 5, 10n6, 50, 234n1, 2
spring, water, 26, 44, 45, 77-9, 208
squatters, 21n1, 23, 25
Ssenoga (RC chairman), 208, 221, 224
Ssewaya, Achilles, 4n3
Stack, C., 10n6
Staugard, F., 11n7, 145
STDs *see* disease
  National Control Programme, 170, 173-5 *passim*
Steptoe, A., 151
stigma, moral, 143, 148-9, 151, 166, 176-8 *passim*, 181, 183, 185, 227
Stren, R., 10
structure:organization relation, 13-14, 231, 233-5 *passim*
students, 63, 64
support, during illness, 106-8
survey, Broad Brush, 15, 24, 35, 74, 114, 122
  Ethnographic, 15, 47, 58, 90-110 *passim*, 114, 168, 169, 208, 214
  Treatment Source, 111, 114-41, 146, 148, 166, 168
  Women's, 15, 90-110 *passim*
Swantz, M.L., 13
symptoms, 2, 8, 12, 103, 115-16, 120-2, 145-6, 148, 153-61, 166, 170-5 *passim*, 178-81, 187-8, 227-9 *passim*
  assessment of, 2, 3, 103, 158-61, 165
syphilis (kabootongo), 167, 169-74, 178-81 *passim*, 185, 187-8

tablets, 103, 104, 183, 192, 193, 200, 202, 204
Talle, A., 11n7
Tamale, N., 21n1
taxis, 28, 34, 76
TB, 98-9
tenants, 218, 230 *see also* rents/renting
toilets, 24-7, 41-3 *passim*
tracks, 23-4
trade, 5, 13, 28, 154 *see also* markets
training, 118, 157, 165
treatment, 2, 8, 14, 102-3, 111-51, 153, 157-9, 161-5, 168-75, 182-7, 205, 220, 222, 227-9 *passim*
  choice/decisions re, 2, 12, 15, 102, 103, 144, 145, 153, 161-3, 165, 185, 190-205 *passim*, 226, 227
  cost of, 192, 194, 197, 200-4 *passim*,

228 *see also* payment
delay in, 153, 161, 184, 197
home, 12, 144-51, 157-8, 165, 191, 192, 194-5, 197, 199, 201, 228
modern *see* health sector
outcomes, 163-4 self-, 150, 151, 174, 177, 182, 192, 194-5, 197, 199, 223
traditional, 112-22, 129-41, 161, 227
see also healers
tribal factors, 10, 28-9, 33, 221, 223
trichomoniasis, 173
Turnham, D., 10
Twaddle, M., 5, 6
Twa-Twa, J.M., 168
typhoid, 101, 178

ulcers, genital (*ekiwo*), 121, 167-74 *passim*, 181, 187 stomach, 148
UN, 9
unemployment, 10, 91, 195, 221
UNICEF, 11, 152, 214n4
urban system, 13-15, 28-36, 227-8, 233-5

vaccination, 192
Valentine, C., 230
video project, 206-25
editing, 214-19, 225
planning, 207-10
shooting, 210-13, 224-5
viewing, 219-24
vomiting, 103, 154-61 *passim*, 164, 165

Wadel, C., 92
wages, 6, 9-10, 70, 147
Wallman, S., 4, 10n6, 12-14 *passim*, 34, 93, 108, 225, 230, 231, 233, 233n1

Wamai, G., 7
warts, genital, 168
water, 22, 24-7 *passim*, 77-9, 91, 98, 152, 156, 209, 211, 212, 214, 216, 217, 220, 221, 229, 230
collection, 11, 77-9
payment for, 26, 77, 77n2
piped, 22, 24, 25, 98
sellers, 26, 27, 77-9, 98
taps, 26, 45
Watts, T., 152
Weeks, J., 10
wellbeing, 11, 15, 90-110, 230, 235
Wellings, K., 232
White, R., 10
WHO, 114, 161
Whyte, Susan, 144, 146-8 *passim*, 150
Wiebe, P.D., 146
Williams, G., 21n1
witchcraft, 89, 101, 143, 149, 156, 182, 199
work, women's, 11, 92-4, 110, 143-4, 223, 235
World Bank, 7
worms, 103, 155, 202
Wrigley, C.C., 5

X-ray services, 124

Yoder, P.S., 155
youth, 17, 56, 60, 68-71 *passim*, 84, 101, 154, 178-85 *passim*, 213, 222
'Youth Alive', 83, 209

Zirabamuzaale, C., 152
Zwi, A., 7